ABOUT US

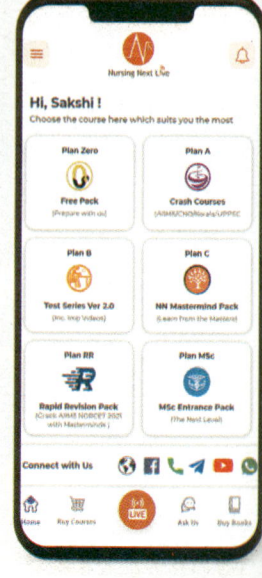

Nursing Next Live has been conceptualized based on the observation that there is a huge gap between the educational services available to the medical graduates and the nursing students. As these two are the strong pillars in providing holistic care to the patients, it is extremely vital that nurses should get equal exposure to access learning. To overcome this issue, we have come forward with the commitment of providing quality education to the nurses in India at their doorstep through Nursing Next Live. And therefore, we say **"We are bringing Learning to the People Instead of People Going for Learning".**

It is India's first and the biggest digital learning platform in the field of Nursing Education. The Nursing Next Live is an interactive self-assessment app, which helps you to build knowledge of nursing specialities any time and anywhere. In a span of one year we have magnified the nursing sector by upscaling it with the strategically designed Quality Content by the Top Medical Faculties of India. We at Nursing Next Live envisage that all students from Kashmir to Kanyakumari should get quality education. We pledge to give the best learning experience to all our students, under one single roof, and that is **"All-in-one and One-in-All platform".**

The Core Values and Principles of Nursing Next Live is:

- First Digital Learning platform for All Nursing Competitive & Undergraduates Exams with Futuristic Approach
- We are bringing Learning to People, Instead of People going for learning!
- Concept Based Teaching by TOP Medical & Nursing Educators (The Masterminds)
- "Quality Content" & "Smart-Study" Approach
- One in All, All in One! Nothing Beyond
- 360 Degree Approach for your complete Preparation
- Most Up to date & updated Content
- Best Guidance & Support at every step
- Best Interface with Unique & Advance Features
- Everything at one Platform ...Buy CBS Nursing Books at Special Discounts/Cashbacks

Nursing Next Live is the fastest-growing Edutech organization in the field of Nursing! With **70k+** downloads, **1200+** total number of selections, **150+** AIIM NORCET 2020 Selections, and many backend achievements it is the Highest Ranked App on the Play Store. The idea was possible to bring into reali because it was backed by the team of best professionals who did not see time; had One vision and One Goal in Mind of providing the students Nothir but The Best! Their trust towards the vision for the brand and their efforts to continuously make it a success helped Nursing Next to reach to this positi

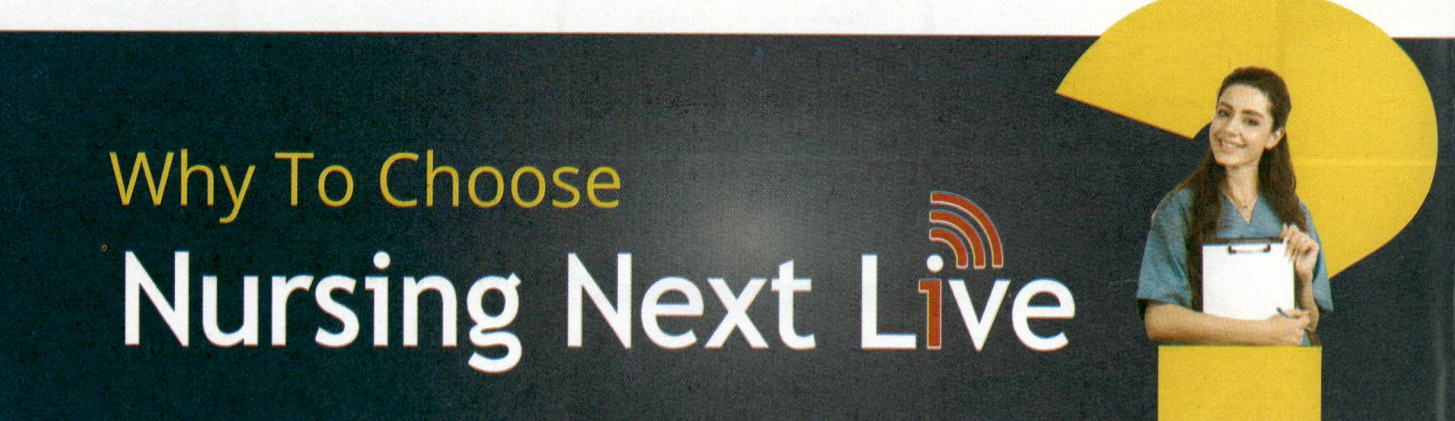

- India's 1st Digital Learning Platform for all nursing competitive, nursing undergraduate and nursing postgraduate exams (One-in-All, All-in-One)
- User friendly interface with unique & advanced features
- Most Up-to-date & Quality Content based on New INC Syllabus
- Conceptual learning with an integrated and futuristic approach
- Smart Study under the guidance of India's Top Educators who are the masterminds of their subjects
- Enhance your learning from Basic To Advance level with a 360-degree approach
- Regular Live Doubt Sessions and Live Tests based on real-time exam pattern
- TOP Selections in AIIMS NORCET, AIIMS MSc, BFUHS, CHO, SGPGI, JIPMER, RRB, DSSSB etc (From Rank 1 to 1000)
- Study Planner that helps you to organize your study
- Faculty-Student Meet (Forthcoming) that provides you an opportunity to meet with faculty and get clarify your doubts
- Printed Booklet: You will get the printed notes of the video lectures that will save your time in notes making and organize your time in a better wa
- Customize Study which helps you to create your own pack depending on your needs and wants
- Daily dose of information keeps you updated everyday with new information
- One-in-all all-in-one: You will get exam oriented plan in the app for whatever exams you are targeting. Simulation Videos

THE COMPLETE PACKAGE

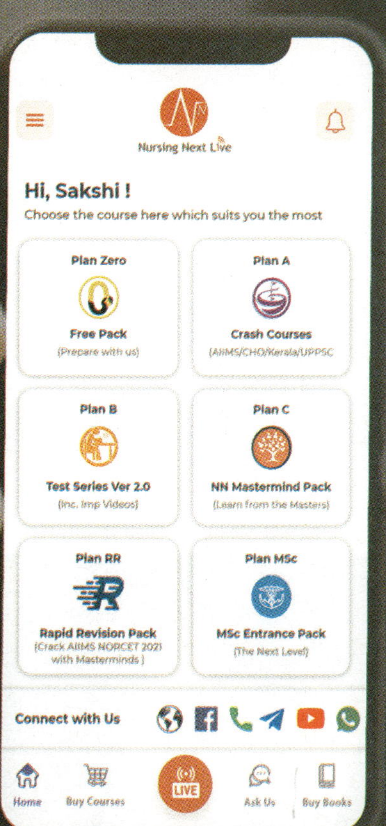

50,000+
MCQs with their Rationale

2000+
Hours of Recorded video lectures (Covering All Subjects/All Topics/ Imp Topics Chanting Videos/Exam Discussions/LMR/IBQ & VBQs Discussions)

150+
Previous years' question papers covering all National & State Level Exams (2021-2010)

Monthly/Weekly/Daily
Live Doubt Sessions & Faculty-Students' Meet (Forthcoming)

1500+
E-Notes/Flash cards of all the subjects for Last-minute Revision

1000+
Image-based Questions with their Rationale

200+
Video-based Questions with their Rationale

Monthly
Special Mega Assessment Tests, National Scholarship Test with up to 100% Scholarship & Reward points

200+
CBS Nursing Books available for purchase

200+
Newly Created Subject-wise cum Topic-wise Test, Mini Test & Grand Tests based on all important National Exams like AIIMS, PGIMER, JIPMER, DSSSB, RRB & ESIC, also State level exams like Kerala PSC

Special Features

Live Classes

Live Doubt Sessions

Mega Assessment Tests

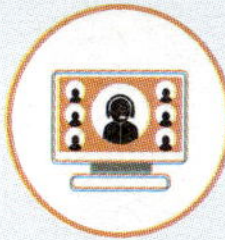
Live Webinars

Faculty-Student Meet on Zoom Sessions

Study Plans

Success Stories

Daily Dose of Knowledge

Blogs

National Scholarship Test with upto 100% scholarship

Any Doubt Ask Us

Exam Notifications

Buy CBS Nursing Books

Bookmark Your Imp Topics

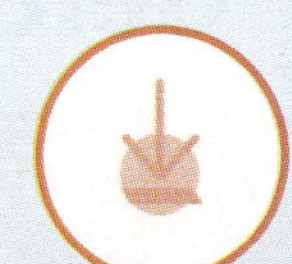
Download Videos/ Notes

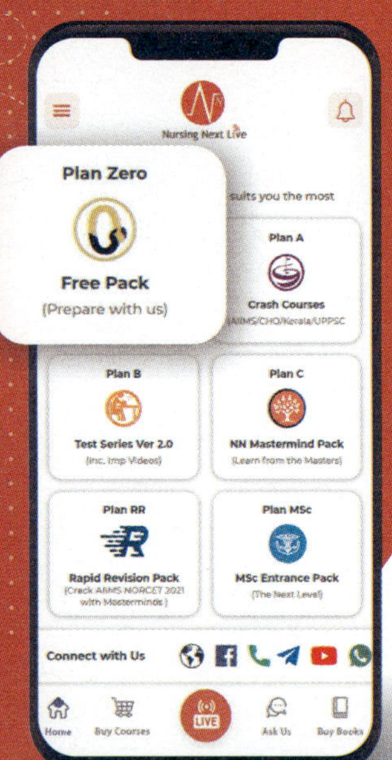

NURSING NEXT LIVE BROCHURE 2021

"जांचो, परखो, फिर खरीदो!"

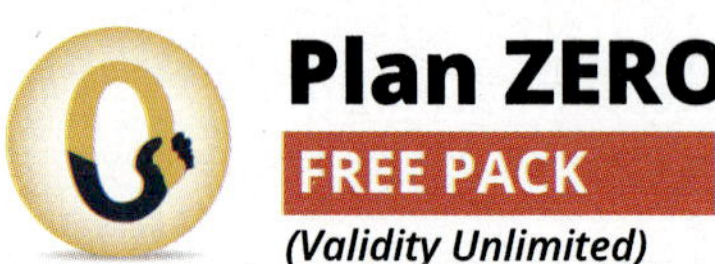

Plan ZERO

FREE PACK

(Validity Unlimited)

Nursing Next Live focuses on providing you the with the best and beyond, nothing less. In Plan ZERO we provide you the glimpse of the content from the various pack that gives you the rights to explore the contents in the App and help in taking the right decisions before selecting the pack.

WHY TO EXPLORE

- Glimpse of the content from the various packs
- TRY-TRUST-OPT. It provides you the rights to first analyze and then go for the best pack
- Enriched content

BEST FOR

- Those who want to explore before selecting the right pack
- Students who have an urge to gain the last momentum by giving a final touch to their preparation.

What all you will get

- **2000+** MCQs with Rationale covering All Subjects, Important Topics
- **150+** E-Notes covering All Subjects, Selective important Topics
- **100+** Hours of Lectures covering All Subjects (Topic-wise/Imp Topics/Chanting/Exam Discussions)
- **100+** IBQs & VBQs of All Subjects
- **15** Most Recent/Previous Years Papers with Rationale
- **5+** Grand Test & Bonus Test based on Real Time Exam Pattern
- **5+** National Scholarship test with negaitive marking, National Level Ranking & Cash Rewards
- Daily Dose of Knowledge— Word of the Day, Fact of the Day, Practice Pearls, Question of the Day
- Unsolved & Solved Question Papers of BSc 1st to 4th Year in a consolidated manner covering all Important Universities (Forthcoming)
- Monthly National Scholarship Test with Special Discount for Top Rankers
- How to Prepare for Exams (in the form of Study Planner/Videos)
- Complete Access to Target High Extra Edge Section – which includes additional MCQs & Golden Points in Video Form

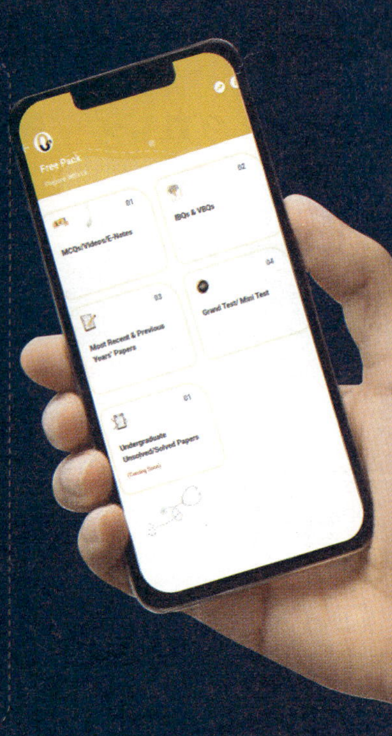

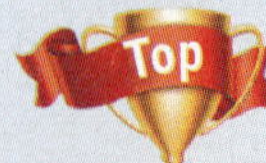

Top Selections in Various Competitive Nursing Exams

What our glorified achievers say about Nursing Next Live

REFURBISHING MY SKILLS WITH THE EXCLUSIVE TESTS!

"MAT and NST helped me in cracking my exams. The regular live sessions by top-notch faculty add to the advantage."

Harjeet Signh
(Rank-1, BFUHS)

CONCEPT BASED LEARNING!

"An effective app in clearing the concepts and doubt of students in very simple terms and the faculty is very professional."

Suresh Kumar
(Rank-1, CHO-MP)

LEARNING MY WAY THROUGH WITH NNLIVE!

"The study content is prepared by the experts, which helped me in polishing my knowledge in all the vital subjects."

Rahul Dahiya
(AIR Rank-3, NORCET'2020)

लक्ष्य तय है, तो PLAN A सही है!"

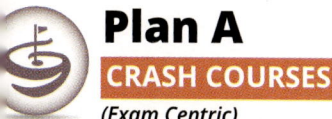

Plan A
CRASH COURSES
(Exam Centric)

you have a set target and working to achieve it then Plan A is the perfect plan for you. We have come up th this plan to help you prepare for a particular exam that includes exam-centric AIIMS NORCET 2020, PGI, CHO & Target Kerala PSC Crash Courses to help you get a hold of every topic in-depth. You get access in-detailed content of Real-Time Pattern of exams and their latest syllabus. Put your hands on the best!

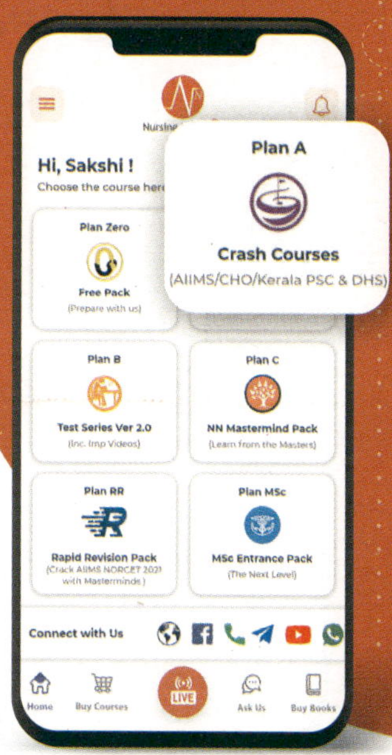

HY TO SUBSCRIBE

- xam specific, it targets the specific exam therefore its pattern syllabus is as per the targeted exam
- et Acquainted with exam pattern that helps you improve your skills
- elps in the last minute revision

EST FOR

- Those who are preparing for specific exams and want to improve their knowledge by practicing
- Those who are working professionals and want to prepare for exams along with their jobs

What all you will get

Plan A1 — CHO Crash Course

- **35+** Subject-wise Tests & Grand Tests (including Bonus Tests & Previous Years Papers)
- **1500+** Questions with rationale
- **70+** E-notes for last-minute revision covering all the important topics as per the syllabus of CHO
- **30+** (Duration of 30+ Hours) Pre-recorded Videos given by top faculties in Hinglish covering every important topic from exam point of view

MRP ₹689/- Validity 2 Months

Plan A2 — AIIMS NORCET 2020 Crash Course

- **60+** Live Tests Subject-wise based on AIIMS Delhi pattern
- **1500+** Qs with Rationale including MCQs, IBQs, VBQs, Clinical skills, Priority setting, and case study
- **15+** Mock Test, Revision Test, and Grand Tests based on Real-time pattern of AIIMS Delhi with Negative Marking and National Level Ranking
- All Subject-wise Tests & Grand Tests are with Detailed Rationale
- **140+** Last-Minute Revision Notes based on Frequently asked Topics of previous Years
- **12+** Videos on Chanting Session by Top Educators/Subject Experts
- **35+** Multiple videos on special tricks for non-nursing subjects, tips on memory retention, strategies to attempt exams, etc.
- Success Guaranteed as we have had 150+ Selections (Rank 3 to 5k) in AIIMS NORCET 2020.

MRP ₹1499/- Validity 2 Months

Plan A3 — Target Kerala PSC Crash Course

- **60+** Subject-wise/Grand Tests with Rationale
- **320+** E-Notes in the form of Subject-wisesynopsis
- **50+** Hours of Videos in English (Important Topics Pre-loaded video + Chanting videos) In association with our Best-Selling Title- Target High Staff Nurse Entrance Exam

MRP ₹945/- Validity 2 Months

Plan A4 — UPPSC Staff Nurse Crash Course

- **40+** subject-wise tests which cover the complete syllabus from basics to advance
- **7** Grand Tests Based on real time exam pattern
- **3** Extra Edge Tests covering Important Positions, Important Nursing Procedures, Drug Calculation, suture techniques & COVID special)
- Previous Year Paper Discussion video helps you how to approach the correct answer
- **25+** Quick Revision videos in one-liner form that covers all the important points from the weightage subject
- 1 **"SUCCESS MANTRA"** video to guide you the right approach for preparation

MRP ₹1499/- Validity 3 Months

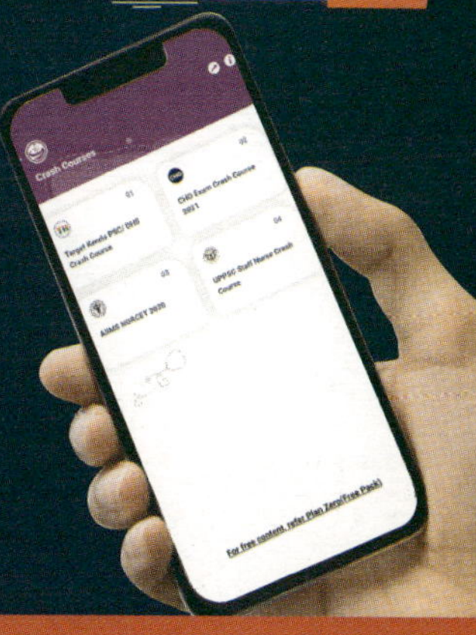

H-END TEST SERIES LEVELS UP THE PROGRESS!
e Test Series helped me get a quick overall analysis of my gress."
Nisha Singla
(AIR Rank-12, NORCET'2020)

COMPREHENSIVE AND INFORMATIVE CONTENT!
"You get to be familiar with the Real-Time exam experience. Also, the content provided is very informative and easy to understand."
Arushi Mittal
(AIR Rank-14, NORCET'2020)

MOVING FORWARD WITH CONFIDENCE!
"This app has helped me boost my confidence, just in my first attempt. The teachers here are superb and deserve a big thumbs up"
Komal Dhull
(AIR Rank-51, NORCET'2020)

COME AN ACHIEVER FROM A DREAMER!
reatly thankful to the NNL team who have helped me ch my preparation targets of achieving my desired rank. neans a lot to me"
Shivani Bourai
(AIR Rank-72, NORCET'2020)

BEST FOR GAINING THE LAST MINUTE MOMENTUM!
"The Image-Based and overall questions of the Nursing Next Live app are very informative and helpful for last-minute revision"
Nivedita Saini
(AIR Rank-79, NORCET'2020)

NN LIVE IS AS PROMISING AS IT CLAIMS!
"Nursing Next Live has helped me achieve great ranks in all the competitive exams that I have attempted. It does what it has promised and guides you through every step needed to succeed."
Rupali Garg
(AIR Rank-89, NORCET'2020)

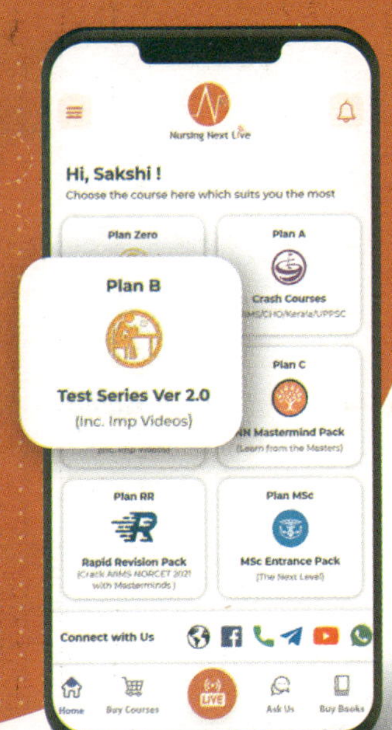

"आज का अभ्यास, आपके कल की सफलता!"

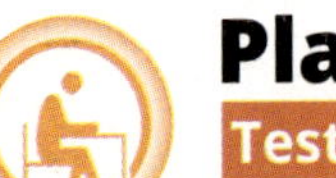

Plan B

Test Series Ver 2.0

(360° Approach)

Test series 2.0, as the name says to excel in any test, you need to base your learnings on two principles 1 is practice, practice, practice, and then 2nd is a 360-degree approach. Variety of subject-wise a topic-wise tests, IBQs, and VBQs that follow the latest exam fashion to help you level up your preparatc work. To give a complete touch to the preparation, we have covered all important national & state le last 15 years papers with important topics/ exam discussion videos.

WHY TO SUBSCRIBE

- Comprehensive test pack with 360 degree approach for those who are targeting any staff nurse examination of National or State level
- Keep track of your progress through test analysis report
- Last-minute revision notes of important topics from all the subjects
- Detailed explanation helps you to enhance your knowledge

BEST FOR

- The students who want to delve into the topic and opt for extensive preparation for any staff nurse entrance exam.
- Who never want to stop learning and always look forward to upgrading their pre-acquired knowledge.
- Working students who don't want to compromise with their preparation and success.

What all you will get

Pre Loaded Content (Phase 1 + Phase 2)

- **190+** Newly Created Subject-wise, Mini Test and Grand Test focusing all important National Exams AIIMS, PGIMER, JIPMER, DSSSB, RRB and ESIC
- **15K+** Qs (MCQs, IBQs, VBQs) with Rationale and updated reference from standard textbooks. All the Tests are designed by the Subject Experts and Topper Students
- **400+** Hours Recorded Video Lectures of Nursing/Non-Nursing Subjects by some of India's best nursing faculties/subject experts. Lectures are in English/Hindi language focusing on concept-based learning.
- **5** Exam Discussion Videos of 2019 Exam papers (Duration 20 Hours)
- **150+** Hours of Recorded Video on Subject-wise Exam Discussion of previous years papers (2017-18) of all nursing exams delivered by subject experts
- **5** Skill Procedure videos demonstrating Nursing Skills in real-time
- **100+** Previous Year Exam Papers of all Nursing Exams from 2020-10 with Rationale (Attempt/View PDF Mode)
- **1500+** Flashcards/E-notes on all the important topics of all the subjects for last minute revision (In 6 months)
- **800+** Image-based Questions with Rationale
- **200+** Video-based Qs with Rationale
- **Complete Access to Plan A-Crash Courses**

New Content (Phase 3) Q Bank Pack

- **8000+** Qs in Q Bank form of all the topics from all the subjects
- **700+** E-Notes covering all subjects/all topics

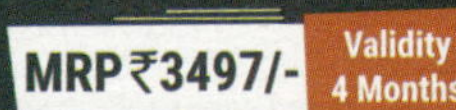

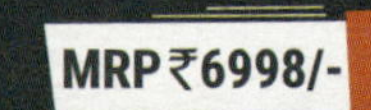

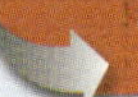

TESTIMONIALS

What our subscribers say about "TEST SERIES PLAN"

RIGHT DECISIONS TO SUCCESS!
"My wise investment in Plan B and continuous practice have proved to be the key to my way to success."
Sabita

LEARNING EFFORTLESSLY!
"Plan B made my understanding better of each vital subject in a very unchallenging manner. I am grateful."
Ritika

GAINING CLARITY WITH PLAN B!
"Plan B covers all the critical and analysis level questions v the rationale that helped me gain clarity of the concepts."
Deeksha B

THOROUGHLY RECOMMENDED PLAN 101!
"The questions with rationales helped me a lot. Highly recommended for all future nursing officers."
Shilpa Kashyap

ADDING JOY IN LEARNING!
"I am heartily grateful to become a part of Nursing Next Live. The faculty helped me thoroughly in this Pandemic by adding a sense of joy to my studies."
Suman Chauhan

PAVED MY WAY TO SUCCESS!
"More than enough time to practice and brace yourself T MCQs and videos with Rationales and topic-wise LMR ha helped me understand the vital subjects in a better way."
Rajkumar Jar

URSING NEXT LIVE BROCHURE 2021

तैयारी आगे की!"

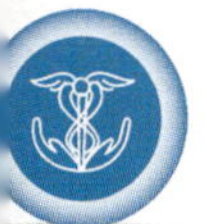

Plan MSc

MSc Digest

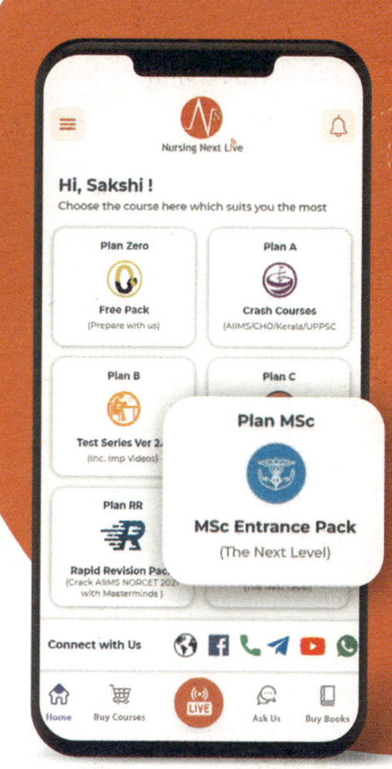

/e cant be louder about It, Nursing Next Live is the only growing platform offering MSc preparations › the aspirants. As we say, that your success is our success, so we always look forward to providing the est and beyond study content with a futuristic approach. MSc Digest contains every vital information oout the subjects in one place so that it gets easy for all to access the content on one platform.

VHY TO SUBSCRIBE

- Make your preparation easy with your job
- Enriched content helps you to prepare, revise and assess
- Content is prepared by the top Medical & Nursing experts
- Guidance and support

BEST FOR

- Who are always hungry to gain more knowledge from anywhere when they get a chance.
- Who believe in focusing on one topic at a time
- Who want to go further and upgrade their study content to the next level.

What all you will get

- Subject-wise synopsis covering image base illustrations and interesting Mnemonics to provide an extra edge preparation
- **3500+** MCQs covering the important topics of all subjects
- **800+** IBQs covering all subjects/topics
- **10+** Milestone papers covering more than 1000 MCQs to imbibe the environment of a real examination
- **3** Tests covering 150 IBQs
- **3** Tests covering 75 VBQs
- **10** Previous year papers (2020-2017) covering questions based on important topics/sub-topics from all subjects
- Exam capsules in the form of flashcards & tables
- **400+** LMR flashcards covering all subjects
- Hard copy of notes will be provided

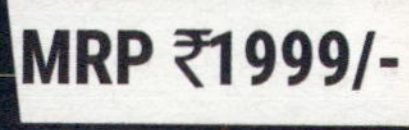

MRP ₹1999/- Validity 90 Days

TESTIMONIALS

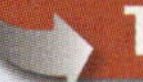

What our glorified achievers of MSc Entrance Exam say about Nursing Next Live

IE APP WITH A COMPLETE GUIDE TO NURSING SUCCESS!
NL has helped me a lot in preparing for MSc entrance exam d get a good rank. I will recommend this for every Nursing pirant out there."
Sabarni
(AIR Rank-21, AIIMS MSc 2021)

TAKING UNDERSTANDING TO THE NEXT LEVEL!
"It has helped me clear every doubt and that made my understanding of the subjects clearer. Thank you, team!"
Ritika Rajpoot
(AIR Rank-23, AIIMS MSc 2021)

THOROUGHLY RECOMMENDED PLAN 101!
"It was a wonderful experience studying from the top educators and getting counseled by them."
Priti Prajapati
(AIR Rank-39, AIIMS MSc 2021)

L FOUND ME WHAT I WAS LOOKING FOR!
helped me to polish my subject knowledge and upgraded preparations. Overall, It is an excellent application for all Nursing Aspirants."
Pritika Thakur
(AIR Rank-119, AIIMS MSc 2021)

AS EFFICIENT AS THE APP CLAIMS TO BE!
"This app is very helpful if you are looking forward to clearing your doubts in a comprehensive way. The faculty is highly professional and informative."
Aditi Yadav
(AIR Rank-133, AIIMS MSc 2021)

STRESS TURNED INTO THE JOY OF STUDYING!
"NN Live has made me admire the study pattern they follow. The way of teaching of the faculty is very helpful and valuable and filled with enthusiasm."
Shivani Shashni
(AIR Rank-173, AIIMS MSc 2021)

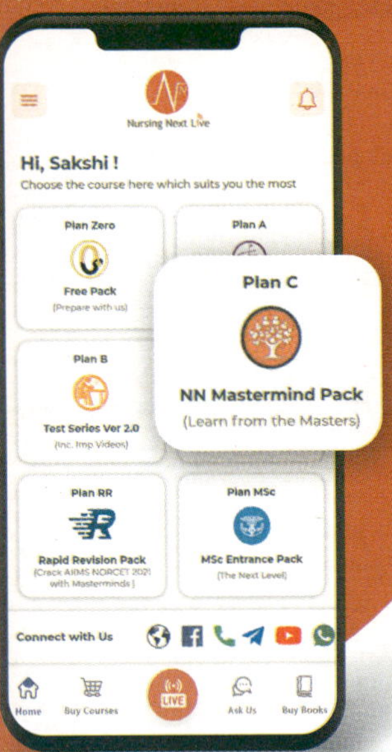

"ज्ञान हो बढ़ाना, तो PLAN C ही लेना!"

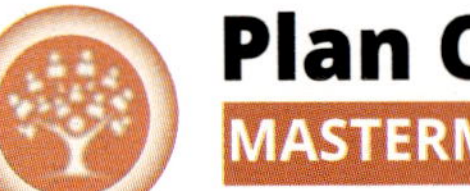

Plan C/C Plus

MASTERMIND Pack *(One-in-All, All-in-One)*

Nursing Next's One in all, all in one Mastermind pack for complete preparation! Plan C plus is a full packa that contains all that you need for your 100% preparation for all the Nursing competitive exams. T content of this package is curated and drafted by the Top-Educators of Nursing Next Live, who are t masterminds of their subjects. NN Mastermind Pack is a gradual phase-wise learning journey with t option of Individual and combined pack and a validity of 12 months!

WHY TO SUBSCRIBE

- Detailed lectures as per the INC syllabus
- Helps you in building the strong foundation
- The MASTERMINDS : India's top medical & nursing faculty is here to guide you
- Sufficient content to cater your undergraduate and entrance exams needs
- Handwritten notes of the lectures that help you to revise the topic
- Question Bank with the topics that help you to assess your understanding in that particular topic

BEST FOR

- Students who are at a good progression level and want to build up their foundation more.
- Those who look forward to studying from the best and beyond educators.
- The students who want to upgrade their knowledge or the one aiming for Staff Nurse Entrance Exam, and also for the Undergraduates.

SPECIAL FEATURES

- Nursing Next's "Mastermind Pack", is a One-Stop solution for all your exam preparation needs for Staff Nurse Entrance Exams & Nursing Undergraduate Exams!
- It is our One-in-All, All-in-One pack for the nursing students of the Digital era!
- NN Mastermind Pack is exactly that 'learning tool' for all the nursing aspirants. It is carefully planned, and strategically designed, under the expertise of TOP Medical/Nursing Educators, just to make learning more authentic and easier for our students.
- Covering All Subjects, All Topics concepts from Basics to Advanced level pattern with the help of Videos/Question Banks & Handwritten Notes
- The Masterminds (TOP EDUCATORS) of NN Live have focused on ALL the upcoming Nursing Exams by giving two convenient options under 'Individual Subject Pack', & 'Combined (NN Mastermind Pack)'
- NN Mastermind Pack is a "road to success" for those who are preparing for any or all staff nurse entrance exams.

What all you will get

Plan C (Including Plan RR)

- **1200+** hours of Video Lectures on All Subject/All Topics
- **11,000+** Questions with Rationale covering All Subject/All Topics
- IBQ/VBQ Video Discussions of All Subjects
- **Monthly Live Doubt Sessions/Live Classes**
- **80+Hours** of Rapid Revision Videos for **AIIMS NORCET**
- **2021** by Mastermind faculty
- **Handwritten Notes** of videos in PDF format integrated in the App
- Focusing on Quality study over quantity study, using the smart-study approach
- Monthly **Mega Assessment** Tests with National LevelRanking
- All upcoming exam's Important Topics & Exam/Discussions will be covered
- Complete **360-degree approach** for preparation
- Unlimited Watch Time, FREE Download Video option, National Level Ranks, Bookmark the content, Pause & Resume video option
- Best Guidance & Support at every stage
- Monthly Live Doubt Sessions/Live Classes/Live Webinars by Mastermind Faculty

Validity: 12 Months

MRP ₹12974/-

Plan C Plus (Including Plan A+B+C+RR)

- Plan A of NN Live (Complete access to Crash Courses—CHO/AIIMS NORCET 2020/KERALA PSC/UPPSC

+

- Plan B of NN Live (Complete access to Test Series Pack Focusing AIIMS NORCET 2021 & Other Staff Nurse Exams)

+

- Plan C of NN Live (Complete access to Plan C by the Mastermind Faculty

+

- Plan RR of NN Live (Complete access to Rapid Revision Pack)

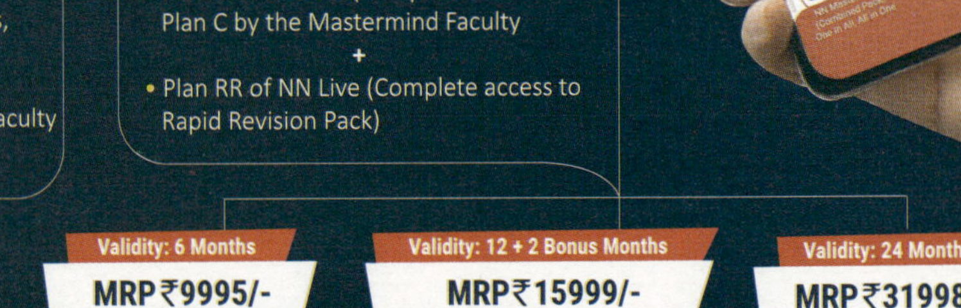

Validity: 6 Months	Validity: 12 + 2 Bonus Months	Validity: 24 Months
MRP ₹9995/-	MRP ₹15999/-	MRP ₹31998/-

Undergraduate Packs (Prof.-wise)

1st Year Students
- ✓ Anatomy
- ✓ Physiology
- ✓ Biochemistry & Nutrition
- ✓ Microbiology
- ✓ Fundamentals of Nursing

2nd Year Students
- ✓ Pharmacology
- ✓ MSN – Medicine
- ✓ MSN – Surgery
- ✓ Community Health Nursing
- ✓ Sociology
- ✓ CET

3rd & 4th Year Students
- ✓ Pediatric Nursing
- ✓ Midwifery & Obstetrical Nursing
- ✓ MSN – Medicine
- ✓ MSN – Surgery
- ✓ Mental Health Nursing
- ✓ Community Health Nursing
- ✓ Nursing Research & Statistics
- ✓ Nursing Management & Administration

Other Mastermind Plan

Mastermind Plan C

For 3rd & 4th Year Students those who are targeting for Sta Nurse Exams

Mastermind Plan C Plus

For Pass out Students those wh are targeting for AIIMS NORCET Staff Nurse Exams

The Masterminds

Learn from the Top Educators of India

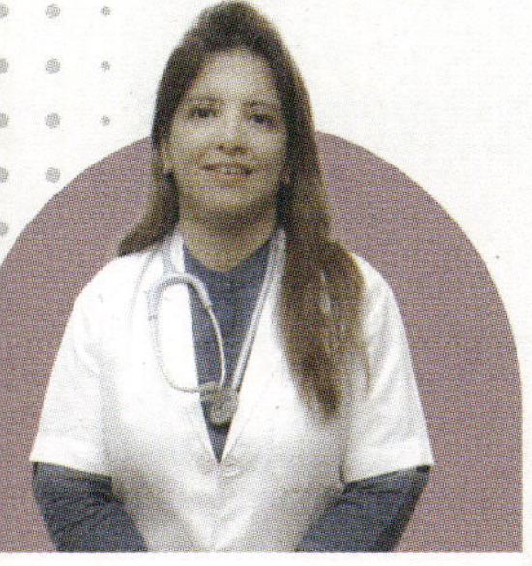

Dr Sakshi Arora Hans

idwifery & Obstetrical Nursing

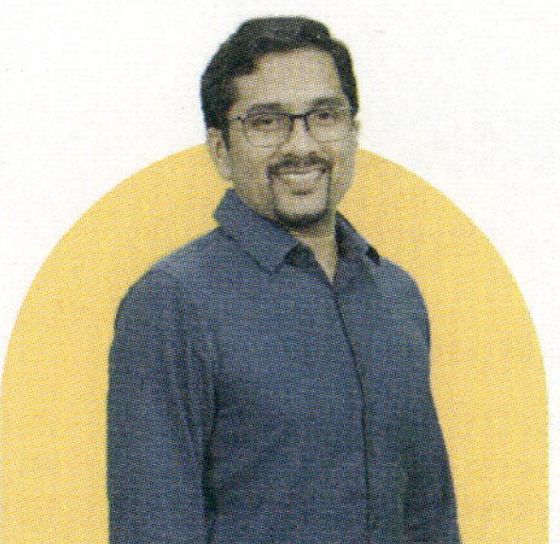

Dr Rohan Khandelwal

MSN - Surgery

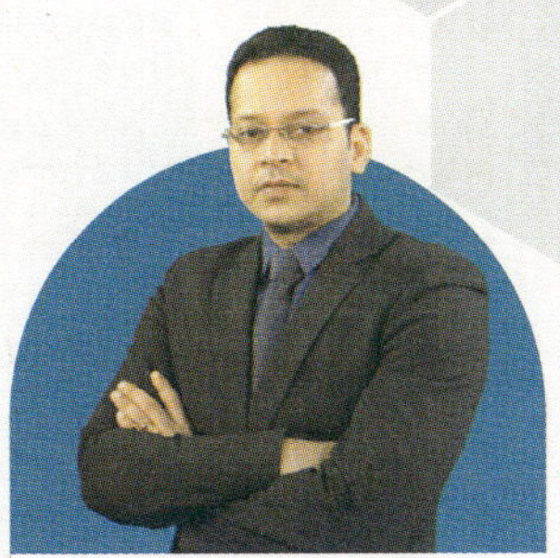

Dr Ranjan Patel

Pharmacology

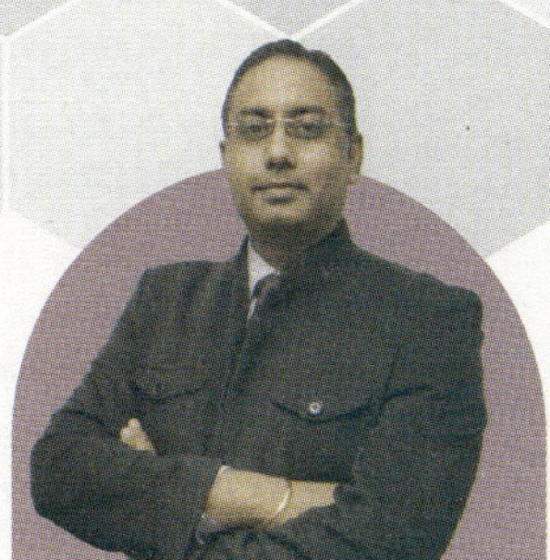

Dr Mukhmohit Singh

Community Health Nursing

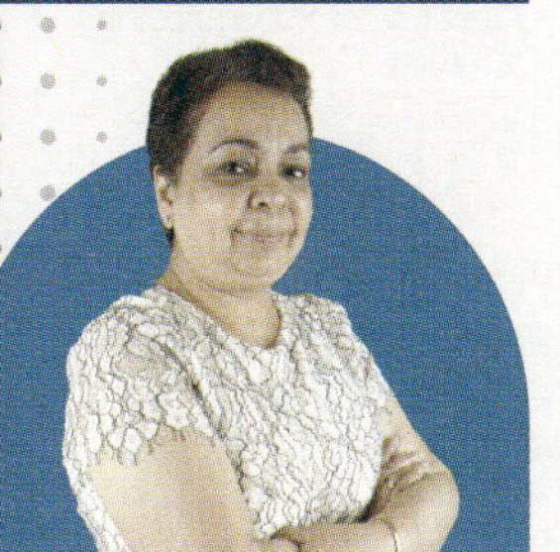

Dr Shivika Sethi

Microbiology

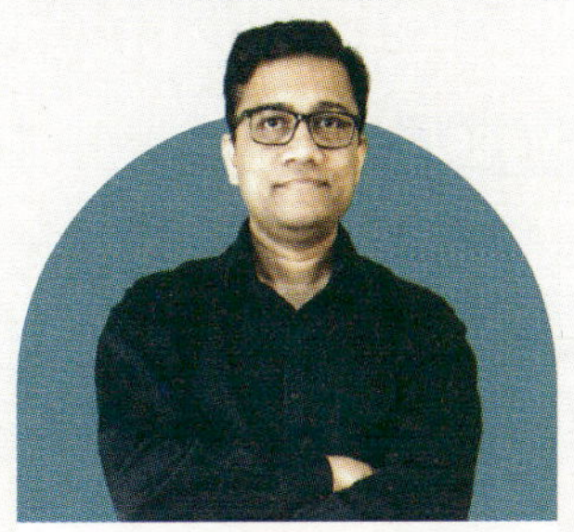

Dr Ashish Kumar

Physiology

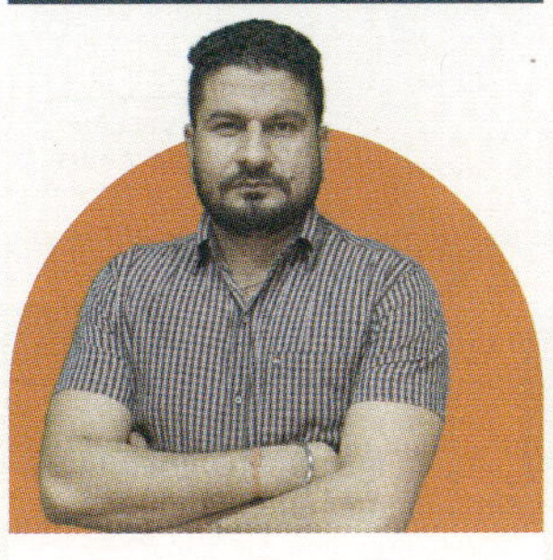

Dr Aman Setiya

MSN - Medicine

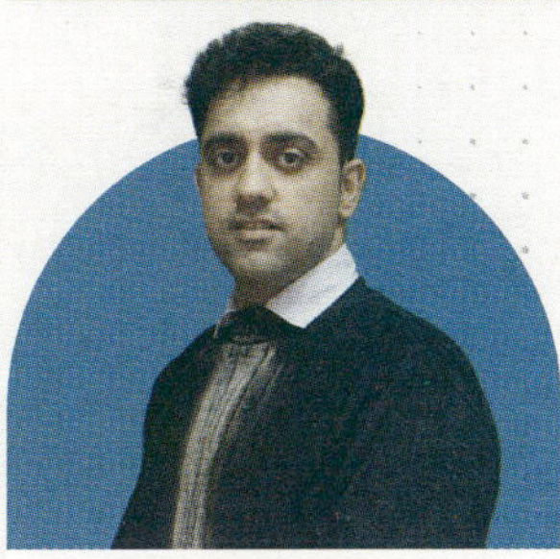

Dr Anand Bhatia

Pediatric Nursing

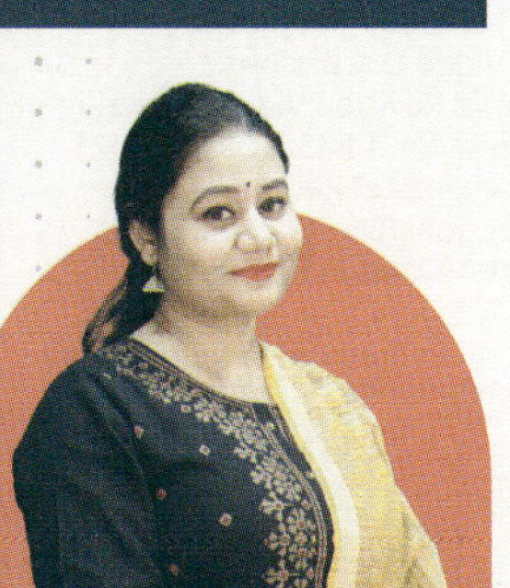

Ms Sabina Ali

Fundamentals of Nursing

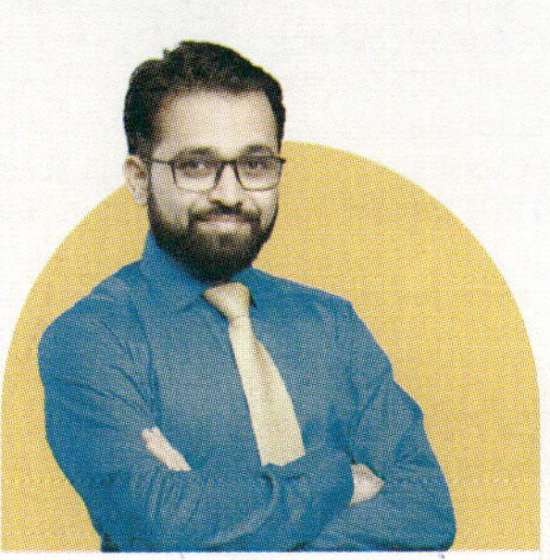

Dr Shrikant Verma

Anatomy

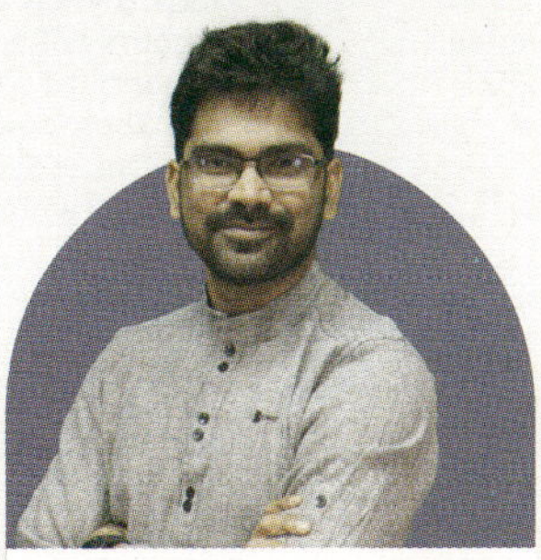

Dr Karthikeyan Pethusamy

Biochemistry & Nutrition

Ms Chetana

Mental Health Nursing

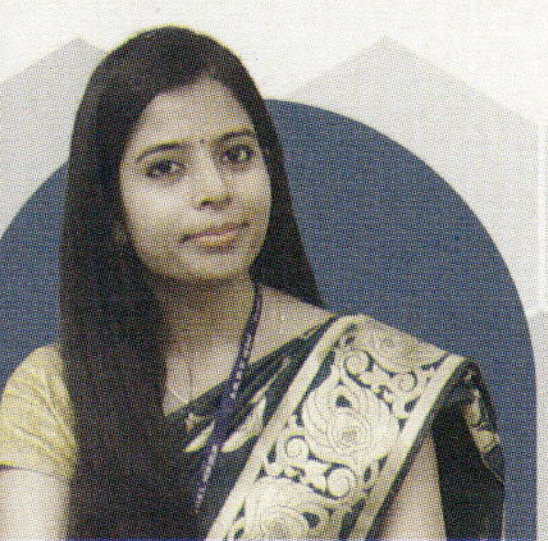

Saumya Srivastava

Nursing Management & Nursing Education

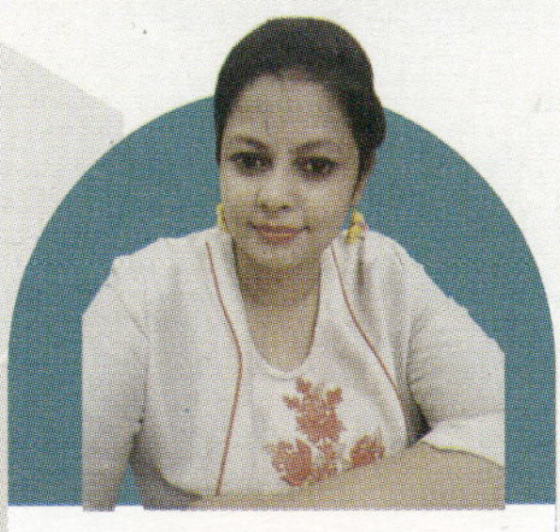

Ms Priyanka Randhir

Sociology & Computers

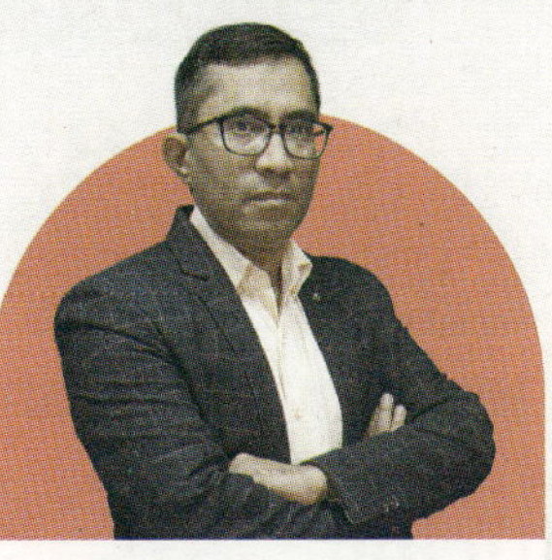

Mr Nitish Dubey

General Arithmetic

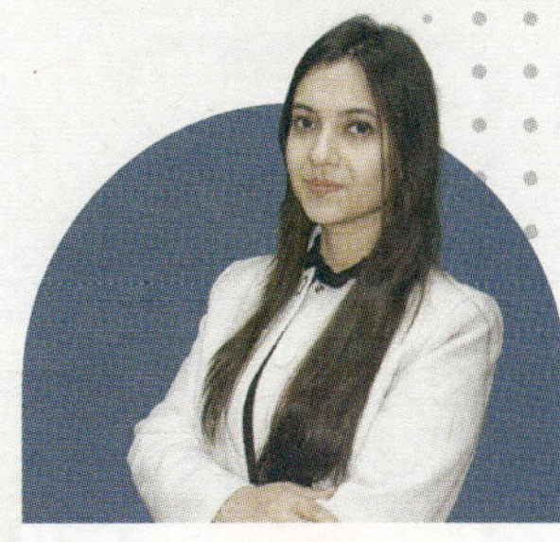

Ms Saloni Sharma

Aptitude & Reasoning

Individual

By TH

Midwifery & Obstetrical Nursing

By Dr Sakshi Arora Hans

What all you will get

- **100** hours of Videos on All topics
- IBQs & VBQs Discussion Videos
- **15** hours of Rapid Revision Videos covering Important Topics for AIIMS NORCET 2021
- **1000** Topic-wise MCQs with Rationale
- Live Doubt Sessions/Live Classes
- **88** Hand written Notes in PDF format

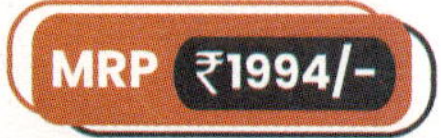

MSN - Surgery

By Dr Rohan Khandelwal

What all you will get

- **50** hours of Videos of All topics
- IBQs & VBQs Video Discussions
- **3** hours of Rapid Revision Videos covering Important Topics for AIIMS NORCET 2021
- **800** Topic-wise Qs with Rationale
- Live Doubt Sessions/Live Classes
- **51** Hand written Notes in PDF format integrated in App

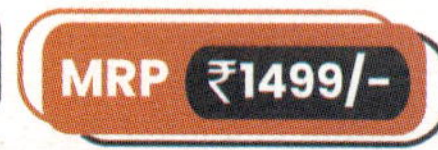

Pharmacology

By Dr Ranjan Patel

What all you will get

- **50** hours of Videos of All topics
- IBQs & VBQs Video Discussions
- **10** hours of Rapid Revision Videos covering Important Topics for AIIMS NORCET 2021
- **800** Topic-wise Qs with Rationale
- Live Doubt Sessions/Live Classes
- **71** Hand written Notes in PDF format integrated in App
- **100** Probable Questions of Pharmacology for AIIMS NORCET 2021

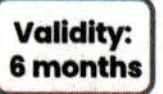

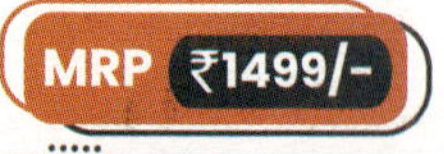

Community Health Nursing

By Dr Mukhmohit Singh

What all you will get

- **90** hours of Videos of All topics
- IBQs & VBQs Video Discussions
- **7** hours of Rapid Revision Videos covering Important Topics forAIIMS NORCET 2021
- **900** Topic-wise Qs with Rationale
- Live Doubt Sessions/Live Classes
- **87** Hand written Notes in PDF format integrated in App
- **300** Probable Questions of CHN for AIIMS NORCET 2021

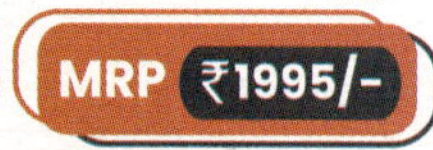

Microbiology

By Dr Shivika J Sethi

What all you will get

- **54** hours of Videos of All topics
- IBQs & VBQs Video Discussions
- **8** hours of Rapid Revision Videos covering Important Topics for AIIMS NORCET 2021
- **800** Topic-wise Qs with Rationale
- Live Doubt Sessions/Live Classes
- **75** Hand written Notes in PDF format integrated in App
- **100** Probable Questions of Microbiology for AIIMS NORCET 2021

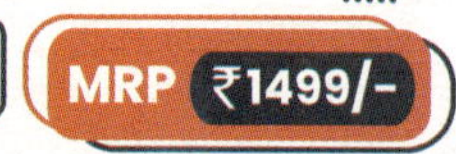

MSN - Medicine

By Dr Aman Setiya

What all you will get

- **90** hours of Videos of All topics
- IBQs & VBQs Video Discussions
- **5** hours of Rapid Revision Videos covering Important Topics for AIIMS NORCET 2021
- **900** Topic-wise Qs with Rationale
- Live Doubt Sessions/Live Classes
- **90** Hand written Notes in PDF format integrated in App
- **400** Probable Questions of MSN - Medicine for AIIMS NORCET 2021

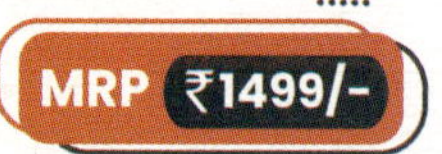

" जितनी जरूरत उतना पढ़ो !"

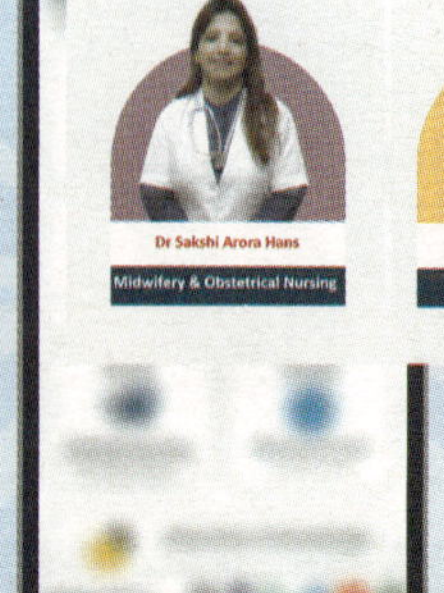
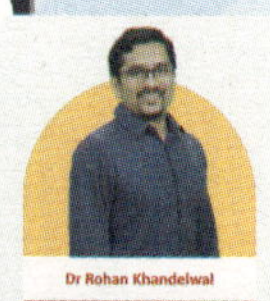

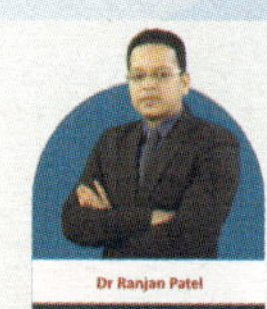

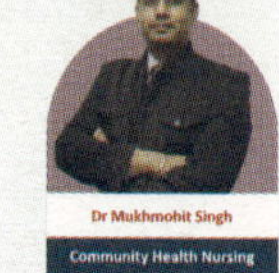

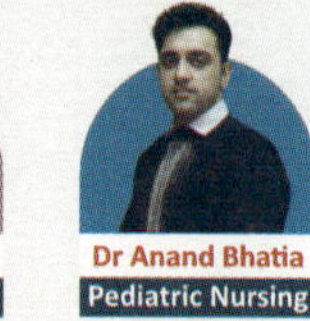
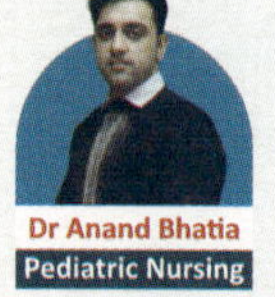

Dr Anand Bhatia
Pediatric Nursing

Now you have
The Freedom to Choose

Introducing

CREATE YOUR PACK

Undergraduate Packs

By THE MASTERMINDS

Undergraduate Pack - 1st Year

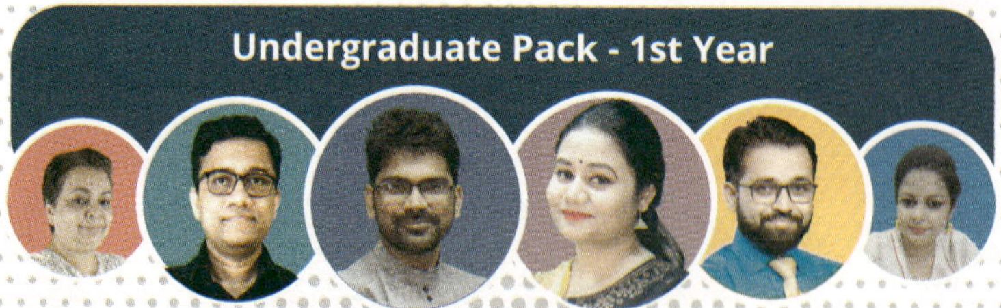

What all you will get

Main Subjects	Video Duration	No. of Questions
Anatomy	**60+** Hours	**600+** Qs
Physiology	**60+** Hours	**600+** Qs
Biochemistry & Nutrition	**50+** Hours	**500+** Qs
Microbiology	**50+** Hours	**500+** Qs
Fundamentals of Nursing	**200+** Hours	**400+** Qs

Bonus Subjects:- Computers & Psychology

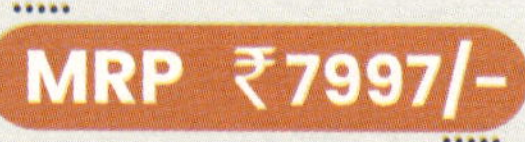

Validity: 18 months

Undergraduate Pack - 2nd Year

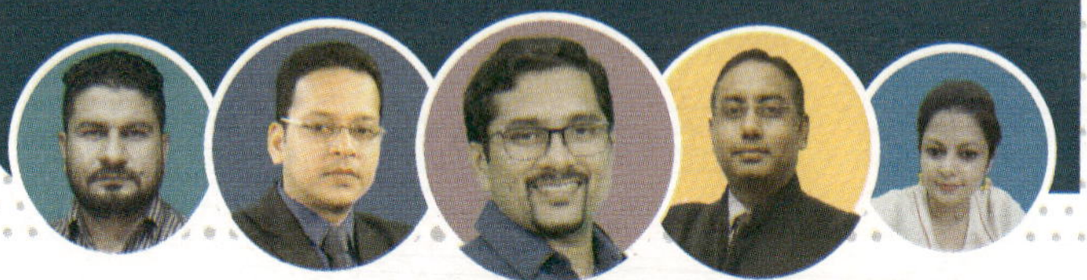

What all you will get

Main Subjects	Video Duration	No. of Questions
Pharmacology	**50+** Hours	**800+** Qs
MSN - Medicine	**90+** Hours	**900+** Qs
MSN - Surgery	**50+** Hours	**600+** Qs
Community Health Nursing	**90+** Hours	**900+** Qs
Sociology	**40+** Hours	**250+** Qs

MRP ₹7997/-

Validity: 18 months

Undergraduate Pack - 3rd & 4th Year

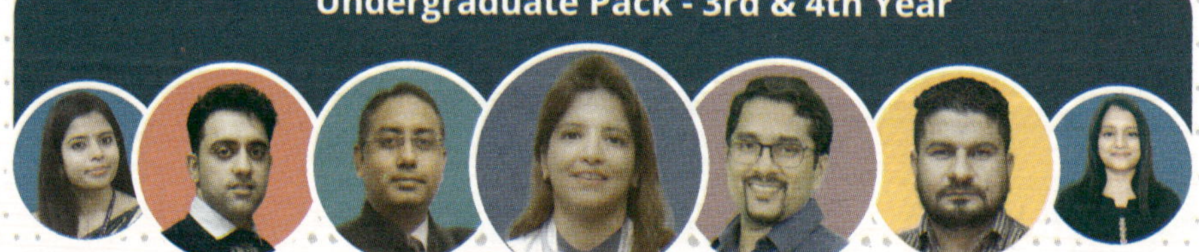

What all you will get

Main Subjects	Video Duration	No. of Questions
Pediatric Nursing	**80+** Hours	**900+** Qs
Midwifery & Obstetrical Nursing	**100+** Hours	**1000+** Qs
MSN - Medicine	**90+** Hours	**900+** Qs
MSN - Surgery	**50+** Hours	**600+** Qs
Mental Health Nursing	**90+** Hours	**900+** Qs
Community Health Nursing	**90+** Hours	**900+** Qs
Nursing Research & Statistics	**35+** Hours	**400+** Qs

Bonus Subjects:- Nursing Managment & Nursing Education

MRP ₹12992/-

Validity: 24 months

Special Features

- Handwritten Notes of Videos in PDF Format
- IBQs/VBQs Discussion Videos of above mentioned Subjects
- Monthly Mega Assessment Tests
- Monthly Live Doubt Session/Live Classes/Live Webinar by MM Faculty
- Best Guidance & Support
- Get your query directly resolved by MM faculty

NURSING NEXT LIVE BROCHURE 2021

"कम समय में जीत पक्की!"

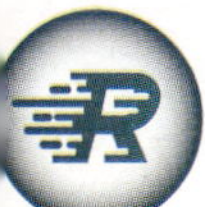

Plan RR

Rapid Revision Pack

(Ready, Steady & Rapid)

We are here to make you a Mastermind for all your Nursing exams, and for that, we believe the last-minute revision works like a wonder. Rapid Revision Pack, as the name says is to make you all ready and rapid for all your Nursing Competetive exams. Learn from basics to advance level and get a hold of every topic. Gain the last-minute momentum with this pack and open the gateway to excellence for yourself.

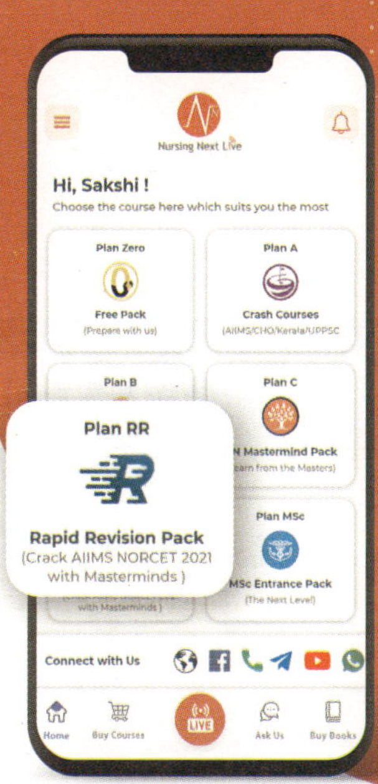

WHY TO SUBSCRIBE

- Rapid and intense course of study
- Covers important topics in concise yet complete form
- Most probable Qs which have large rate of incidence in exam
- If your foundation is good, then this is good pack to revise before the exam

BEST FOR

- Those who believe in doing extensive preparation for their Nursing competitive exams.
- The students who want to clear all of their last moment doubts.
- Working professionals who never want to compromise with their learnings for the competitive exams.

What all you will get

Plan RR

- **80-100 Hours of Rapid Revision Videos** covering Most Imp Topics for NORCET 2021 (Major Subjects including Nursing Management & Nursing Education)
- **2000+** Probable Qs with Rationale (MCQs + NCLEX Pattern)
- IBQ & VBQ Video Discussions by Master Mind Faculties (Relevant Subjects)
- **10 Special Mega Assessment Test** based on AIIMS NORCET Pattern
- Various Imp Tips/Trick & How to Prepare for NORCET 2021 Videos
- **15+** Imp Videos on COVID 19/Test & Discussion covering MCQ & NCLEX Pattern Qs
- COVID-19 Capsule (MCQs & Videos)
- Rapid Revision eBook in PDF format

MRP ₹2777/- Validity: 2.5 Months

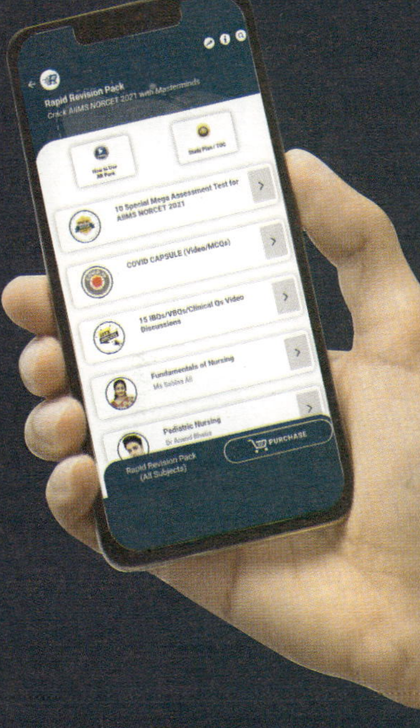

Plan RR+Mini TSP

Complete Ccontent of RR Pack + Mini TSP:

- **15k** Questions with Rationale
- **1000+** IBQs/VBQs with Rationale Subject-wise/System-wise approach
- **190+** Tests (Subject-wise/Grand Test)
- **1500** E-notes/Clinical Gems
- **400+** Hours of videos Lectures/Subject-wise Exam discussion/Skill Procedure Videos

MRP ₹7520/- Validity: 3+1 Months

TESTIMONIALS

What our Subscribers say about our Rapid Revision Pack

SELF-EVALUATION IS THE KEY!
"It has proved the best plan if you look forward to self evaluate before your exams. Great initiative."
Sushma Rani

LESS TIME CONSUMING AND MORE LEARNING!
"Through the Rapid revision pack and test series 2.0, I learned from excellent educators in a time-saving way"
Usha Rani

EXPERIENCE REAL-TIME EXAM VIBE!
"Rapid Revision Pack has helped me clear my doubts by providing real-time exam experience preparation. I gained an overall improvement in my studies."
Akansha Sharma

INNOVATIONS DETERMINES EFFECTIVENESS!
"Excellent pack if you want to do a quick revision effectively. The lectures are in a very comprehensive manner which makes it one of the best initiatives by NNL."
B. Snegha Varshini

NN LIVE BECAME MY PARTNER-IN-LEARNING!
"Mastermind C Plus Pack became an amazing opportunity for me as I got everything from MCQs to High Standard Questions. Got the RR plan as a bonus too. Also, the faculty is always there to boost you up!"
Rahul Sain

IMPROVING RESULTS AND CHANGING STUDY PERSPECTIVES!
"Even the micro-content helped me to study in a macro way. With NNL, it has become very simple for me to understand the topics in a very comprehensive way. The Live sessions just work as an advantage. Thank you Nursing Next Live!"
Yashpal Vishvakarma

GLORIFIED ACHIEVER

With over 150+ AIIMS NORCET 2020/100+ CHO &

AIIMS NORCET 2020

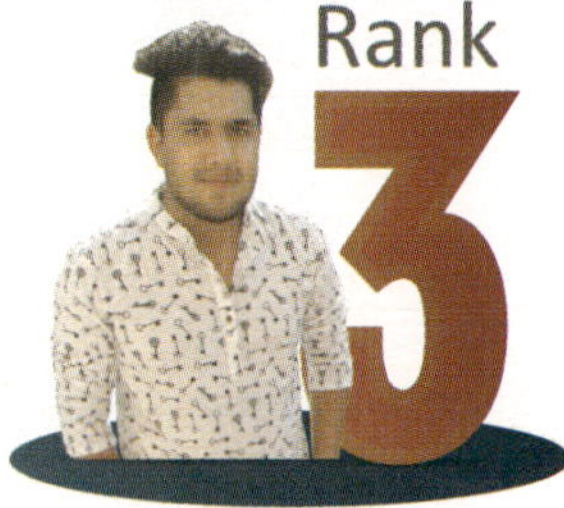

Rahul Dahiya
Roll No. 9016060

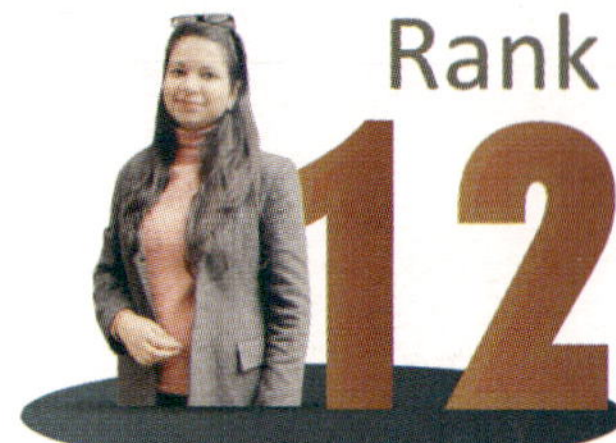

Nisha Singla
Roll No. 9101820

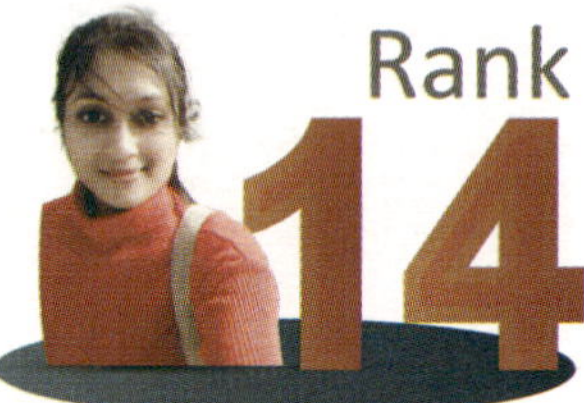

Arushi Mittal
Roll No. 9079646

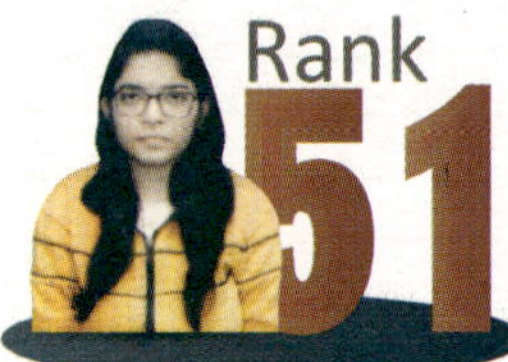

Komal Dhull
Roll No. 9024458

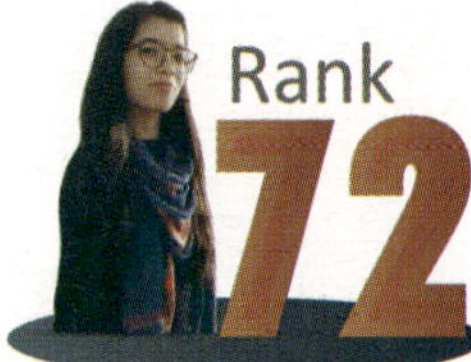

Shivani Bourai
Roll No. 9092877

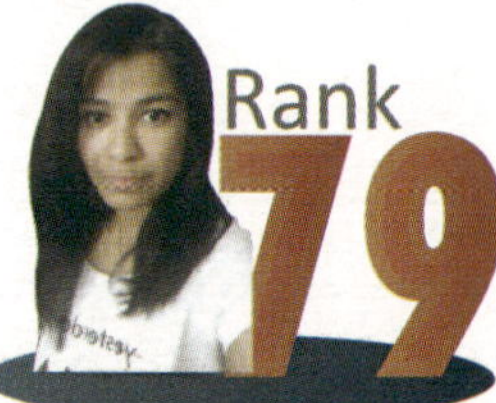

Nivedita Saini
Roll No. 9004587

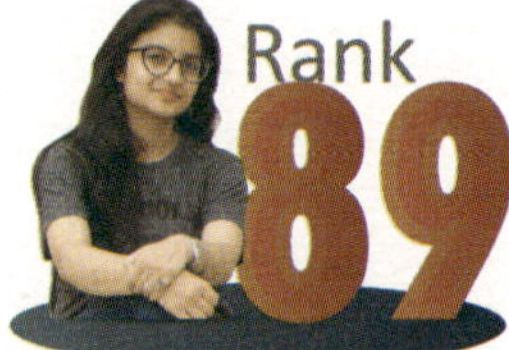

Rupali Garg
Roll No. 9054544

And many mo

CHO 2020

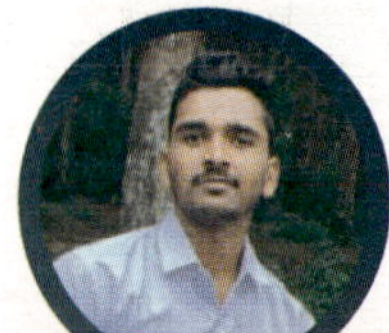
Suresh Kumsr
Rank- 1
Roll No. 12090
MP

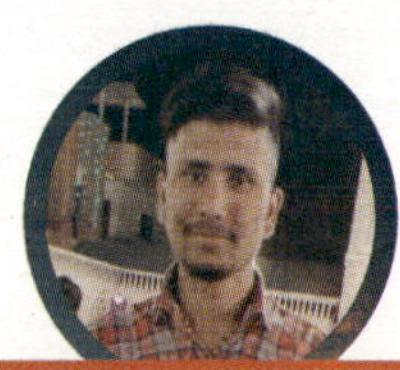
Vikas Kumar Sahu
Rank- 14
Roll No. 10011
MP

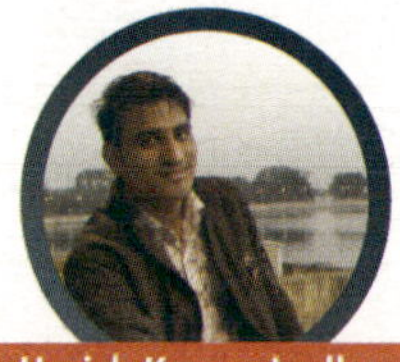
Harish Kumar Lodha
Rank- 18
Roll No. 7930
MP

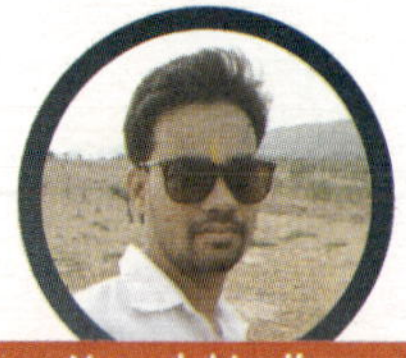
Heeralal Lodha
Rank- 33
Roll No. 10009
MP

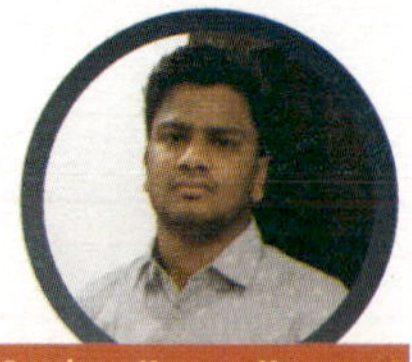
Sandeep Krumar Kumawat
Rank- 44
Roll No. 12585
MP

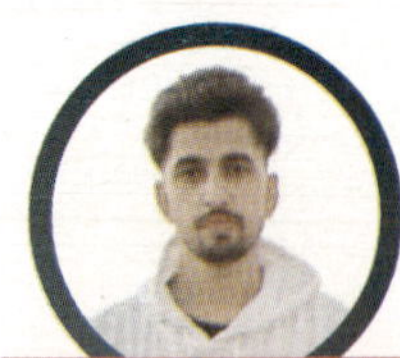
Mahadev Aanjan
Rank- 50
Roll No. 10130
MP

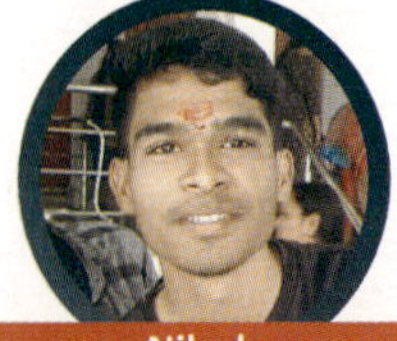
Nilesh
Rank- 81
Roll No. 10572
MP

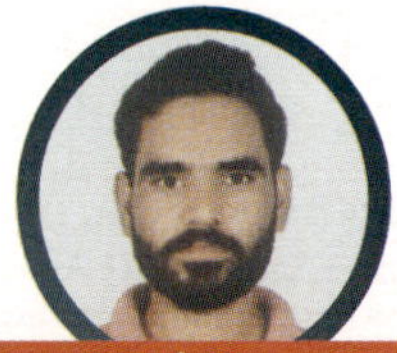
Balveer
Roll No. 619175
RAJASTHAN

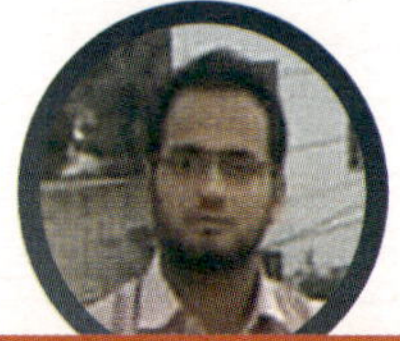
Mahendra Singh Gurjar
Roll No. 626167
RAJASTHAN

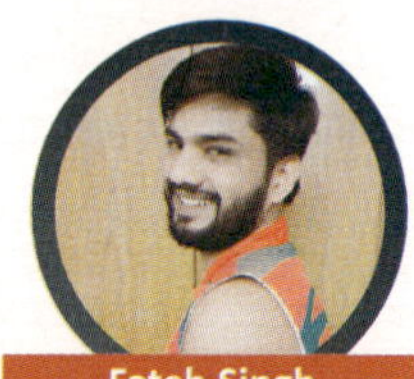
Fateh Singh
Roll No. 108169
RAJASTHAN

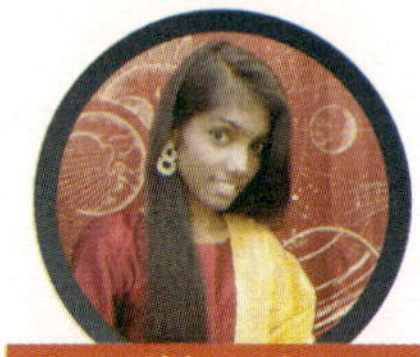
Shivangi
Roll No. 406105
RAJASTHAN

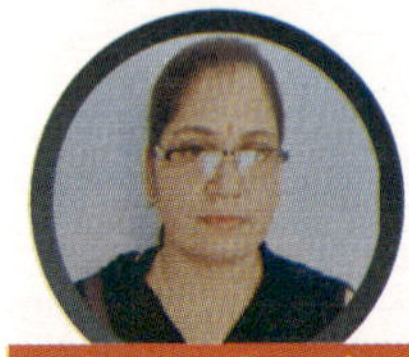
Suneeta Swami
Roll No. 619378
RAJASTHAN

And many mo

OF NURSING NEXT LIVE

200+ STUDENTS who cleared Various National/State Level Nursing Exams

BFUHS 2021

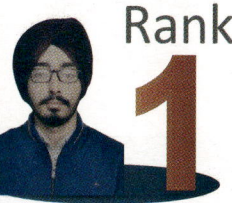
Rank 1
Harjeet Singh
Roll No- 472478

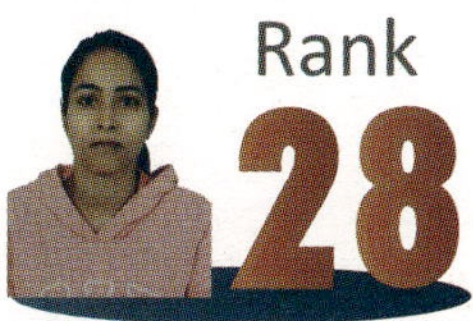
Rank 28
Kuljit Kaur
Roll No. 473956

Rank 32
Karan Sharma
Roll No. 469134

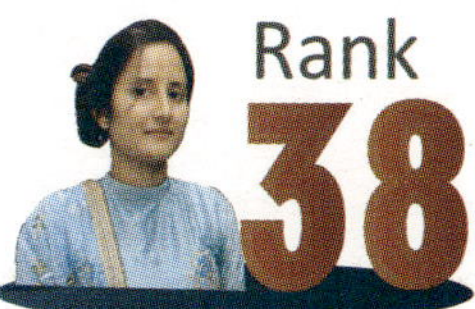
Rank 38
Smriti Rana
Roll No. 463342

Rank 107
Harpreet Kaur
Roll No. 474125

And many more

AIIMS MSc ENTRANCE EXAM 2021

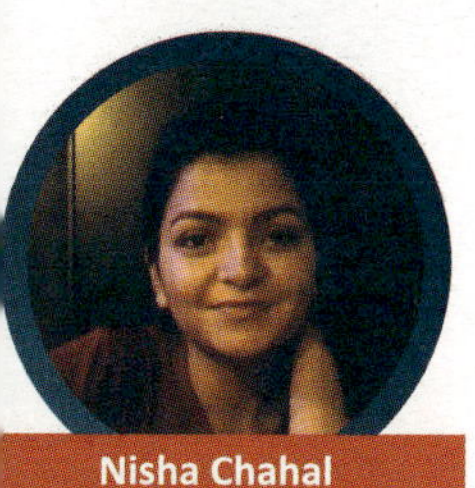
Nisha Chahal
AIIMS AIR-18

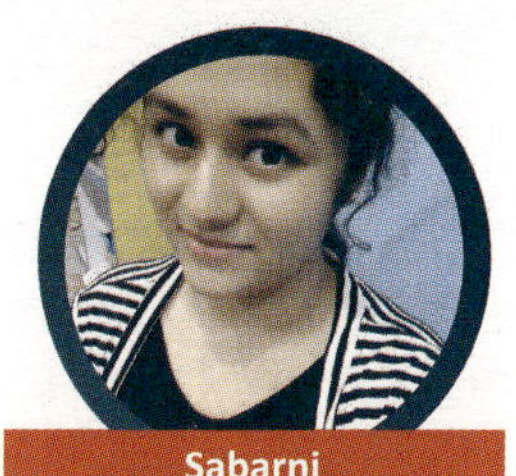
Sabarni
AIIMS AIR-21

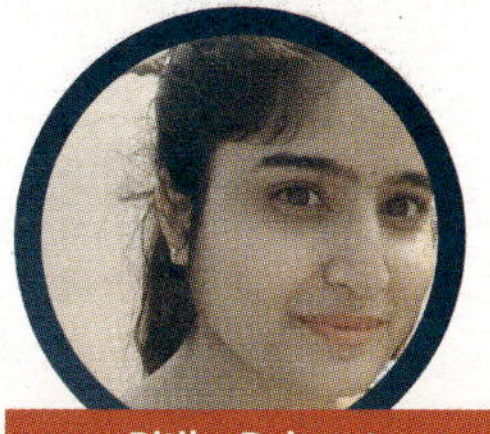
Ritika Rajpoot
AIIMS AIR-23

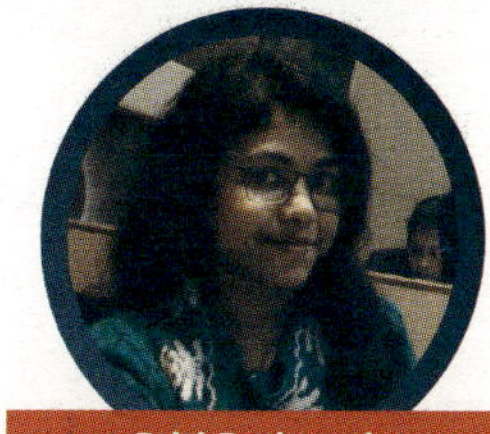
Priti Prajapati
AIIMS AIR-39

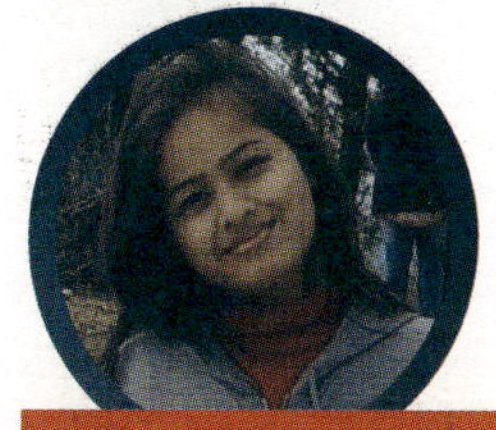
Shivangi Patwal
AIIMS AIR-64

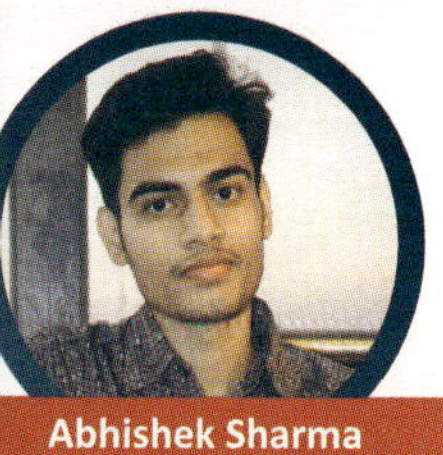
Abhishek Sharma
AIIMS AIR-97

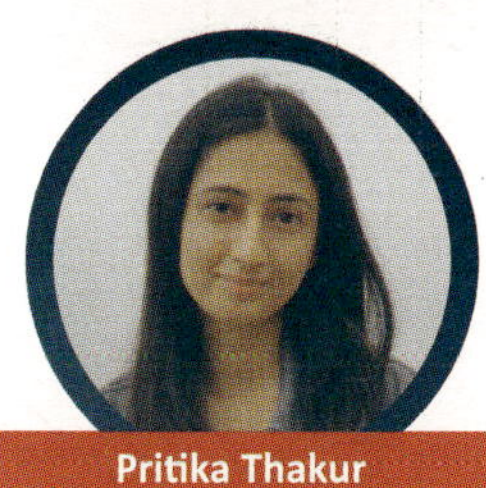
Pritika Thakur
AIIMS AIR-119

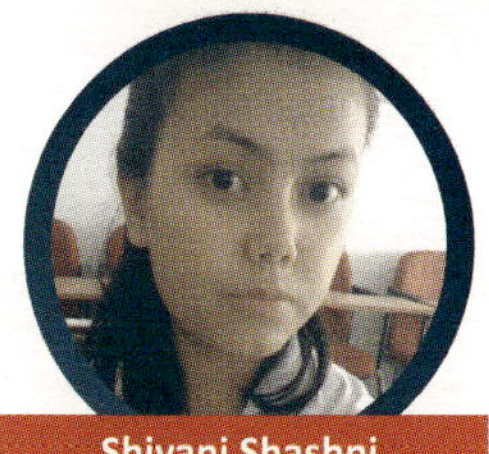
Shivani Shashni
AIIMS AIR-173

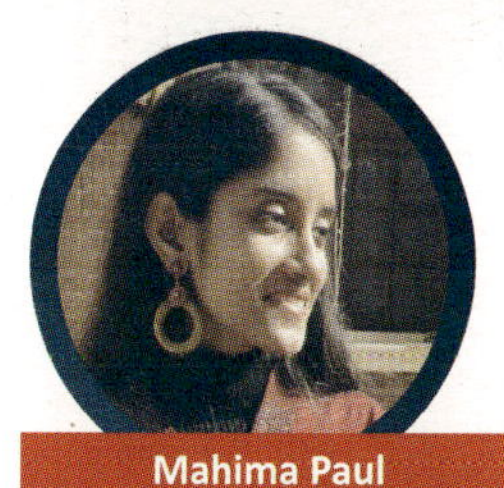
Mahima Paul
AIIMS AIR-175

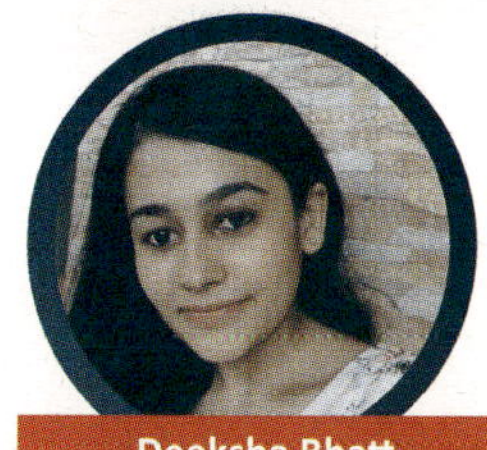
Deeksha Bhatt
AIIMS AIR-281

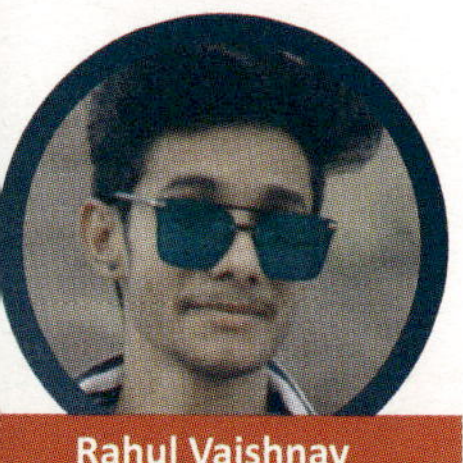
Rahul Vaishnav
AIIMS AIR-301

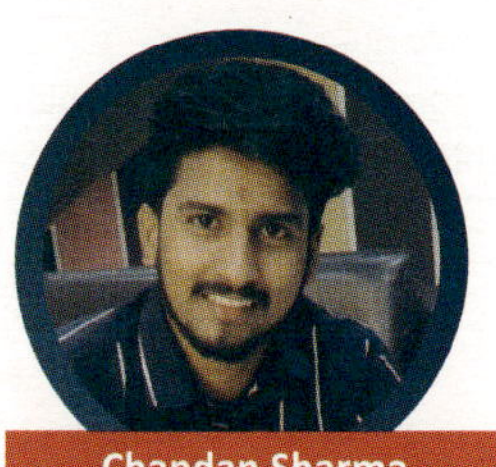
Chandan Sharma
AIIMS AIR-310

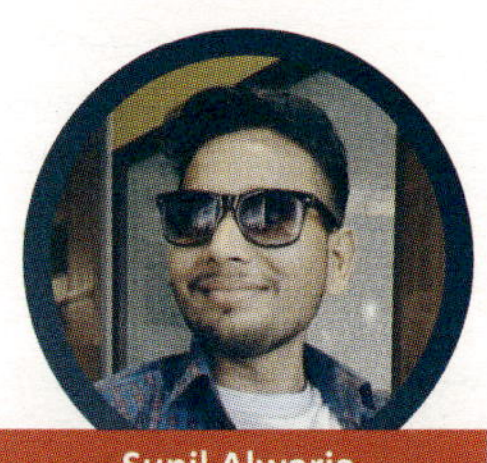
Sunil Alwaria
AIIMS AIR-677

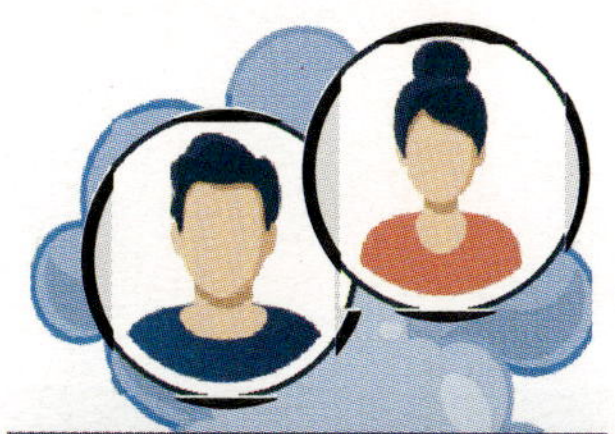
You Will Be The Next...

Scan the QR code to visit to our YouTube Channel to hear their success stories.

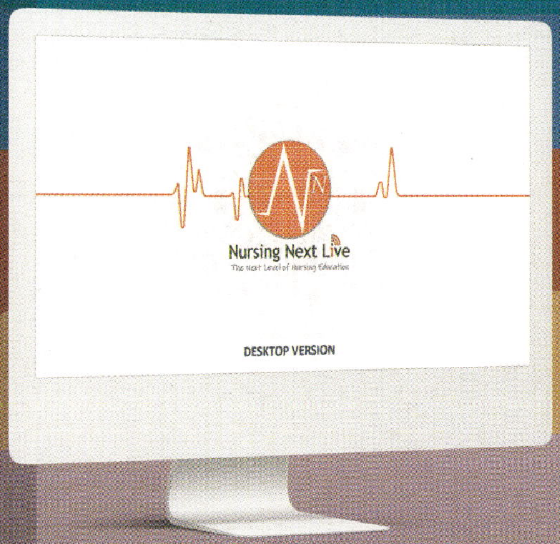

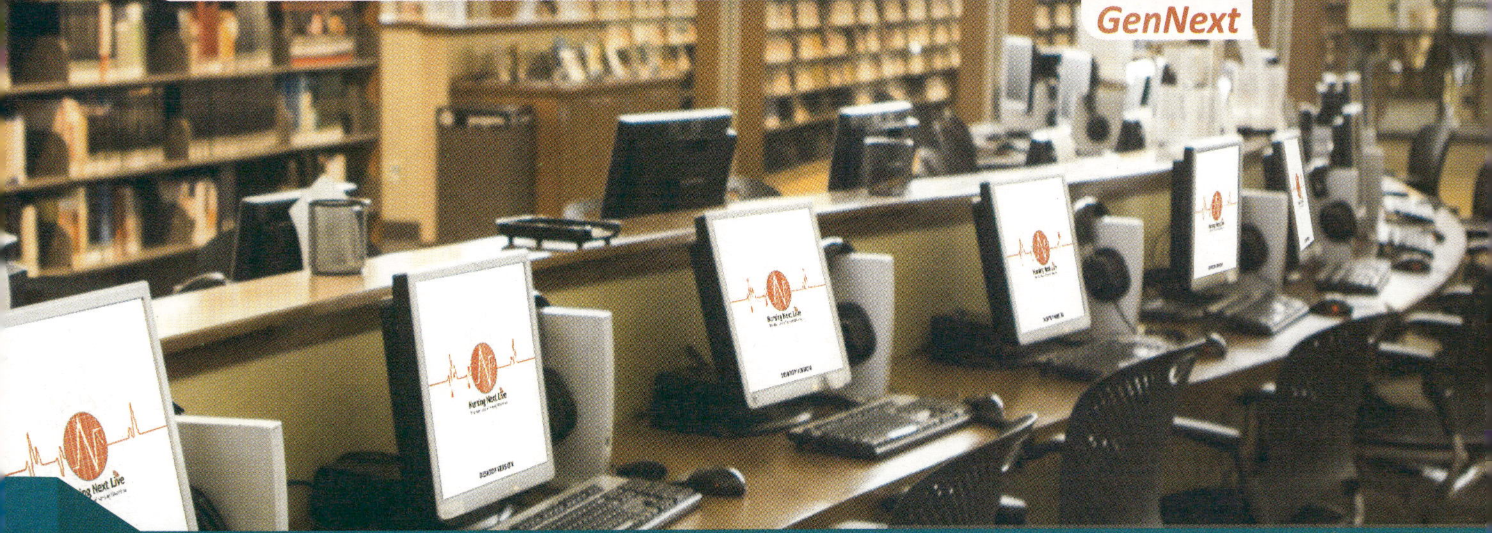

Plan-wise Comparison Chart

Compare and Choose the Best Suited to You

	Plan Zero	Crash Course	Test Series	Rapid Revision	Mastermind Plan C	Mastermind Plan C Plus
Videos						
1. All Subjects /Topics Videos	–	–	–	–	✓	✓
2. Video Lectures of Imp Topics	✓	–	✓	✓	–	✓
3. Exam Discussion Videos	–	–	✓	–	–	✓
4. Procedure Videos	–	–	–	–	–	✓
5. Rapid Revision Videos	–	–	–	✓	–	✓
6. IBQ/VBQ/Clinical Qs Discussion	–	–	✓	✓	–	✓
7. Live Doubt Sessions	–	–	–	–	✓	✓
8. Student-faculty Meet	–	–	–	–	✓	✓
9. Zoom Sessions/Webinar	–	–	–	–	✓	✓
10. Youtube Videos	–	–	✓	✓	✓	✓
Tests						
11. Special Mega Assessment Tests	–	–	✓	✓	✓	✓
12. Grand Tests	✓	✓	✓	–	–	✓
13. Subject-wise Tests	✓	✓	✓	–	–	✓
14. Mini Tests	✓	–	✓	–	–	✓
15. IBQs/VBQs	✓	–	✓	–	–	✓
16. Most Recent Papers	✓	✓	✓	–	–	✓
17. Previous Years Papers	✓	✓	✓	–	–	✓
18. Kerala Psc Crash Course	–	✓	✓	–	–	✓
19. CHO Exams Crash Course	–	✓	✓	–	–	✓
20. AIIMS NORCET 2020 Crash Course	–	✓	✓	–	–	✓
21. UPPSC Crash Course	–	✓	✓	–	–	✓
22. Most Probable Qs	–	–	–	✓	✓	✓
23. National Scholarship Test	✓	✓	✓	✓	✓	✓
24. Subject-wise Qs of All Topics	–	–	–	–	✓	✓
Notes						
25. Handwritten Notes Integrated With Lectures	–	–	–	–	✓	✓
26. Last-minute Revision Notes	✓	✓	✓	–	–	✓
27. Notes Integrated With Rapid Revision Videos	–	–	–	✓	✓	✓
28. Printed Booklets(*Forthcoming*)	–	–	–	–	✓	✓
Features						
29. Desktop Version	–	–	–	✓	✓	✓
30. Any Doubt Ask Us	✓	✓	✓	✓	✓	✓
31. Report A Query	✓	✓	✓	✓	✓	✓
32. National Level Ranking	✓	✓	✓	✓	✓	✓
33. Blogs	✓	✓	✓	✓	✓	✓
34. Daily Dose Of Knowledge	✓	✓	✓	✓	✓	✓
35. Forums Get Latest Info	✓	✓	✓	✓	✓	✓
36. Resume Learning	✓	✓	✓	✓	✓	✓
37. Buy Books	✓	✓	✓	✓	✓	✓
Supports						
38. Guidance & Counseling	–	–	–	✓	✓	✓
39. Faculty Telegram Channel	–	–	–	✓	✓	✓
40. Faculty Facebook Page	–	–	–	✓	✓	✓

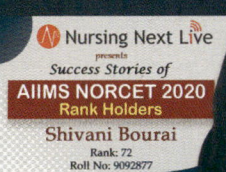

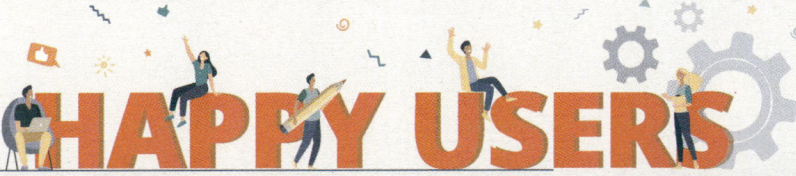

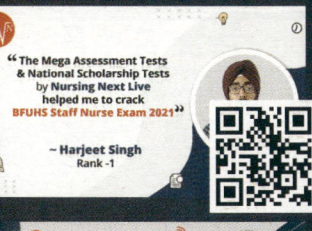

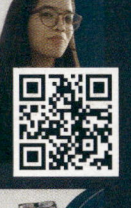

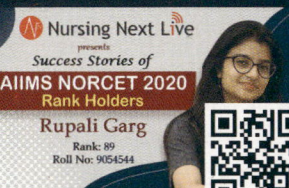

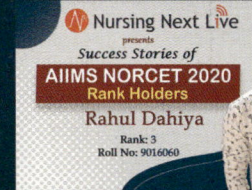

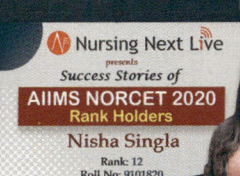

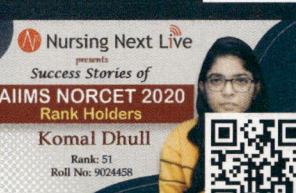

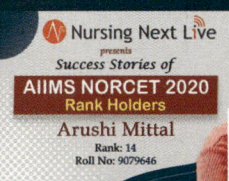

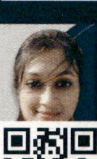

Clinical Case Record
for the Students of
Obstetrical Nursing

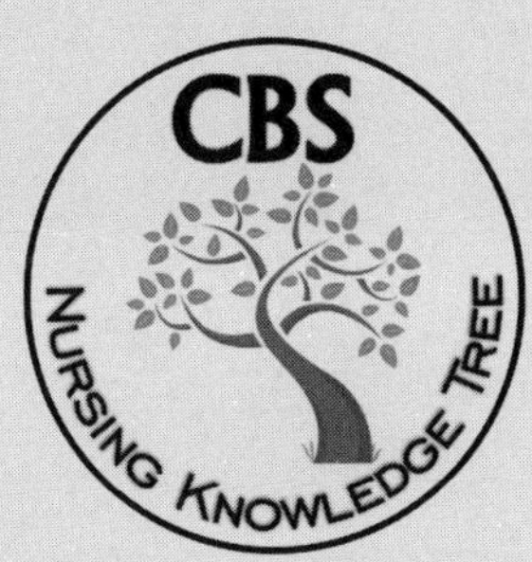

(As per the New Syllabus of Indian Nursing Council)

Second Edition

Soni Kumari MSc (N), OBG

Tutor

Indira Gandhi Institute of Medical Sciences
College of Nursing
Patna, Bihar

Foreword

Anuja Daniel

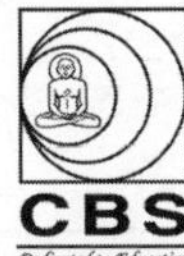

CBS Publishers and Distributors Pvt Ltd

• New Delhi • Bengaluru • Chennai • Kochi • Mumbai
• Hyderabad • Kolkata • Nagpur • Patna • Vijayawada

Clinical Case Record
for the Students of
Obstetrical Nursing

ISBN: 978-93-88178-51-8

Second Edition: 2019

First Edition: 2016

Published by **Satish Kumar Jain** and produced by **Varun Jain** for

CBS Publishers and Distributors Pvt Ltd

4819/XI Prahlad Street, 24 Ansari Road, Daryaganj, New Delhi 110 002, India.

Ph: 23289259, 23266861, 23266867 Website: www.cbspd.com

Fax: 011-23243014

e-mail: delhi@cbspd.com; cbspubs@airtelmail.in.

Corporate Office: 204 FIE, Industrial Area, Patparganj, Delhi 110 092

Ph: 4934 4934 Fax: 4934 4935

e-mail: bhupesharora@cbspd.com

Branches

- ***Bengaluru:*** Seema House 2975, 17th Cross, K.R. Road, Banasankari 2nd Stage, Bengaluru 560 070, Karnataka
  Ph: +91-80-26771678/79 Fax: +91-80-26771680
  e-mail: bangalore@cbspd.com
- ***Chennai:*** No. 7, Subbaraya Street, Shenoy Nagar, Chennai 600 030, Tamil Nadu
  Ph: +91-44-42032115 Fax: +91-44-42032115
  e-mail: chennai@cbspd.com
- ***Kochi:*** Ashana House, 39/1904, AM Thomas Road, Valanjambalam, Eranakulam 682 018, Kochi, Kerala
  Ph: +91-484-4059061-62-64-65 Fax: +91-484-4059065
  e-mail: kochi@cbspd.com
- ***Kolkata:*** No. 6/B, Ground Floor, Rameswar Shaw Road, Kolkata-700014 (West Bengal), India
  Ph: +91-33-2289-1126, 2289-1127
  e-mail: kolkata@cbspd.com
- ***Mumbai:*** 83-C, Dr E Moses Road, Worli, Mumbai-400018, Maharashtra
  Ph: +91-22-24902340/41 Fax: +91-22-24902342
  e-mail: mumbai@cbspd.com

Representatives

- Hyderabad +91-9885175004
- Nagpur +91-9021734563
- Patna +91-9334159340
- Vijaywada +91-74069-04007
- Mangalore +91-9741432102

Printed At : Goyal Offset Printers

From Publisher's Desk

"Gaining knowledge is the first step to wisdom. Sharing it is the first step to humanity."

The above mentioned lines form the foundation stone of CBS publishers and Distributors Pvt Ltd, the flag bearer in medical publishing. Headquartered in New Delhi, the national capital of India, CBS was established in the year 1972 and it has expanded its roots to grow as a pioneer in the field of medical publishing in Asia. CBS is one of the largest and the fastest growing publishers of medical books in Southeast Asia. We are partners in the education of undergraduate and postgraduate students for we believe in nurturing the brains of medicos since the beginning of their careers in medicine. CBS joins the hands with the medical students as their first choice since the very moment they enter the college with BD Chaurasia's Human Anatomy and CC Chatterjee's Human Physiology. CBS is the proud owner of many bestselling titles like OP Ghai's Textbook of Pediatrics, Manipal's Surgery, KD Chatterjee's Textbook of Parasitology, and the list goes on. CBS has successfully partnered in sculpting the careers of millions of medicos across the world.

Since establishment of "CBS Nursing Knowledge Tree", we have published many successful titles in the field of nursing and we have proved ourselves in the nursing fraternity in providing Quality Education.

Vision and Mission of CBS Nursing Knowledge Tree

CBS Nursing Knowledge Tree is conceptualized with a vision of being the first of its kind to bring the best quality books for education of Nurses. Keeping in mind the changing trends in the Nursing Education, we at CBS have taken up a mission to bring student-friendly and syllabus-based books written by Subject Experts from PAN India without compromising on the Quality of content and presenting it in a Unique manner.

Foundation Stones of CBS Nursing Knowledge Tree

- **Strong editorial support by the leading subject experts and faculties in Nursing from PAN India.** Every manuscript/proposal that is received is critically reviewed by our Editorial Board at various levels to ensure the Quality of content. A book is published only after all the parameters in our process management are satisfied.
- **Special care taken to publish Plagiarism-free matter.** With the copyright laws being highly strict these days, we at CBS are paying extra attention at various stages of publishing a book to crosscheck and avoid any copyright infringement.
- **Books authored by Subject Experts and Senior Faculties all over India.** Every title owned by CBS Nursing Knowledge Tree is written by the senior-most faculties and subject masters from every nook and corner of the country to provide them a bigger platform to share their knowledge and experience amongst budding nursing fraternity.
- **All the books developed as per INC syllabus and needs of the students without compromising on the Quality of the content.** Often students complain that some books are either not covering the complete syllabus or have too much content as compared to the syllabus. In this series, extra care is being taken to develop books strictly as per INC syllabus in the most student-friendly manner.
- **All books being reviewed by Top-notch faculties and Subject Experts to maintain high standards of Quality.** Every title goes through tough grilling regarding the content and the overall presentation by various top subject experts as reviewers. This ensures that only the Quality content gets published.
- **Best International standard layouts for every book.** Every title in CBS Nursing Knowledge Tree is designed and formatted in the best layouts of international standards because we strongly believe that every book deserves to be treated the Best!

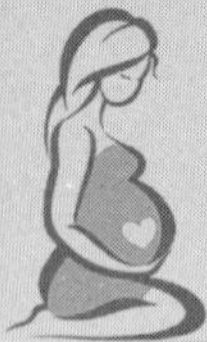

- **Additional and Unique features given with every title.** Every title is accompanied by one or the other additional feature to complement the learning of students like—*Workbook, DVD, Last Minute Revision Notes*. We have also included many features like *How to make Most out of this Book, Assess Yourself* that contains questions and MCQs and other special boxes according to the need of the content.

Let's Join Our Hands Together

We can only bring the change that we want to see in Nursing Education with the support and cooperation of leading faculties in all Nursing specialties. If you envision the same, we are happy to welcome you to our panel of contributors and reviewers and let's take up this mission together of creating a Change in Nursing Education.

We crave cooperation from all the students and faculties to provide their genuine feedback on the quality of the books and how we can improve upon the deficiencies in future on the following email id: cbsvpdesk@yahoo.com . Constructive criticism with concrete suggestions for improvement for all our books will be highly appreciated.

Expanding Horizons

We are also highly active in attending various National Level Conferences and Meets organized by various Nursing Societies. We are keenly working to expand our horizons of associations by participating in conferences organized by **SOCHNI, ISPN, NRSI, ICMR, SOMI,** etc. every year. CBS has always been a forerunner and a big supporter of all National level Nursing Conferences. *If you have any National and State level conference proposals, we are happy to be the part of these conferences.*

Being Social is Our Aspiration

In this era of Social Media, we are happy being social as well by bringing you our Facebook page **facebook.com/cbsnursingtree** of "CBS Nursing Knowledge Tree" to expand our reach to the maximum people in Nursing. It is a platform purely dedicated to bring the important aspects and latest updates and developments in various domains and fields of Nursing. It will be our privilege if you could connect with us and share your knowledge and experiences as well on our Facebook page.

I would like to invite all the readers to come and join us on our facebook page and share some input, information and literature.

With this vision and above features we are happy to announce the release of Clinical Case Record for the Students of Obstetrical Nursing by Soni Kumari!

Bhupesh Arora
Vice President-Publishing and Marketing
(NURSING Division)
CBS Publishers and Distributors (Delhi) Pvt. Ltd.
Email: bhupesharora@cbspd.com
Mobile: (+91) 9555590180

Foreword

I am feeling too pleased to give foreword for the clinical case record for midwifery notes based on maternal and newborn care written by Soni Kumari.

This set of *Clinical Case Record for the Students of Obstetrical Nursing* is well planned and written in such a way that it could help the students of nursing as practical guide and also in planning and implementing antenatal, intranatal and postnatal cares. It is easy-to-understand, for the basic skills in delivering safe and thoughtful planned care to both mother and child.

The *Clinical Case Record for the Students of Obstetrical Nursing* consists of basic contents of midwifery and it could support as a very good practical guide and helps the students in attending their viva.

So I suggest this book to nursing students. It would be very supportive in providing comprehensive care to mother and child. Hope this will help our students to achieve the practical for midwifery and obstetrical nursing requirements as peer INC syllabus for BSc Nursing/General Midwifery Nursing.

Professor Anuja Daniel MSc (N), MCH

Principal

IGIMS College of Nursing

Patna, Bihar

Preface

It gives me immense pleasure to introduce "Clinical Case Record for the Students of Obstetrical Nursing" which will help the nursing students to meet their practical requirement as per INC Syllabus for ANM, GNM and BSc Nursing.

The main purpose behind writing this casebook is to develop skill of midwives, to handle all types of pregnancies from normal to high risk, assessment and proper care to them. This casebook is designed to meet the current demands of the midwifery students in all aspects.

Soni Kumari

Name of the Institution

Certificate

Department of Midwifery

This is to certify that Mr/Ms .... with Registration no. .... has satisfactorily completed his/her requirements of Midwifery as prescribed by **Indian Nursing Council, New Delhi**, and ....
....
University/Board during the years ....

Date:

Place:

Signature of Subject in Charge **Signature of HOD**

Signature of Principal

Internal Examiner

1. ....
2. ....
3. ....

External Examiner

1. ....
2. ....
3. ....

Name of the Institution

Certificate of Clinical Training

Department of Midwifery

This is to certify that Mr/Ms .... has satisfactorily completed his/her clinical postings of Midwifery as prescribed by **Indian Nursing Council, New Delhi**, and .... University/Board at .... hospital from .... / .... /201.............. to .... / .... /201.............. .

Date:

Place:

Signature of Principal
of
Hospital/Departmental Head

Acknowledgements

The success was possible due to the collective efforts of so many personality to whom I express my gratitude

I would like to express a deep sense of gratitude to God Almighty for his adding grace and blessing which gave us moral support, strength and guidance for the successful completion of the casebook.

It is indeed gratifying that this book has been successfully completed because of favorable environment, continuous support and motivation of my colleague.

I extent my deep sense of gratitude and respect to the Principal, Ms Anuja Danial MSc (Maternal and Child Health Nursing) for her constant guidance, highly instructive suggestion, advice, as well as providing all possible facilities for successfully carrying out this study, in spite of her busy schedule of work.

It is a great pleasure to express my deep gratitude and thanks to Assistant Professor Mrs Fauzia Kazi, MSc (Pediatric Nursing), for her personal interest, and encouragement for the completion of this project.

I thank to all the nursing faculty members of IGIMS, College of Nursing for their guidance and encouragement.

My whole-hearted thanks to My Family for their love and blessing to complete this midwifery casebook.

Mr Anup Ghosh, Manager-Sales and promotions for their meticulous efforts in the direction of bringing out this book.

I express my warm appreciation to all those who have helped me directly and indirectly to make the fruition of this project possible.

I appreciate support of **Mr Satish Kumar Jain** *(Chairman)* and **Mr Varun Jain** *(Managing Director)*, M/s CBS Publishers and Distributors Pvt Ltd. for their whole-hearted support in publication of this book. No amount of words can describe role, efforts, inputs and initiatives undertaken by **Mr Bhupesh Arora**, *(Vice President-Publishing and Marketing, PGMEE and Nursing Division)*, for his endeavor toward the development of the book.

I thank Dr Mrinalini Bakshi (Sr Content Developer and Editor) for her editorial support and Ms Nitasha Arora (Project Manager), Ms Neetu Jindal (Asst. Production Manager), Mr Nitish K Dubey (Senior Editor) and all the production team members Mr Ashutosh Pathak, Mr Bunty Kashyap, Mr Phool Kumar, Mr Chaman Lal, Mr Prakash Gaur, Ms Tahira Praveen, Ms Babita Verma, Mr Raju Sharma, Vikram Chaudhary, Manoj Chaudhary and Manoj Malakar for devoting laborious hours in designing and typesetting of this book. I convey thanks to all those who are associated with this book.

Contents

Midwifery Casebook Record

Name of the Student : ....

Name of the Institute : ....

Batch Number/Session : ....

Registration Number/Roll No. : ....

Paste your passport size photo

ESSENTIAL REQUIREMENTS

Contents	Recommended	Page nos	Completed
Antenatal examination	30		
Conduction normal deliveries	20		
Vaginal examination	5		
Episiotomy and suturing	5		
Neonatal resuscitation	5		
Assisted with cesarean section	2		
Witness/assisted abnormal deliveries	5		
Postnatal case nursed	20		
Insertion of IUCD	5		

Signature of Student **Signature of Class Coordinator** **Signature of Principal**

Signature of External Examiner **Signature of Internal Examiner**

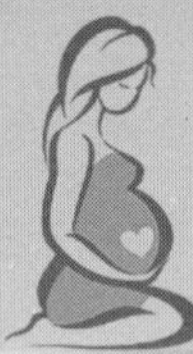

Midwifery and Obstetrical Nursing

General Objectives

Upon completion of the midwifery casebook the student shall be able to:

- Identify health needs of woman during pregnancy, labor and puerperium
- Identify deviation from normal pregnancy and take appropriate nursing care
- List different reproductive problem demonstrate skill in providing nursing care
- Demonstrate the skill in providing care to antepartum, intrapartum and postpartum period
- Give postnatal nursing care to the mother
- Practice administration of drug as per protocol
- Perform immediate nursing care of newborn
- Counsel and teach family planning methods for parenthood
- Educate woman for improving quality of life of the family
- Participate in maintaining the record.

Specific Objectives

- **Antenatal Clinic/OPD:**
  - Perform antenatal assessment
  - Assist/perform Hb and urine test for albumin and sugar
  - Identify risk status
  - Provide immunization and maintain health record
  - Maintenance of antenatal care (ANC) record
  - Counsel antenatal mother.
- **Labor room**

  Mother
  - Assess woman in labor room
  - Monitoring and caring of woman in labor room
  - Maintenance of partograph
  - Carry out pervaginal examination
  - Conduct normal deliveries
  - Perform episiotomy and repair it
  - Maintenance of labor and birth records.

  Newborn
  - Newborn assessment
  - Immediate newborn care
  - Resuscitation of newborn.
- **Operation theater**
  - Arrange for cesarean section.
  - Assist for medical termination of pregnancy (MTP) and other surgical procedure.
  - Assist with cesarean section.
  - Care of woman and baby after surgery.
- **Postnatal ward**

  Mother
  - Prepare for providing nursing care to postnatal mother and baby
  - Assessment of postnatal mother
  - Identification of deviation from normal puerperium
  - Demonstrate perineal care
  - Demonstrate breastfeeding technique
  - Practice to counsel and teach mother and family for parenthood
  - Educate postnatal mother regarding mother craft, postnatal care exercise and immunization.

  Newborn
  - Assessment of baby
  - Perform baby bath
  - Follow immunization schedule
  - Participate in lactation management.
- **Newborn**
  - Asses newborn
  - Identify newborn at risk
  - Provide nursing care to newborn at risk
  - Assist feeding at risk neonates
  - Practice administration of medication
  - Assisting in diagnostic procedure
  - Assisting with exchange transfusion
  - Follow infection control technique
  - Perform monitoring and care of neonates
  - Organize for teaching and counseling of parents
  - Practice thermal management of neonate
  - Teaching and counseling of parents regarding newborn care
  - Maintenance of neonatal records and reports.
- **Family planning clinic**
  - Counsel and provide family welfare services
  - Follow counseling technique
  - Assist/perform insertion of intrauterine device (IUD)
  - Arrange for and assist with family planning operation
  - Maintenance of family planning records and reports.

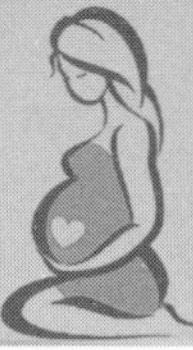

Short Notes on Midwifery

FEMALE PELVIS AND FETAL SKULL

Female Pelvis

Structure of Pelvis–Made up of Mainly four Parts

- Two innominate bone or hip bones (Ileum, Ischium and Pubis)
- One sacrum (Five fused vertebrae)
- One coccyx (fusing of four vertebrae)

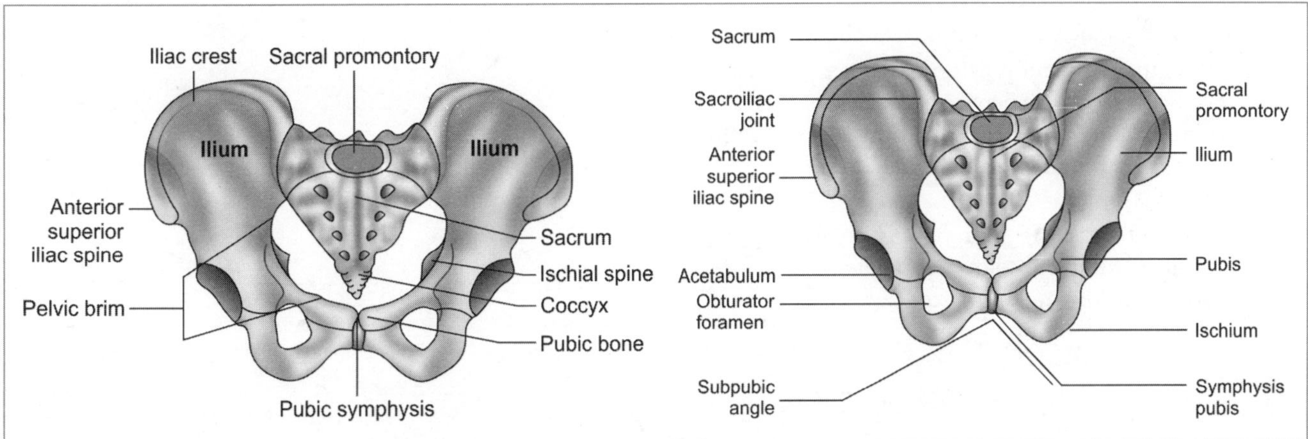

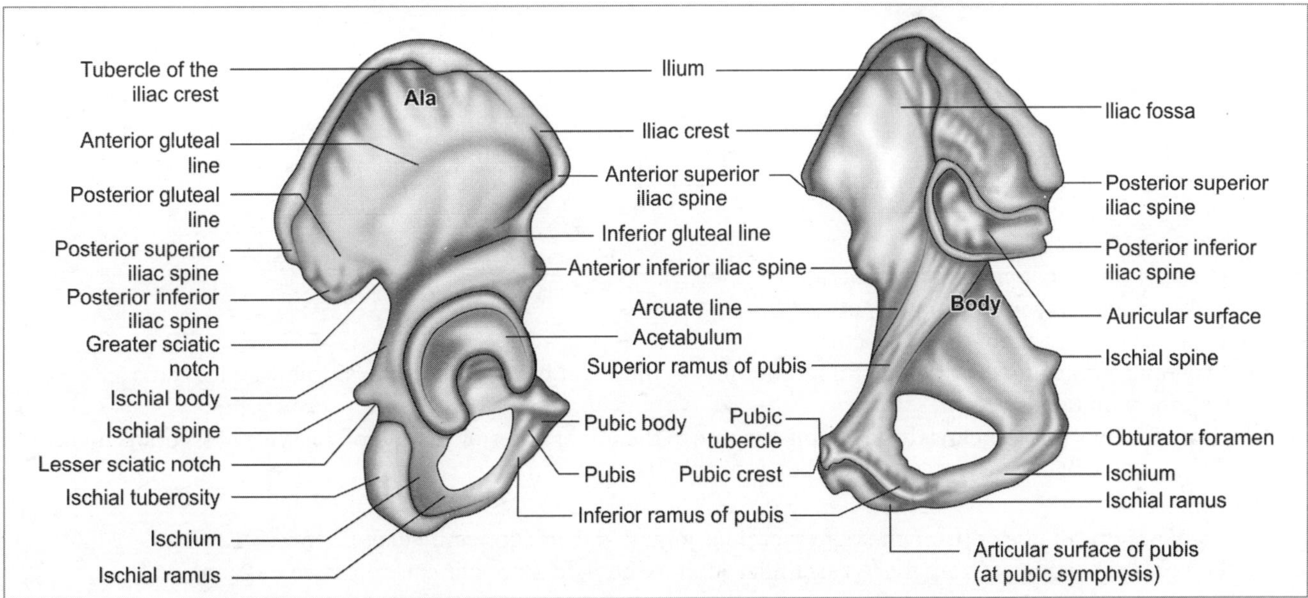

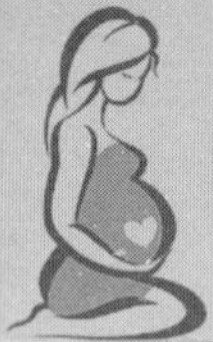

Joints in Pelvis

- Two sacroiliac joints
- One sacrococcygeal joint
- One symphysispubic.

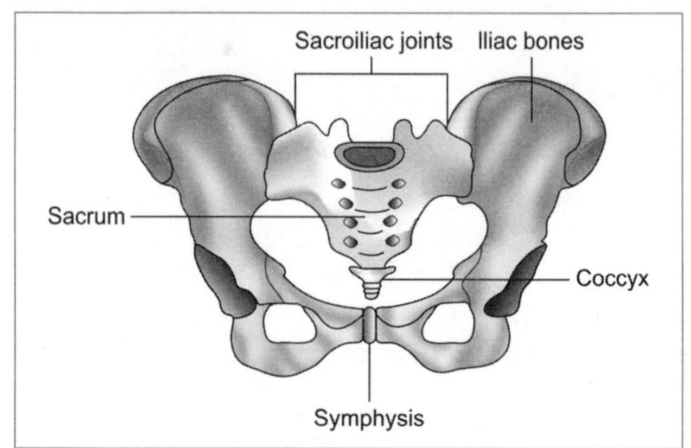

The Pelvis Ligament

- The sacroiliac ligaments
- The sacrotuberous ligaments
- The sacrospinous ligaments
- The sacrococcygeal ligaments
- Interpubis ligaments

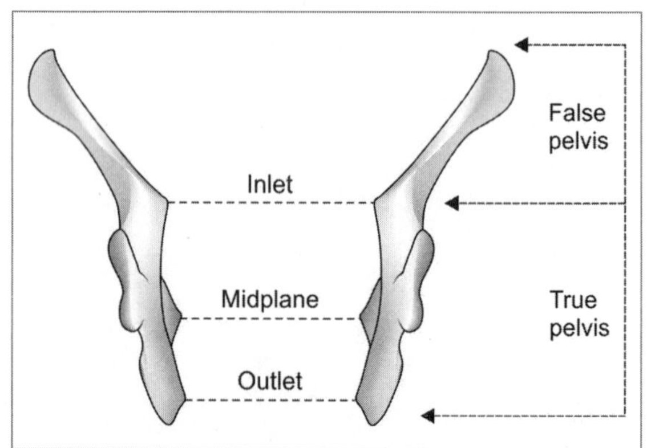

Anatomically Pelvis is Divided into Two Types

- **False pelvis** (iliac part of innominate bone-above brim)
  - The upper broader portion of the pelvic cavity called false pelvis or false pelvic cavity
  - It is formed by the iliac portion of the innominate bones and limited above by iliac crest.
- **True pelvis**
  - True pelvis is the part of the pelvis important in childbirth and lies below the pelvic inlet.
  - True pelvis divided into three parts
    - Inlet/brim (upper part of pelvis, round in shape)
    - Cavity (middle part of pelvis, round in shape)
    - Outlet (lower part of true pelvis)

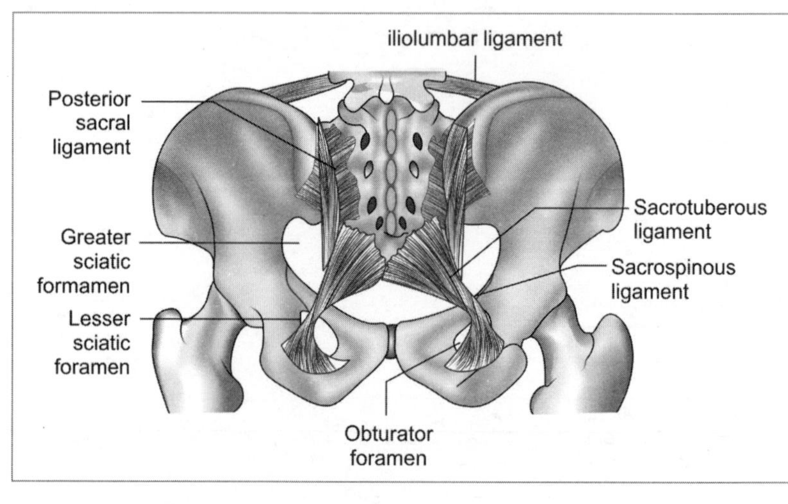

Diameter of Pelvic Inlet

- **Anteroposterior diameters:**
  - Anatomical anterior-posterior diameter/true conjugate (sacral promontory to the upper border of the symphysis pubis. = 11 cm)
  - Obstetric conjugate (sacral promontory to symphysis pubis, i.e. 1 cm below its upper border = 10.5 cm)
  - Diagonal conjugate (the tip of sacral promontory to the lower border of symphysis pubis. = 12.5 cm)
  - External conjugate = 20 cm
  - From the depression below the last lumbar spine to the upper anterior margin of the symphysis pubis measured from outside by the pelvimeter. It has not a true obstetric importance.
- **Oblique diameters**
  - Right oblique diameter (from the right sacroiliac joint to the left iliopectineal eminence. = 12 cm
  - Left oblique diameter (from the left sacroiliac joint to the right iliopectineal eminence = 12 cm)
  - Sacrocotyloid diameters (from the promontory of the sacrum to the right and left iliopectineal eminence, so the right diameter ends at the right eminence and vice versa= 9–9.5 cm)

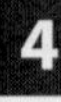

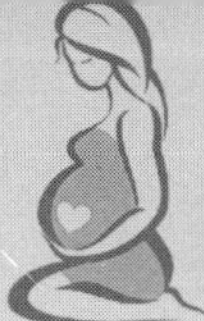

- **Transverse diameters:**
  - Anatomical transverse diameter (between the farthest two points on the iliopectineal lines = 13 cm, It is the largest diameter in the pelvis.)
  - Obstetric transverse diameter (true conjugate and is slightly shorter than the anatomical transverse diameter.)

Diameter of Pelvic Cavity

- Antero-posterior diameter =12 cm
  - From midpoint on the posterior surface of the symphysis pubis to the junction of 2nd and 3rd sacral vertebrae.
- Transverse: 12cm
  - It cannot be precisely measured as the point lies over the soft tissues covering the sacrosciatic notches and obturator foramen.

Diameters of Pelvic Outlet

- Anteroposterior diameters
  - Anatomical anterior-posterior diameter = 11 cm
    - From the tip of the coccyx to the lower border of symphysis pubis
  - Obstetric anteroposterior diameter = 13 cm
    - From the tip of the sacrum to the lower border of symphysis pubis as the coccyx moves backward during the second stage of labor.
- **Transverse diameters**
  - Bituberous diameter = 11 cm
    - Between the inner aspects of the ischial tuberosities
  - Bispinous diameter = 10.5 cm
    - Between the tips of ischial spines.

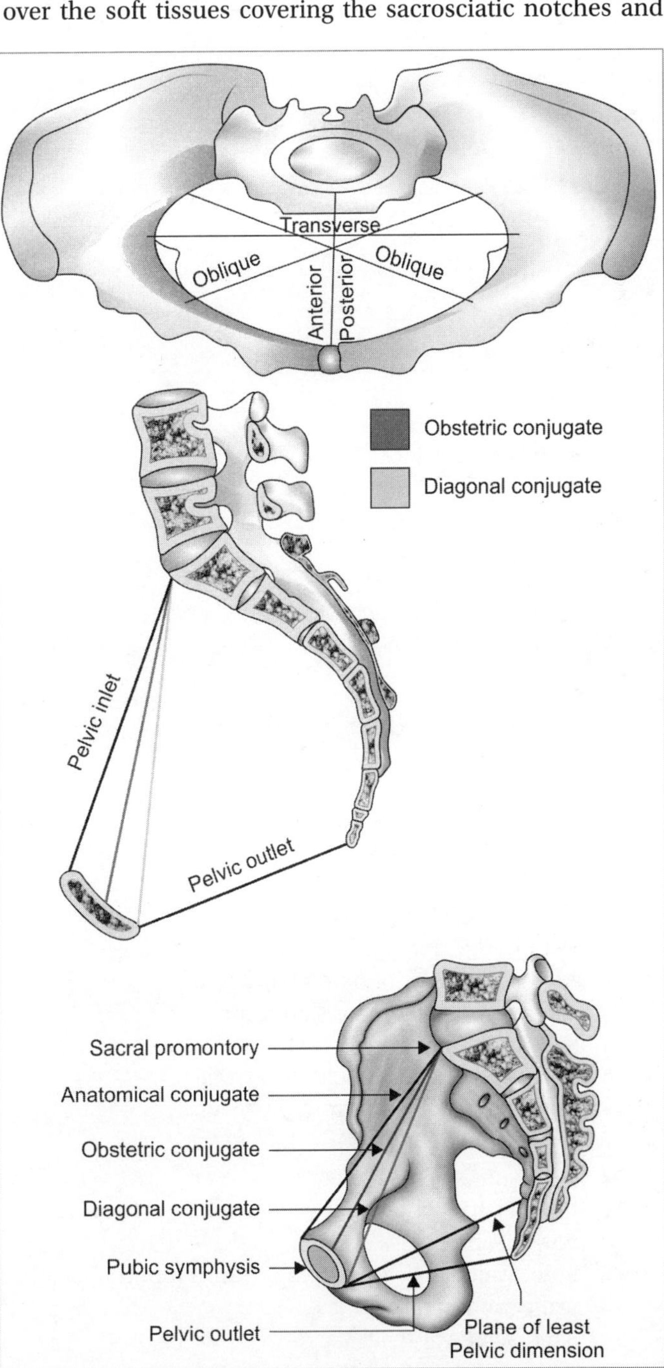

Land mark of the Pelvis/Inlet

- Sacrum promontory
- Ala of sacrum
- Sacroiliac joints/articulation
- Iliopectineal line
- Iliopubic eminence
- Pectineal line/upper border of the superior pubic ram
- Pubic tubercle
- Pubic crest
- Symphysis pubis/upper border of symphysis pubis

The Pelvic Outlet

Anatomical outlet

It is lozenge-shaped bounded by:

- The lower border of symphysis pubis
- Pubic arch
- Ischial tuberosities

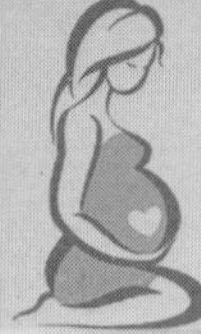

- Sacrotuberous and sacrospinous ligaments and
- Tip of the coccyx.

Obstetric outlet

It is a segment, the boundaries of which are:

- The roof is the plane of least pelvic dimension
- The floor is the anatomical outlet
- Anteriorly the lower border of symphysis pubis
- Posteriorly the coccyx
- Laterally the ischial spines.

Types of Female Pelvis

Four types of female pelvis are described

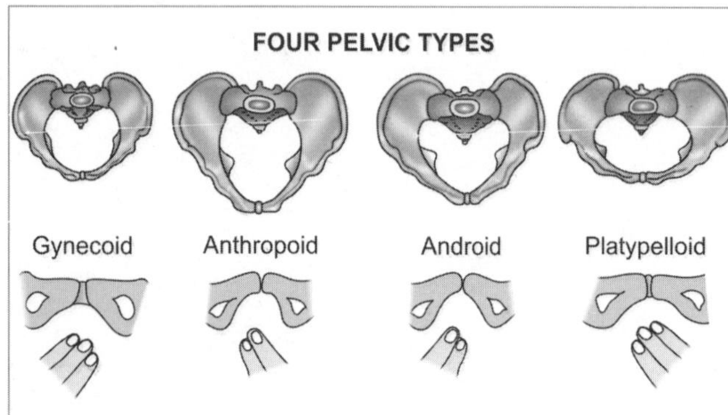

Actually, the majority of pelvis is of mixed types:

- **Gynecoid pelvis (50%)**
    - It is the normal female type
    - Inlet is slightly transverse oval
    - Sacrum is wide with average concavity and inclination.
    - Side walls are straight with blunt ischial spines
    - Sacrosciatic notch is wide
    - Subpubic angle is 90–100°.
- **Anthropoid pelvis (25%)**
    - It is ape-like type.
    - All anteroposterior diameters are long
    - All transverse diameters are short
    - Sacrum is long and narrow
    - Sacrosciatic notch is wide
    - Subpubic angle is narrow.
- **Android pelvis (20%)**
    - It is a male type
    - Inlet is triangular or heart-shaped with anterior narrow apex
    - Side walls are converging (funnel pelvis) with projecting ischial spines
    - Sacrosciatic notch is narrow
    - Subpubic angle is narrow 90°.
- **Platypelloid pelvis (5%)**
    - It is a flat female type
    - All anteroposterior diameters are short
    - All transverse diameters are long
    - Sacrosciatic notch is narrow
    - Subpubic angle is wide.

FETAL SKULL

Area of Skull

- **Vertex:** It is the quadrangular area bounded anteriorly by the bregma and coronal sutures behind by the lambda and the lambdoid sutures and laterally by the line passing through the parietal eminences.
- **Brow:** It is an area bounded on one side by the anterior fontanel and the coronal sutures and on the other side by the root of the nose and supra-orbital ridges of the either side.
- **Face:** It is an area bounded on one side by the root of the nose and the supra-orbital ridges and on the other by the junction of the floor of mouth with neck.

Landmark of Fetal Skull

- **Occiput:** It is the occipital bone/external occipital protuberance
- **Sinciput:** It is the forehead region of fetal head
- **Parietal eminences:** These are the eminences of parietal bone on either side
- **Mentum:** It is the chin
- **Vertical point:** It is the center of sagittal suture
- **Frontal point:** It is the root of nose
- **Sub occiput:** It it is the junction fetal neck and occiput
- **Submentum:** It it is the junction between neck and chin
- **Biparietal:** It is the transverse distance between two parietal eminences
- **Bitemporal:** It is the distance between two lower end of coronal suture.

Sutures

- **Frontal suture:** This lies in between two frontal bone.
- **Sagittal suture:** This lies in between two parietal bone.

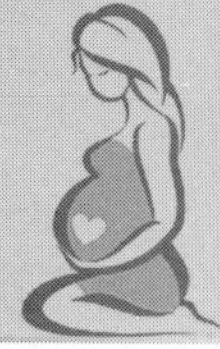

- **Coronal suture:** This lies in between the frontal and parietal bone on either side.
- **Lambdoid suture:** It lies in between the parietal and occipital bone on either side.

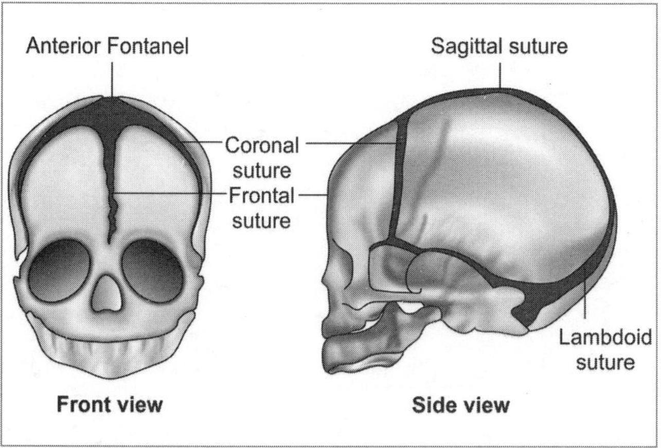

Clinical Importance of Suture

- These suture permit gliding movement of one bone over other during molding of the head in the vertex presentation, as a result the diameter of the head get smaller so passage of head through the birth canal become easier
- Position of fontanel and sagittal suture can identify attitude and position of vertex
- From the digital palpation of the sagittal suture during labor, degree of internal rotation and degree of molding of the head can be noticed
- In deep transverse arrest, this sagittal suture lies transversely at the level of the ischial spines.

Area of Skull

- **Vertex:** It is the quadrangular area bounded anteriorly by the bregma and coronal sutures behind by the lambda and the lambdoid sutures and laterally by the line passing through the parietal eminences
- **Brow:** It is an area bounded on one side by the anterior fontanel and the coronal sutures and on the other side by the root of the nose and supraorbital ridges of the either side
- **Face:** It is an area bounded on one side by the root of the nose and the supraorbital ridges and on the other by the junction of the floor of mouth with neck.

Diameter of Skull

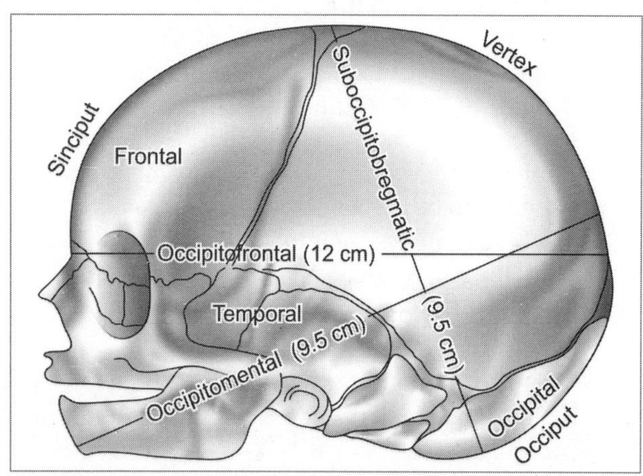

The engaging diameter of the fetal skull depends on the degree of the flexion of the presenting part.

- The anteroposterior diameter, which may be engaged are:
  - **Suboccipitobregmatic**
    It extends from the nape of the neck to the center of anterior fontanel .
    Length: 9.5 cm, Attitude: complete flexion
  - **Suboccipitofrontal**
    It extends from the nape of the neck to root of nose.
    Length—10 cm, Attitude incomplete flexion, Presentation—vertex
  - **Occipitofrontal**
    Extends from the occipital eminence to the root of the nose (glabella)
    Length—11.5 cm, attitude—marked deflexion, presentation—vertex.
    Clinical importance: This engaging diameter may give rise to prolonged labor.
  - **Mentovertical**
    It extends from the mid—point of the chin to the center of the sagittal suture
    Length—14 cm, Attitude—partial extension, presentation—brow.
    Clinical importance-in this engaging diameter, baby has delivered by cesarean section.

- **Submento vertical:**
  It extends from the junction of the floor of the mouth and neck to the center of the sagittal suture.
  Length—15.5 cm, attitude— incomplete extension, Presentation—face
  Clinical importance: In this engaging diameter, baby has to be delivered by cesarean section.
- **Submento bregmatic:**
  It extends from the junction of the floor of the mouth and neck to the center of bregma.
  Length—9.5cm, attitude—complete extension, presentation—face
  Clinical importance: In this engaging diameter, baby has to be delivered by cesarean section.

- **Transverse diameter of fetal skull**
  - **Biparietal diameter**
    It extends between two parietal eminences.
    Length—9.5 cm
  - **Bitemporal diameter**
    Distance between the anterior—inferior ends of the coronal suture.
    Length—8.5 cm

Fetal Skull Changes in Labor

- **Molding:** It is the changes in shape of the head in vertex presentation during labor while passing through the resistant birth canal.
- **Mechanism:**
  - Overlapping of cranial bones at the membranous joints due to compression of the engaging diameter of the head.
  - It is physiological, harmless and disappears within a few hours after birth.

Grading

Grade 0: The bones lie side by side having an intervening membrane.

Grade +: The bone touching but not overlapping

Grade++: Overlapping but easily separated by pressure.

Grade+++: Fixed overlapping and cannot be separated.

Differences Between Caput Succedaneum and Cephalic Hematoma

Caput succedaneum	Cephalic hematoma
• Present at birth on normal vaginal delivery	• Appears within a few days after birth on normal or forceps delivery
• May lie on suture, not well defined	• Well defined by suture, gradually developing, and hard edge
• Soft, pits on pressure	• Soft, elastic but does not pit on pressure
• Skin ecchymotic	• No skin change
• Size largest at birth, gradually subsides within a day	• Become largest after birth and then disappears within 6–8 weeks to few months
• No underlying skull bone fracture	• May underlying skull bone fracture
• No treatment required	• No treatment required

ANTENATAL ASSESSMENT

Diagnosis of Pregnancy

1st Trimester (1st–12th Week)

- Subjective symptoms
  - Amenorrhea and morning sickness
  - Pregnancy of micturition
  - Breast discomfort
  - Fatigue
- Objective signs
  - Breast changes (pronounced pigmentation, secondary areola, montgomery tubercles and increase vascularity)
  - Abdomen (uterus pelvic organ till 12th week)
  - Pelvic organ (Jacquemier/Chadwick sign, Osiander sign, Goodles sign)
  - Uterus (Piskackek's sign, Hegar's sign, Palmer sign)
  - Intradecidual gestation sac (29–35 days of gestation)

Second Trimester (13–28 Weeks)

- Quickening
- Progressive enlargement of the lower abdomen
- Chloasma
- Linea nigra
- Striae
- Uterus - ovoid in shape
- Braxton hicks contraction
- Palpation of fetal part

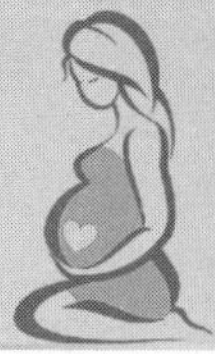

- Active fatal movement
- External ballottement/internal ballottement
- FSH, uterine souffle

3rd Trimester (29–40 Weeks)

- Amenorrhea
- Enlargement of the abdomen
- Lightening
- Increase frequency of maturation
- Fetal movement (more pronounced)
- Increase pigmentation and striae
- Uterine shape (cylindrical to spherical -36 weeks)
- Fundal height (increase/decrease) depends on weeks
- Braxton hicks contraction (more evident)
- Fetal movement easily felt
- FHS (heard distinctly)

Estimation of the Number of Pregnancies to be Registered Annually

Example for Estimation of the Number of Pregnancies Annually

Birth rate = 25/1000 population

Population under the subcenter = 5,000

Therefore,

Expected number of live births	=	(25 × 5000)/1000
	=	125 births
Correction factor	=	10% of 125 (i.e. [10/100] × 125)
	=	13

Therefore,

Total number of expected pregnancies in a year in that subcenter = 125 + 13 = 138

Component of Antenatal Checkup/History Taking

- Client's Profile
- Menstrual history to calculate the EDD (estimated date of delivery)

  EDD = date of LMP + 9 month + 7 days
- Menstrual history (to calculate the EDD), LMP, EDD menstrual cycle, duration of period, blood flow, dysmenorrheal/menstrual problem.
- History of present pregnancy-GPLAS, LMP, EDD, symptom, discomfort, symptom indicating complication (nausea and vomiting, heart burn, constipation, increase frequency of urination, fever, persistent vomiting, abnormal vaginal discharge/ itching, palpitation, easy fatigability, breathlessness at rest/on mild exertion, generalized swelling of the body, puffiness of the face, severe headache and burning of vision, passing smaller amounts of urine and burning sensation during micturition, vaginal bleeding, decreased or absent of movement, leaking of watery fluid per vaginal)
- Obstetric history: Term/preterm delivery, abortion. Stillbirth, nature of delivery, immunization, growth and development of baby, nature of puerperium
- Indication for high risk pregnancy - (stillbirth or neonatal loss, three or more spontaneous consecutive abortion, obstructed labor, premature births, twins or multiple pregnancies, weight of the previous baby <2,500 g or >4,500g, admission for hypertension or pre-eclampsia/eclampsia in the previous pregnancy, surgery on reproductive tract, congenital anomaly, treatment for fertility, spinal deformities/scoliosis/ kyphosis/polio, Rh-negative in the previous pregnancy)
- Personal history
- Present and past medical history
- Family history of systematic illness
- History of drug intake/allergies- she is taking any drug that might be harmful to the fetus.
- Examinations of the patient
  - General examination
  - Physical examination
  - Abdominal examination
- Risk factors for pregnant woman

  Malpresentation, multiple pregnancy, any bleeding P/V during pregnancy and after delivery (more than 500 mL blood loss), severe headache with blurred vision, hemoglobin<7 g, convulsion or loss of consciousness, decreased or absent fetal movement, active labor lasting longer than 12 hours in a primipara and more than 8 hours in multipara, continuous severe abdominal pain, PROM (before 37 weeks), high protein with proteins in urine, increase temperature more than 38°C, foul smelling discharge before or after delivery or abortion, rupture membrane more than 18 hours, FHR>160/minute or 120/minute, perineal tear (2nd, 3rd and 4th degree).
- Nursing diagnosis
- Health education
  - Antenatal visit (1st visit- within 12 week, 2nd visit- between 14 and 26 weeks, 3rd visit - between 28 and 34 weeks, 4th visit-between 36 weeks and term)

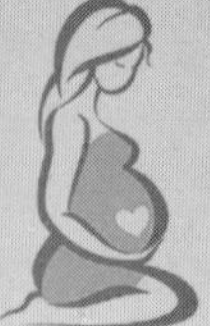

- Micro birth planning
- Birth preparedness
- Diet and rest
- Breastfeeding
- Sex during pregnancy
- Family planning

INTRAPARTUM ASSESSMENT

Deciding the Stages of Labor

- **1st stage:** This is the period from the onset of labor pain to the full dilatation of the cervix, i.e. to 10 cm. 1st stage takes about 12 hours in primigravidas and 8 hours in multipara.
  - **Latent stage:**
    - Cervix is dilated < 4 cm.
    - Contraction weak (less than 2 contraction in 10 minute).
  - **Active stage:** Cervix is dilated > 4 cm.
- **Second stage:** This is the period from full dilatation of the cervix to the delivery of the baby; this stage takes about 2 hours for primigravida about half an hour for multigravida.
- **Third stage:** This is the period from after delivery of the baby till the delivery of the placenta and membranes. This stage takes about 15 minutes to half an hour.
- **Fourth stage:** This is the first one hour after the delivery of the placenta. This is a critical period as PPH, a potentially fatal complication, is likely to occur during this stage.

True and False Labor Pain

True Labor Pain

- Begins irregular but becomes regular and predictable
- Felt first in the lower back and sweep around to the abdomen in a wave pattern
- Continues no matter what the woman's activity
- Increases in duration, frequency and intensity with passage of time
- Show/blood stained mucous discharge
- Cervical effacement and cervical dilatation.

False Labor Pain

- Begins irregular and remains irregular
- Felt first abdominally and remains confined to the abdomen and groin
- Often disappear with ambulation or sleep
- Does not increase in duration, frequency or intensity with passage of time
- Show absent
- No Cervical effacement and cervical dilatation.

Fetal Head Movement During Labor/ Mechanism of Labor

- Head floating, before engagement
- Engagement, flexion, descent
- Further descent, internal rotation
- Complete rotation and beginning of extension
- Complete extension
- External rotation of head and internal rotation of shoulder
- Delivery of anterior shoulder
- Delivery of posterior shoulder.

Care During Labor/Monitoring and Managing the Stages of Labor

1st Stage of Labor

Oxytocin drug for inducing/accelerating labor should not be administered before delivery as their use is associated with high incidence of rupture of the uterus.

Monitoring and Managing 1st Stage of Labor

- **Monitoring**
  - Monitor the following every hour.
    - **Contraction:**
      — Frequency: How many contraction in 10 minute.
      — Duration: For how many seconds each contraction lasts.
    - **FHR:** Normal FHR is between 120–160 beats/ minute.
      — Presence of any sign of an emergency. (Difficult in breathing, shock, vaginal bleeding convulsion and unconsciousness.)
  - Monitor the following every four hours:
    - Cervical dilation
    - Temperature

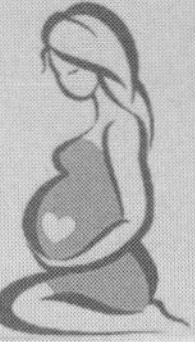

    - Pulse
    - Blood pressure
  - Monitor the following every 30 minutes
    - Maternal pulse
    - Contraction—frequency and duration
    - FHR
    - Presence of signs such as meconium blood stained amniotic fluid and prolapsed cord
- **Action/management**
  - Record time of rupture of membrane and color of amniotic fluid.
  - Never leave the woman alone
  - Allow her to remain mobile (Only **If membranes are intact**)
  - Let her choose the position in which she is comfortable
  - If after 8 hours, the contraction are stronger and more frequent but there is no progress in cervical dilatation, with or without rupture of membranes, it indicates nonprogress of labor
  - Start monitoring a partograph when the woman reaches active labor
  - Reassess the woman
  - Call senior person, if available
  - Encourage the woman to empty her bladder
  - Ensure adequate hydration but omit solid foods
  - Encourage her to maintain an upright position and walk, if she wishes
  - Monitor intensively, using the partograph.

Plotting Partograph

Note

- Start plotting the partograph in active labor (4 cm dilated)
- First recording of cervical dilatation on alert line
- Each of small boxes of partograph represents a half hour interval.

Plotting

- Identification of data
- Name, W/O, age, parity, reg. no, date and time of admission, date and time of ROM.
- ***Fetal condition***
  - **FHR count**
    - Every half an hour
    - For one full minute.
    - Immediately after a uterine contraction
  - **Amniotic fluid**
    - Condition of membrane and color of amniotic fluid
    - Record in
      - — Membrane intact
      - — Membrane rupture
      - — Clear liquor
      - — Meconium-stained liquor
  - **Labor progress and cervical dilatation**
    - Begins plotting when cervical dilatation 4 cm/ more
    - Check cervical dilatation every 4 hours.
    - 1st recording on the alert line using a sign (x).
    - Write time accordingly corresponding row for time.
  - **Uterine contraction**
    - Record the contraction every half an hour.
    - Contraction is less than 20 seconds fill the box with dots.
    - Contraction is between 20 and 40 second, draw diagonal lines in the box.
    - Contraction is more than 40, darken the box.
  - **Intervention**
    - Mention dose, route and time of drug administer.
    - Include the food items and liquid consumed.
  - **Maternal condition**
    - Maternal pulse on graph every half hours mark with a dot (.)
    - Record BP on the every 4 hour, using vertical arrow (↑)
    - Record temperature every 4 hour and in centigrade.

Second Stage of Labor

It begins with complete dilatation of the cervix and ends with the birth of the baby.

Sign and Symptom

- Expulsive contraction
- Rupture of membrane
- Vaginal stretching
- Dilatation and gaping of the anus and perineal bulging
- Progressive visibility of the fetal head at the introitus
- Congestion of the vulva.

Maternal Physiological Changes

- Blood pressure (may rise 5 to 20 mm Hg with contraction)
- Metabolism (steady rise in metabolism)
- Pulse rate (increase during pushing effort)
- Temperature (increase during delivery time, increase 0.5 to 10°C is consider normal)
- Gastrointestinal changes (decrease in gastric motility).

Mechanism of Normal Labor

- Positional movements are as follows
- Engagement
- Descend throughout
- Flexion
- Internal rotation of the head
- Crowning
- Birth of the head by extension
- Restitution
- Internal rotation of the shoulder
- External rotation of the head
- Birth of the shoulders and body by lateral flexion.

Episiotomy

An episiotomy is an incision of the perineum during delivery to:

- Substitute a straight surgical incision for the laceration that may otherwise occur
- Facilitate repair of laceration and promote healing
- Spare the neonate's head from prolonged pressure and pushing against the rigid perineum, which may result in brain damage, especially in the premature neonate
- Shorten the second stage of labor

Types of Episiotomies

Median (Midline)

- Incision is made in the middle of the perineum and directed toward the rectum.
- If proper perineal pressure does not apply during delivery, there may be chances of rectum tear.

Mediolateral

- This type is commonly used now a days.
- Firstly, Incision is made longitudinally about 1 cm and then 1.5 cm laterally towards thighs (either Right/Left).
- This method avoids the tear of anal sphincter if enlargement is needed. Women find it extremely uncomfortable during healing.
- More difficult to repair. Associated with increased blood loss

Management

- Pain relief
  - The stretching of the perineum and pressure from the fetal head may provide a natural numbing effect.
  - Local perineal infiltration with lidocaine provides anesthesia for performing and repairing the episiotomy.
  - A pudendal block provides anesthesia to the lower two-thirds of the perineum and vagina using lidocaine injection into the vaginal walls.
    - Epidural anesthesia provides anesthesia from the level of the umbilicus to the midthigh area.
- The episiotomy is performed when the fetal head is about 3 to 4 cm visible with a contraction.
- The repair of the episiotomy usually begins after the delivery of the placenta.

Nursing assessment

During the recovery period, the episiotomy should be evaluated every 15 minutes and three times a day after this.

- Describe and document the degree of healing
- Assess for infection, which may be indicated by edema, redness, purulent drainage at the site; increased temperature —delete it and write
- Assess episiotomy wound healing by using REEDA Scale (R-Redness, E-Edema, E-Ecchymosis, D-Discharge, A-Approximation)
- Monitor for hematoma formation.

Nursing diagnoses

- Risk for infection related to traumatized tissue
- Acute pain related to surgical procedure.

Third Stage of Labor

The 3rd stage of labor begins upon completion of the birth of the baby and ends with the birth of the placenta.

- Physiological process of the placental separation and expulsion:
  - Placental separation
  - Descent of the placenta
  - Expulsion of the placenta
  - Hemostasis.
- Active MTSL consists of the following three activities:
  - Uterotonic drug
  - Controlled cord traction
  - Uterine massage.

Immediate Postpartum Care

- The 1st two hours after the delivery of the placenta are the 4th stage.
- This stage comprises of both observation and care of the mother and newborn.
- **Evaluation and inspection of the**
  - Uterus
  - Hemostasis

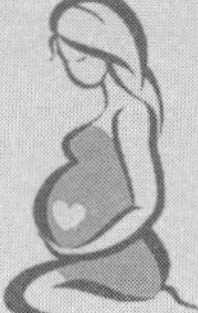

- Inspection of the cervix and upper vaginal vault
  - Repair
  - Perineal cleansing and positioning of leg.
- **Care and monitoring**
  - Vital sign.
  - Palpation of the fundus for contractility.
  - Massage the uterus and expression of the clot
  - Measurement of the fundus
  - Inspection of the perineum
  - Inspection of the bladder
  - Inspection and changes of perineal pad
  - Fluid and foods.

CARE OF NEWBORN

- Place an identity label with mother name and any identification information
- Give IM, Vitamin 'K' injection (1mg- 1,500 g or above newborn, 0.5 mg - less than 1,500 mg newborn)
- Notify health care provider if bleeding occurs, other than slight oozing
- Check baby breathing and color, every 5 minutes
- If the baby cyanotic/breathing less than 30 or more than 60 breath per minute, make initial attempts at resuscitation
- Check if the baby is warm, by feeling his/her feet every 5 minutes
- Check cord for bleeding every 15 minutes
- Wipe off any meconium/blood stain from baby's skin
- Encourage the mother for breast feeding within half an hour of birth
- Weight every baby before leaving delivery room
- Delay baby 1st bath (24 hours)
- Ensure baby is dressed warmly
- Watch for any complication (convulsion, coma and feeding problem).

RESUSCITATION OF NEWBORN

- The goal of newborn resuscitations are to
  - Establish and maintain a clear air way
  - To ensure effective circulation
  - To correct acidosis
  - To prevent hypothermia, hypoglycemia, and hemorrhage.
- Risk of complication in newborn may occur as
  - Preterm
  - Born after long traumatic labor
  - Born to mothers who received sedation during the late stages of labor.
- Equipment used for resuscitation
  - Bag and mask equipment (self inflating bag-volume 250/500 mL, face mask-0 and 1 size)
  - Suction equipment (mucous extractor/mechanical suction and tubing)
  - Miscellaneous: Radiant warmer, firm padded surface, warm linen, clock with second hand, oxygen source with flow meter, gloves, shoulder roll, cord tie/clamp, sterile blade/scissors
- Steps of resuscitation-
  - Provide warmth
  - Position the baby
  - Clear airway
  - Dry, stimulate to breathe and reposition
  - Ventilation
    - Positioning the bag and mask on the face
    - Frequency of squeezing the bag
  - Assess breathing
  - Assess heart rate:
- Prepare for discharge
  - The following should be kept in mind before the baby is discharge:

Baby	Mother
Ensure the baby is warm, breathing normally, accepting and retaining breast milk, and cord is clean	Ensure uterus is hard and not bleeding
The baby should receive BCG OPV-0 Hepatitis B-0	Counsel mother regarding diet and rest, exclusive BF, iron tablets, FP, Hygiene, avoid sexual intercourse til perineal wound heals, follow-up, complete immunization of baby
Dander sign Breastfeeding poorly Fever/cold to touch Breath fast/difficult in breathing Blood in stool Palm/soles are yellow Convulsion	Danger sign Increase vaginal bleeding Convulsion Fever/too weak Severe abdominal pain Swollen, red or tender breast Dribbling of urine Pain in perineum/pus discharge Foul-smelling lochia

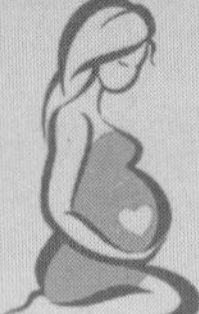

NORMAL PUERPERIUM

Puerperium

Puerperium is the period following childbirth during which the body tissue, especially the pelvic organs, revert approximately to the prepregnant state both anatomically and physiologically.

- Duration
  - Delivery of the placenta to the return of the woman, approximately 6 weeks.
    - Immediate - the 1st 24 hours.
    - Early - up to 7 days.
    - Remote - up to 6 weeks.
- Anatomy and physiological changes of the puerperium:
  - Uterus, cervix, lochia, vagina and puerperium, breast, physiology of lactation.
- General physiological changes:
  - Vital sign, gastrointestinal, weight loss, fluid loss, abdominal wall, hematological changes, menstruation and ovulation.
- Postpartum care:
  - Rest and ambulation, diet, perineal care, care of bladder, care of bowel, sleep, care of breast, uterus and involution, rooming in or bedding in, immunization, monitoring and charting postpartum event, postpartum exercise.
- Danger signs
  - Excessive leaking, i.e. soaking more than 2-3 pads in 20-30 minutes after delivery
  - Convulsion
  - Fever
  - Severe abdominal pain
  - Difficulty in breathing
  - Foul smelling lochia

CESAREAN DELIVERY

Cesarean delivery or birth is the surgical removal of the infant from the uterus through an incision made in the abdominal wall and an incision made in the uterus.

Types of cesarean delivery

- Uterine incisions
  - Low segment transverse incision
    - It is the incision of choice.
  - Classical vertical incision
  - T-extension (low transverse with vertical cut made in the middle of the horizontal incision)
- Abdominal incisions
  - A horizontal incision right above the pubic hair line
  - A vertical incision made in the midline of the abdomen below the umbilicus to the pubis
- Indications for cesarean delivery
  - CPD
  - Uterine dysfunction, inertia and failure to progress
  - Neoplasm obstructing birth canal or pelvis
  - Hypertensive disorders of pregnancy
  - Severe diabetes mellitus
  - Uteroplacental insufficiency and oligohydramnios
  - Malposition and malpresentation
  - Previous uterine surgery (cesarean delivery, myomectomy, hysterotomy) or cervical surgery evaluated on an individual basis
  - Complete or partial placenta previa
  - Abruptio placentae
  - Prolapse of the umbilical cord
  - Fetal compromise
  - Active genital herpes simplex
  - Breech or shoulder presentation
  - Multiple gestation more than three fetuses
  - Conjoined twins
  - Indications for cesarean hysterectomy:
    - Ruptured uterus
    - Intrauterine infection
    - Hemorrhage due to uterine atony that does not respond to oxytocin, prostaglandin or massage
    - Laceration of major uterine vessel
    - Severe dysplasia or carcinoma in situ of the cervix
    - Placenta accreta
    - Gross multiple fibromyomas

FETAL STAGE: 9 WEEKS TO BIRTH

- Development by month
- **First lunar month**
  - Fertilization to 2 weeks of embryonic growth
  - Implantation is complete
  - Primary chorionic villi forming
  - Embryo develops into two cell layers (trophoblast and blastocyst)
  - Amniotic cavity appears.
- **Second lunar month**
  - 3 to 6 weeks of embryonic growth
  - At the end of 6 weeks of growth, the embryo is approximately 1.2 cm long
  - Arm and leg buds are visible; arm buds are more developed with finger ridges beginning to appear
  - Rudiments of the eyes, ears, and nose appear

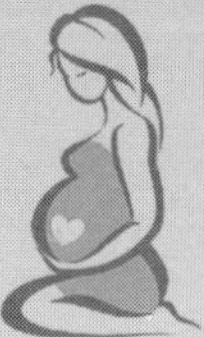

- Lung buds are developing
- Primitive intestinal tract is developing
- Primitive cardiovascular system is functioning
- Neural tube, which forms the brain and spinal cord, closes by the 4th week.

- **Third lunar month**
  - 7 to 10 weeks of growth
  - The middle of this period (9 weeks) marks the end of the embryonic period and the beginning of the fetal period
  - At the end of 10 weeks of growth, the fetus is approximately 6.3 cm from crown to rump and weighs 14 g
  - Appearance of external genitalia
  - By the middle of this month, all major organ systems have formed
  - The membrane over the anus has broken down
  - The heart has formed four chambers (by 7th week)
  - The fetus assumes a human appearance
  - Bone ossification begins
  - Rudimentary kidney begins to secrete urine.
- **Fourth lunar month**
  - 11- to 14-week-old fetus
  - At the end of 14 weeks of growth, the fetus is approximately (12 cm crown-rump length and 110 g
  - Head erect; lower extremities well developed
  - Hard palate and nasal septum have fused
  - External genitalia of male and female can now be differentiated
  - Eyelids are sealed.
- **Fifth lunar month**
  - 15- to 18-week-old fetus
  - At the end of 18 weeks of growth, the fetus is approximately 16 cm crown-rump length and 320 g
  - Ossification of fetal skeleton can be seen on X-ray
  - Ears stand out from head
  - Meconium is present in the intestinal tract
  - Fetus makes sucking motions and swallows amniotic fluid
  - Fetal movements may be felt by the mother (end of month).
- **Sixth lunar month**
  - 19- to 22-week-old fetus
  - At the end of 22 weeks of growth, the fetus is approximately 21 cm crown-rump length and 1 lb 630 g
  - Vernix caseosa covers the skin
  - Head and body (lanugo) hair visible
  - Skin is wrinkled and red
  - Brown fat, an important site of heat production, is present in neck and sternal area
  - Nipples are apparent on the breasts.
- **Seventh lunar month**
  - 23- to 26-week-old fetus
  - At the end of 26 weeks of growth, the fetus is approximately 10 inches (25 cm) crown-rump length and 1,000 g
  - Fingernails present
  - Lean body
  - Eyes partially open; eyelashes present
  - Bronchioles are present; primitive alveoli are forming
  - Skin begins to thicken on hands and feet
  - Startle reflex present; grasp reflex is strong.
- **Eighth lunar month**
  - 27- to 30-week-old fetus
  - At the end of 30 weeks of growth, the fetus is approximately 11 inches (28 cm) crown-rump length and 3 lb 12 oz (1,700 g)
  - Eyes open
  - Ample hair on head; lanugo begins to fade
  - Skin slightly wrinkled
  - Toe nails present
  - Testes in inguinal canal, begin descent to scrotal sac
  - Surfactant coats much of the alveolar epithelium.
- **Ninth lunar month**
  - 31- to 34-week-old fetus
  - At the end of 34 weeks of growth, the fetus is approximately 32 cm crown-rump length and 5 lb 8 oz (2,500 g)
  - Fingernails reach fingertips
  - Skin pink and smooth
  - Testes in scrotal sac.
- **Tenth lunar month**
  - 35- to 38-week-old fetus; end of this month is also 40 weeks from onset of last menstrual period
  - End of 38 weeks of growth, fetus is approximately 36 cm crown-rump length and 7 lb 8 oz (3,400 g)
  - Ample subcutaneous fat
  - Lanugo almost absent
  - Toe nails reach toe tips
  - Testes in scrotum
  - Vernix caseosa mainly on the back
  - Breasts are firm.

OBSTETRIC EMERGENCIES

Ectopic pregnancy: Ectopic pregnancy is gestation located outside the uterine cavity (i.e. implantation occurs at a site other than the endometrium).

Hydatidiform mole: Hydatidiform mole (gestational trophoblastic disease) is an abnormal pregnancy resulting from a developmental anomaly of the placenta.

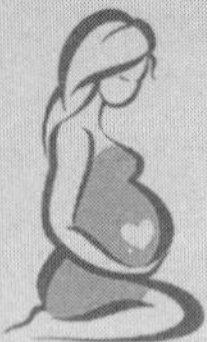

Spontaneous abortion: Spontaneous abortion is the unintended termination of pregnancy at any time before the fetus has attained viability (20 weeks' gestation or fetal weight of more than 500 g).

Hyperemesis gravidarum: Hyperemesis gravidarum is exaggerated nausea and vomiting that persists during pregnancy.

Placenta previa: Placenta previa is the abnormal implantation of the placenta in the lower uterine segment, partially or completely covering the internal cervical os

Abruptio placentae: This is premature separation of the normally implanted placenta before the birth of the fetus.

Hypertensive disorders of pregnancy: Hypertensive disorders of pregnancy, which affect the placenta, are considered the most common medical complications of pregnancy

Polyhydramnios: Polyhydramnios or hydramnios is an excessive amount of amniotic fluid in the amniotic sac. At 36 weeks gestation, approximately 1 L of fluid is present. The amount of amniotic fluid normally decreases after this time.

Oligohydramnios: Oligohydramnios is the marked decrease of amniotic fluid in the amniotic sac of less than 0.5 L between 32 and 36 weeks' gestation. Usually, the fluid is extremely concentrated

Multiple gestation: Multiple gestation or multifetal pregnancy results when two or more fetuses are present in the uterus at the same time.

Vasa previa: Vasa previa, is a condition in which fetal blood vessels cross or run near the internal opening of the uterus. These vessels are at risk of rupture when the supporting membranes rupture, as they are unsupported by the umbilical cord or placental tissue.

Amniotic fluid embolism: An amniotic fluid embolism (AFE) is a rare childbirth (obstetric) emergency in which amniotic fluid, enters the blood stream of the mother to trigger a serious reaction.

Obstetric shock: Shock is a condition resulting from inability of the circulatory system to provide the tissues requirements from oxygen and nutrients and to remove metabolites in pregnant mother.

Cord prolapse: Umbilical cord prolapse occurs when the umbilical cord comes out of the uterus with or before the presenting part of the fetus.

Cord presentation: A cord presentation (also known as a funic presentation) is a variation in fetal presentation where the umbilical cord points towards the internal cervical os or lower uterine segment.

COMPLICATIONS OF LABOR

Preterm labor: Preterm labor is defined as cervical change or effacement and uterine contractions occurring after 20 weeks' gestation and prior to 37 completed weeks of gestation

Premature rupture of membranes: Premature rupture of membranes (PROM) is defined as rupture of the membranes before the onset of labor.

Preterm premature rupture of membranes: Preterm premature rupture of membranes (PPROM) is defined as rupture of membranes before 37 completed weeks' gestation with or without the onset of spontaneous labor

Induction of labor: Induction of labor refers to measures used for the deliberate initiation (stimulation) of uterine contractions before the spontaneous onset of labor for the purpose of achieving a vaginal birth

Dystocia: Dystocia is abnormal labor resulting from abnormalities of uterine contractions or maternal expulsive forces (power), the fetal position, size, or presentation (passenger), or the pelvis or soft tissues (passage)

Shoulder dystocia: Shoulder dystocia is the arrest of spontaneous delivery of shoulders secondary to impaction of the anterior shoulder against the symphysis pubis

Uterine rupture: Uterine rupture is a spontaneous or traumatic rupture of the uterus, i.e. the actual separation of the uterine myometrium or previous uterine scar, with rupture of membranes and extrusion of the fetus or fetal parts into the peritoneal cavity

Anaphylactic syndrome of pregnancy: Anaphylactic syndrome of pregnancy, previously known as amniotic fluid embolism (AFE), is the escape of amniotic fluid containing debris, such as meconium, lanugo, and vernix caseosa, into the maternal circulation, usually resulting in deposition of fluid or debris in the pulmonary arterioles, resulting rapidly in respiratory distress, shock, and the possible development of DIC

Prolapsed umbilical cord: A prolapsed umbilical cord slips in front of or alongside the fetal presenting part

Inversion of the uterus: Inversion of the uterus is a potentially life-threatening complication in which the uterus turns inside out during the third stage of delivery

Forceps delivery: Obstetric forceps are designed for rotating or extracting the fetal head

Vacuum extraction: A vacuum extractor applies suction to the fetal head with a suction cup, thus allowing adequate traction for delivery of the infant's head.

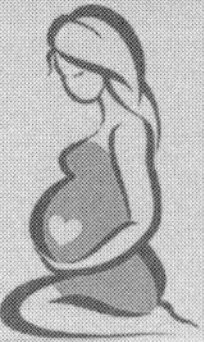

POSTPARTUM COMPLICATIONS

Postpartum infection: Postpartum (puerperal) infection is a postpartum infection of the genital tract, usually of the endometrium (endometritis) that may remain localized or may extend to various parts of the body such as the connective tissue by lymphatic spread (parametritis).

Postpartum hemorrhage: Postpartum hemorrhage involves a loss of 500 mL or more of blood; it occurs early (first 24 hours) or late (after 24 hours and less than 6 weeks after birth). The greatest risk is during the first hour after birth.

Postpartum hematomas: Postpartum hematomas are localized collections of blood in loose connective tissue beneath the skin that covers the external genitalia, beneath the vaginal mucosa, or in the broad ligaments.

Postpartum depression: There is no consensus regarding the classification of postpartum depression.

PROBLEMS OF THE NEWBORN

Premature infant: The premature neonate is a neonate born before the completion of 37 weeks' gestation.

Postmature infant: The postmature newborn infant is one whose gestation is 42 weeks or longer and who may show signs of weight loss with placental insufficiency.

Jaundice in the newborn (hyperbilirubinemia): Hyperbilirubinemia (jaundice) in the neonate is an accumulation of serum bilirubin above normal levels. Onset of clinical jaundice seen when serum bilirubin levels are 5 to 7 mg/100 dL.

Septicemia neonatorum: Septicemia neonatorum (sepsis of the neonate) is a generalized infection that may occur in the neonate and is characterized by the proliferation of bacteria in the bloodstream and frequently involves the meninges.

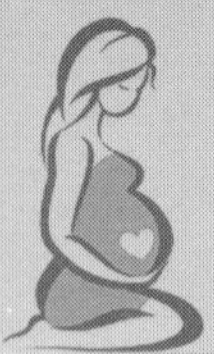

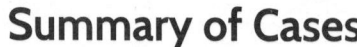

Summary of Cases

ANTENATAL ASSESSMENT

Case nos	Name of Client	Date of Assessment	Register No	Age	GPLAS	LMP, EDD	Weeks of Gestation	Fundal Height (cm)	Abdominal Girth (cm)	Presentation	Position	Engagement	FHS (bpm)	Blood group	Hb %	Urine Albumin/ Sugar	BP (mmHg)	Weight (kg) /Height (cm)	Signature of Supervisor/ Teacher
1.																			
2.																			
3.																			
4.																			
5.																			
6.																			
7.																			
8.																			
9.																			
10.																			
11.																			
12.																			
13.																			
14.																			
15.																			

Contd...

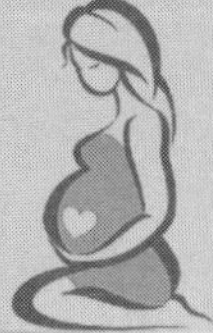

Case nos	Name of Client	Date of Assessment	Register No	Age	GPLAS	LMP, EDD	Weeks of Gestation	Fundal Height (cm)	Abdominal Girth (cm)	Presentation	Position	Engagement	FHS (bpm)	Blood group	Hb %	Urine Albumin/ Sugar	BP (mmHg)	Weight (kg) /Height (cm)	Signature of Supervisor/ Teacher
16.																			
17.																			
18.																			
19.																			
20.																			
21.																			
22.																			
23.																			
24.																			
25.																			
26.																			
27.																			
28.																			
29.																			
30.																			

Signature of Student

____

Signature of Supervisor

____

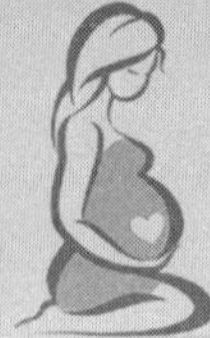

NORMAL DELIVERY WITNESSED

Case Nos	Name of Client	Date of Assessment	Register No.	GPLAS	LMP, EDD	Weeks of Gestation	Fundal Height (cm)	Presentation	Position	BABY			Condition of Baby/Mother	Treatment Advice	Conducted by	Signature of Supervisor/ Teacher
										Sex of Baby	Weight of Baby (kg)	Apgar Score				
1.																
2.																
3.																
4.																
5.																
6.																
7.																
8.																
9.																
10.																
11.																
12.																
13.																
14.																
15.																
16.																
17.																
18.																
19.																
20.																

Signature of Student ____________________

Signature of Supervisor ____________________

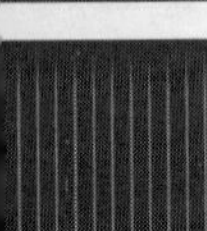

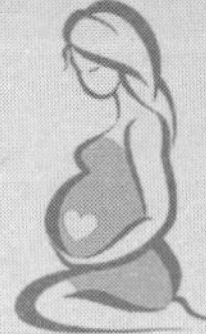

VAGINAL EXAMINATION PERFORMED IN LABOR

Case Nos	Name of Client	Date of Assessment	Register No.	Date of examination	Age	GPLAS	Weeks of gestation	Indication for episiotomy	Cervix		Membranes	Presentation	Position	Station of head	Pelvis Adequacy	Remark	Signature of Supervisor/ Teacher
									Effacement	Dilatation							
1.																	
2.																	
3.																	
4.																	
5.																	

Signature of Student **Signature of Supervisor**

EPISIOTOMY AND SUTURING CASES

Case Nos	Register No	Name of client	Date of delivery	Age	GPLAS	Indication for episiotomy	Type of episiotomy	Number of suture	Condition of episiotomy (REEDA Scale)	Remarks	Signature of Supervisor/ Teacher
1.											
2.											
3.											
4.											
5.											

Signature of Student

Signature of Supervisor

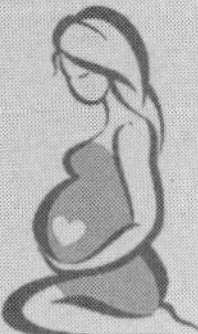

POSTNATAL CASES NURSED

Case Nos	Name of Client	Date of Assessment	Register No.	Age	GPLAS	LMP/EDD	Date/Time of Delivery	Type of Delivery	Perineum	Lochia	Fundus cm	Health status			Treatments Remark	Signature of Supervisor/ Teacher
												Mother	Baby	Apgar Score		
1.																
2.																
3.																
4.																
5.																
6.																
7.																

Contd...

Case Nos	Name of Client	Date of Assessment	Register No.	Age	GPLAS	LMP/EDD	Date/Time of Delivery	Type of Delivery	Perineum	Lochia	Fundus cm	Health status			Treatments Remark	Signature of Supervisor/ Teacher
												Mother	Baby	Apgar Score		
8.																
9.																
10.																
11.																
12.																
13.																
14.																

Contd...

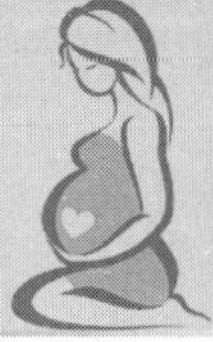

Case Nos	Name of Client	Date of Assessment	Register No.	Age	GPLAS	LMP/EDD	Date/Time of Delivery	Type of Delivery	Perineum	Lochia	Fundus cm	Health status			Treatments Remark	Signature of Supervisor/ Teacher
												Mother	Baby	Apgar Score		
15.																
16.																
17.																
18.																
19.																
20.																

Signature of Student **Signature of Supervisor**

ABNORMAL DELIVERY WITNESSED/ASSISTED

Case No	Date and Time of delivery	Register.No	Name of Client	GPLAS	LMP, EDD	Weeks of Gestation	Fundal Height (cm)	Presentation	Position	BABY			Condition of Baby/Mother	Treatment Advice	Conducted by	Signature of Supervisor/ Teacher
										Sex of Baby	Weight of Baby (kg)	Apgar Score				
1.																
2.																
3.																
4.																
5.																

Signature of Student ____________

Signature of Supervisor ____________

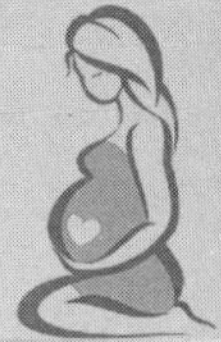

ASSISTED WITH CESAREAN SECTION

Case nos	Name of Client	Date of Assessment	Register No.	GPLAS	Age	LMP/EDD	Weeks of gestation	Presenta-tion/position	Indication for CS	Type of CS	Sex of baby	Weight of baby (kg)	Apgar score	Condition of		Treatment and remark	Signature of supervisor/ teacher
														Mother	Baby		
1.																	
2.																	
3.																	
4.																	
5.																	

Signature of Student

Signature of Supervisor

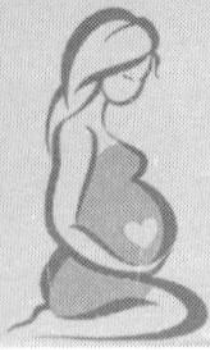

NEWBORN RESUSCITATION

Case Nos	Date	Register No.	Baby of (Mother's Name)	Date and Time of birth	Birthweight	Apgar Score at 1st Minute	Apgar Score at 2nd Minute	Indication for Resuscitation	Resuscitation					Condition after Resuscitation of Baby	Signature of Supervisor/ Teacher
									Suction	Oxygen	Medication	Intubation	CPR		
1.															
2.															
3.															
4.															
5.															

Signature of Student ______________ **Signature of Supervisor** ______________

INSERTION OF IUCD

Case no s	Date	Register No.	Name of the Client	Age	Para	Date of Delivery	No. of Living Children	Contraceptive Used Before	LMP	Type of IUCD Inserted	Remarks	Signature of Supervisor/Teacher
1.												
2.												
3.												
4.												
5.												

Signature of Student

Signature of Supervisor

Antenatal Assessment (Case No. 1)

Client's Profile

Name	:	Education	: ....
Age	:	Occupation	: ....
Hospital name	:	Income per month	: ....
Date of booking	:	Marriage duration	: ....
Reg. No.	:	W/o	: ....
Religion	:	LMP	: ....
Parity	:	EDD	: ....

Address : ....

Period of gestation : ....

Menstrual History

Age at menarche	:	year of age	Blood flow :	average/scanty/heavy ....
Cycle of	:	days	Dysmenorrhea :	....
Period duration of	:	days		

History of Present Pregnancy

No. of antenatal visits : .... Immunization Status : ....

Tick mark (√), if present

Nausea/Vomiting/Back ache/Constipation/Frequency of Micturition/Leaking of watery fluid through vagina/Vaginal bleeding/Severe headache/Blurred vision/Difficulty in breathing/Palpitation/Decrease or absent fetal movement/Acidity/generalized swelling of body or face/Fever

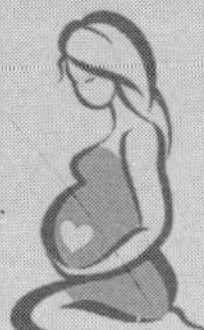

Obstetric History

S. No	Year	Term/ preterm	Abortion/ stillbirth	Nature of delivery	Child		Immunization	Growth and development	Nature of puerperium	Remark
					Alive	Sex/ weight				

Personal History

Allergies to drug : .... Body built : ....

Habit : Smoking/alcohol/betel chewing/any drug addiction : ....

Dietary habits : Vegetarian/nonvegetarian : ....

Hobbies : .... Diet per day - 2/3/4/5/6 : ....

Present and Past Medical History

Hypertension/diabetes/breathlessness on exertion/palpitation/tuberculosis/asthma/renal disease/convulsion/jaundice/malaria/RTI/STI/HIV/AIDS/no any/if any other specify ....

Family History

Family history of systemic illness: Hypertension/Diabetes/Tuberculosis/No any ....

Blood disorder: Thalassemia/Repeated blood transfusion

Delivery of: Twins/Congenital abnormalities

Examinations of Client

General Examinations

Height : ....cm Temperature : ......F Respiration : ....breath/mint

Weight : ....kg Pulse : ....beats/mint BP : ....mm Hg

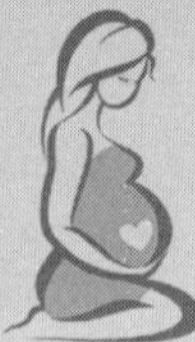

Physical Examinations

General appearance	:	Sick/active/anemic/pallor
Body built	:	Moderate/thin/obsess
Head	:	Dandruff/pediculosis/flakes/dryness/itching/normal
Eye	:	Pupil—normal/dilated/constricted, Conjunctiva—pink/white
Ear	:	Normal/wax impaction/abnormal auricle development
Nose	:	Normal/nasal septum deviation/polyps/rhinitis
Lips	:	Normal/cheilosis/dry/pale lips
Tongue	:	White and smooth/pallor
Nail	:	Pink/pallor
Breast examination	:	Breast—normal/lump/tenderness
Nipple	:	Normal/inverted or flat nipples/crust or sore nipple
Micturition	:	Scanty/retention/incontinence/painful/frequent/normal
Digestion	:	Heart burn/constipation/diarrhea/hemorrhoids/normal

Abdominal Examinations

Inspection

Abdomen : Size : .... Shape : ....

Counter : Fundal notching/convex/flattened anterior wall/cylindrical/spherical ....

Umbilicus : Striae gravidarum: ....

Linea nigra : ....

Palpation

Abdominal girth : ....cm

Fundal height of uterus : ....cm ....weeks

Fetal lie and presentation :

- Fundal palpation/grip
  Presentation—hard and globular (head)/soft and irregular (breech)
- Lateral palpation/grip
  Left—continuous hard/irregular small knobs
  Right—continuous hard/irregular small knobs
- Superficial pelvic grip
  Head (hard and globular)/breech (soft and irregular)/empty
- Deep pelvic grip (only in 3rd trimester)
  Head engagement—head engaged/not engaged

Auscultation

Fetal heart rate (FHR) :... Beats/Mint : ....

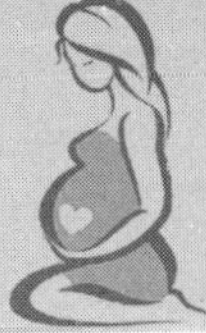

Laboratory Investigations

Date: .... Blood: Hb .... Group .... Sugar .... Urine: Albumin ....

HIV: .... HbsAg :..................... Malaria: VDRL .... Any other specify ....

Treatment

Drugs: .... Dose/Route: ....

Health Education

....

....

....

....

Remark

....

....

....

....

....

....

Signature of Sister in Charge

____

Signature of Supervisor

____

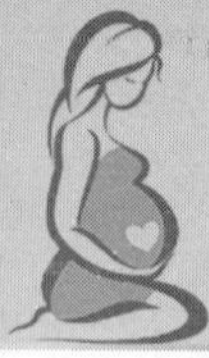

Antenatal Assessment (Case No. 2)

Client's Profile

Name	:	Education	: ....
Age	:	Occupation	: ....
Hospital name	:	Income per month	: ....
Date of booking	:	Marriage duration	: ....
Reg. No.	:	W/o	: ....
Religion	:	LMP	: ....
Parity	:	EDD	: ....

Address : ....

Period of gestation : ....

Menstrual History

Age at menarche	:..............................	year of age	Blood flow :	average/scanty/heavy ....
Cycle of	:..............................	days	Dysmenorrhea :	....
Period duration of	:..............................	days		

History of Present Pregnancy

No. of antenatal visits : .... Immunization Status : ....

Tick mark (√), if present

Nausea/Vomiting/Back ache/Constipation/Frequency of Micturition/Leaking of watery fluid through vagina/Vaginal bleeding/Severe headache/Blurred vision/Difficulty in breathing/Palpitation/Decrease or absent fetal movement/Acidity/generalized swelling of body or face/Fever

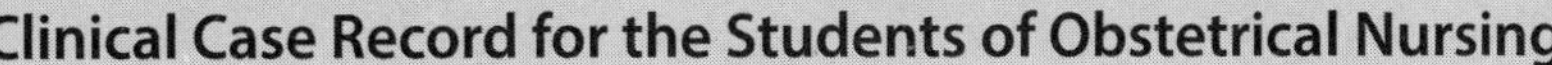

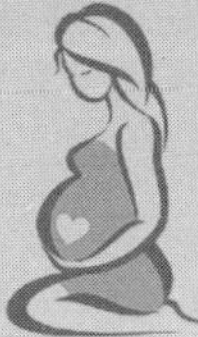

Obstetric History

S. No	Year	Term/ preterm	Abortion/ stillbirth	Nature of delivery	Child		Immunization	Growth and development	Nature of puerperium	Remark
					Alive	Sex/ weight				

Personal History

Allergies to drug : .... Body built : ....
Habit : Smoking/alcohol/betel chewing/any drug addiction : ....
Dietary habits : Vegetarian/nonvegetarian : ....
Hobbies : .... Diet per day - 2/3/4/5/6 : ....

Present and Past Medical History

Hypertension/diabetes/breathlessness on exertion/palpitation/tuberculosis/asthma/renal disease/convulsion/jaundice/malaria/RTI/STI/HIV/AIDS/no any/if any other specify ....

Family History

Family history of systemic illness: Hypertension/Diabetes/Tuberculosis/No any ....
Blood disorder: Thalassemia/Repeated blood transfusion
Delivery of: Twins/Congenital abnormalities

Examinations of Client

General Examinations

Height : ....cm Temperature : ......F Respiration : ....breath/mint
Weight : ....kg Pulse : ....beats/mint BP : ....mm Hg

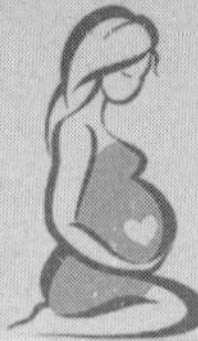

Physical Examinations

General appearance	:	Sick/active/anemic/pallor
Body built	:	Moderate/thin/obsess
Head	:	Dandruff/pediculosis/flakes/dryness/itching/normal
Eye	:	Pupil—normal/dilated/constricted, Conjunctiva—pink/white
Ear	:	Normal/wax impaction/abnormal auricle development
Nose	:	Normal/nasal septum deviation/polyps/rhinitis
Lips	:	Normal/cheilosis/dry/pale lips
Tongue	:	White and smooth/pallor
Nail	:	Pink/pallor
Breast examination	:	Breast—normal/lump/tenderness
Nipple	:	Normal/inverted or flat nipples/crust or sore nipple
Micturition	:	Scanty/retention/incontinence/painful/frequent/normal
Digestion	:	Heart burn/constipation/diarrhea/hemorrhoids/normal

Abdominal Examinations

Inspection

Abdomen : Size : .... Shape : ....

Counter : Fundal notching/convex/flattened anterior wall/cylindrical/spherical ....

Umbilicus : Striae gravidarum: ....

Linea nigra : ....

Palpation

Abdominal girth : ....cm

Fundal height of uterus : ....cm ....weeks

Fetal lie and presentation :

- Fundal palpation/grip
  Presentation—hard and globular (head)/soft and irregular (breech)
- Lateral palpation/grip
  Left—continuous hard/irregular small knobs
  Right—continuous hard/irregular small knobs
- Superficial pelvic grip
  Head (hard and globular)/breech (soft and irregular)/empty
- Deep pelvic grip (only in 3rd trimester)
  Head engagement—head engaged/not engaged

Auscultation

Fetal heart rate (FHR) :.. Beats/Mint : ....

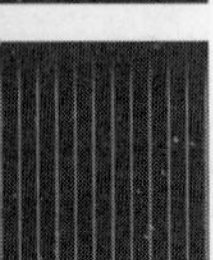

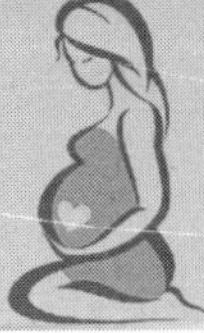

Laboratory Investigations

Date: .... Blood: Hb .... Group .... Sugar .... Urine: Albumin ....
HIV: .... HbsAg :..................... Malaria: VDRL .... Any other specify ....

Treatment

Drugs: .... Dose/Route: ....

Health Education

....

....

....

....

Remark

....

....

....

....

....

....

Signature of Sister in Charge **Signature of Supervisor**

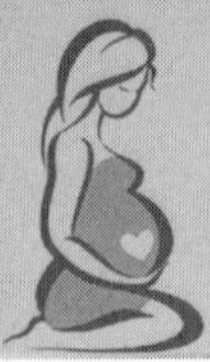

Antenatal Assessment (Case No. 3)

Client's Profile

Name	:	Education	: ....
Age	:	Occupation	: ....
Hospital name	:	Income per month	: ....
Date of booking	:	Marriage duration	: ....
Reg. No.	:	W/o	: ....
Religion	:	LMP	: ....
Parity	:	EDD	: ....

Address : ....

Period of gestation : ....

Menstrual History

Age at menarche	:..............................	year of age	Blood flow :	average/scanty/heavy ....
Cycle of	:..............................	days	Dysmenorrhea :	....
Period duration of	:..............................	days		

History of Present Pregnancy

No. of antenatal visits : .... Immunization Status : ....

Tick mark (√), if present

Nausea/Vomiting/Back ache/Constipation/Frequency of Micturition/Leaking of watery fluid through vagina/Vaginal bleeding/Severe headache/Blurred vision/Difficulty in breathing/Palpitation/Decrease or absent fetal movement/Acidity/generalized swelling of body or face/Fever

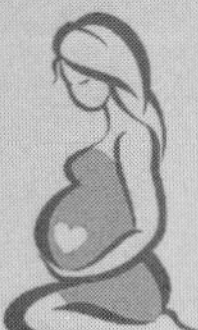

Obstetric History

S. No	Year	Term/ preterm	Abortion/ stillbirth	Nature of delivery	Child		Immunization	Growth and development	Nature of puerperium	Remark
					Alive	Sex/ weight				

Personal History

Allergies to drug : .... Body built : ....

Habit : Smoking/alcohol/betel chewing/any drug addiction : ....

Dietary habits : Vegetarian/nonvegetarian : ....

Hobbies : .... Diet per day - 2/3/4/5/6 : ....

Present and Past Medical History

Hypertension/diabetes/breathlessness on exertion/palpitation/tuberculosis/asthma/renal disease/convulsion/jaundice/malaria/RTI/STI/HIV/AIDS/no any/if any other specify ....

Family History

Family history of systemic illness: Hypertension/Diabetes/Tuberculosis/No any ....

Blood disorder: Thalassemia/Repeated blood transfusion

Delivery of: Twins/Congenital abnormalities

Examinations of Client

General Examinations

Height : ....cm Temperature : ......F Respiration : ....breath/mint

Weight : ....kg Pulse : ....beats/mint BP : ....mm Hg

Physical Examinations

General appearance	:	Sick/active/anemic/pallor
Body built	:	Moderate/thin/obsess
Head	:	Dandruff/pediculosis/flakes/dryness/itching/normal
Eye	:	Pupil—normal/dilated/constricted, Conjunctiva—pink/white
Ear	:	Normal/wax impaction/abnormal auricle development
Nose	:	Normal/nasal septum deviation/polyps/rhinitis
Lips	:	Normal/cheilosis/dry/pale lips
Tongue	:	White and smooth/pallor
Nail	:	Pink/pallor
Breast examination	:	Breast—normal/lump/tenderness
Nipple	:	Normal/inverted or flat nipples/crust or sore nipple
Micturition	:	Scanty/retention/incontinence/painful/frequent/normal
Digestion	:	Heart burn/constipation/diarrhea/hemorrhoids/normal

Abdominal Examinations

Inspection

Abdomen : Size : .... Shape : ....

Counter : Fundal notching/convex/flattened anterior wall/cylindrical/spherical ....

Umbilicus : Striae gravidarum: ....

Linea nigra : ....

Palpation

Abdominal girth : ....cm

Fundal height of uterus : ....cm ....weeks

Fetal lie and presentation :

- Fundal palpation/grip
  Presentation—hard and globular (head)/soft and irregular (breech)
- Lateral palpation/grip
  Left—continuous hard/irregular small knobs
  Right—continuous hard/irregular small knobs
- Superficial pelvic grip
  Head (hard and globular)/breech (soft and irregular)/empty
- Deep pelvic grip (only in 3rd trimester)
  Head engagement—head engaged/not engaged

Auscultation

Fetal heart rate (FHR) :... Beats/Mint : ....

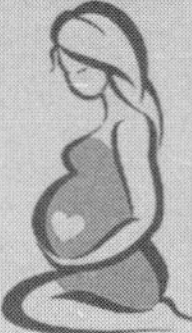

Laboratory Investigations

Date: .... Blood: Hb .... Group .... Sugar .... Urine: Albumin ....
HIV: .... HbsAg :..................... Malaria: VDRL .... Any other specify ....

Treatment

Drugs: .... Dose/Route: ....

Health Education

....

....

....

....

Remark

....

....

....

....

....

....

Signature of Sister in Charge

Signature of Supervisor

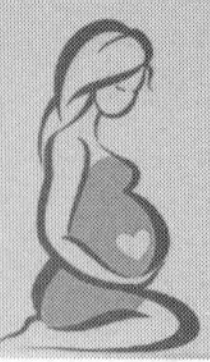

Antenatal Assessment (Case No. 4)

Client's Profile

Name	:	Education	: ....
Age	:	Occupation	: ....
Hospital name	:	Income per month	: ....
Date of booking	:	Marriage duration	: ....
Reg. No.	:	W/o	: ....
Religion	:	LMP	: ....
Parity	:	EDD	:..

Address : ....

Period of gestation : ....

Menstrual History

Age at menarche	:............................	year of age	Blood flow :	average/scanty/heavy ....
Cycle of	:............................	days	Dysmenorrhea :	....
Period duration of	:............................	days		

History of Present Pregnancy

No. of antenatal visits : .... Immunization Status : ....

Tick mark (√), if present

Nausea/Vomiting/Back ache/Constipation/Frequency of Micturition/Leaking of watery fluid through vagina/Vaginal bleeding/Severe headache/Blurred vision/Difficulty in breathing/Palpitation/Decrease or absent fetal movement/Acidity/generalized swelling of body or face/Fever

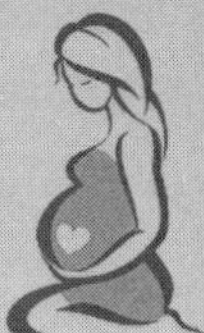

Obstetric History

S. No	Year	Term/ preterm	Abortion/ stillbirth	Nature of delivery	Child		Immunization	Growth and development	Nature of puerperium	Remark
					Alive	Sex/ weight				

Personal History

Allergies to drug : .... Body built : ....

Habit : Smoking/alcohol/betel chewing/any drug addiction : ....

Dietary habits : Vegetarian/nonvegetarian : ....

Hobbies : .... Diet per day - 2/3/4/5/6 : ....

Present and Past Medical History

Hypertension/diabetes/breathlessness on exertion/palpitation/tuberculosis/asthma/renal disease/convulsion/jaundice/malaria/RTI/STI/HIV/AIDS/no any/if any other specify ....

Family History

Family history of systemic illness: Hypertension/Diabetes/Tuberculosis/No any ....

Blood disorder: Thalassemia/Repeated blood transfusion

Delivery of: Twins/Congenital abnormalities

Examinations of Client

General Examinations

Height : ....cm Temperature : ......F Respiration : ....breath/mint

Weight : ....kg Pulse : ....beats/mint BP : ....mm Hg

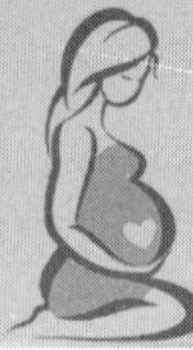

Physical Examinations

General appearance : Sick/active/anemic/pallor
Body built : Moderate/thin/obsess
Head : Dandruff/pediculosis/flakes/dryness/itching/normal
Eye : Pupil—normal/dilated/constricted, Conjunctiva—pink/white
Ear : Normal/wax impaction/abnormal auricle development
Nose : Normal/nasal septum deviation/polyps/rhinitis
Lips : Normal/cheilosis/dry/pale lips
Tongue : White and smooth/pallor
Nail : Pink/pallor
Breast examination : Breast—normal/lump/tenderness
Nipple : Normal/inverted or flat nipples/crust or sore nipple
Micturition : Scanty/retention/incontinence/painful/frequent/normal
Digestion : Heart burn/constipation/diarrhea/hemorrhoids/normal

Abdominal Examinations

Inspection

Abdomen : Size :.. Shape :..
Counter : Fundal notching/convex/flattened anterior wall/cylindrical/spherical ....
Umbilicus : Striae gravidarum: ....
Linea nigra : ....

Palpation

Abdominal girth : ....cm
Fundal height of uterus : ....cm ....weeks
Fetal lie and presentation :

- Fundal palpation/grip
  Presentation—hard and globular (head)/soft and irregular (breech)
- Lateral palpation/grip
  Left—continuous hard/irregular small knobs
  Right—continuous hard/irregular small knobs
- Superficial pelvic grip
  Head (hard and globular)/breech (soft and irregular)/empty
- Deep pelvic grip (only in 3rd trimester)
  Head engagement—head engaged/not engaged

Auscultation

Fetal heart rate (FHR) :.. Beats/Mint :..

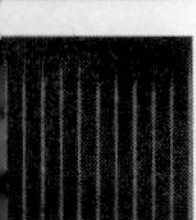

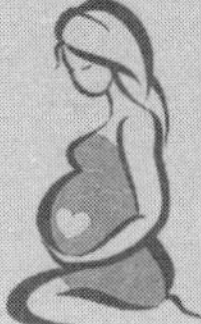

Laboratory Investigations

Date: .... Blood: Hb .... Group .... Sugar .... Urine: Albumin ....
HIV: .... HbsAg :..................... Malaria: VDRL .... Any other specify ....

Treatment

Drugs: .... Dose/Route: ....

Health Education

....

....

....

....

Remark

....

....

....

....

....

....

Signature of Sister in Charge

Signature of Supervisor

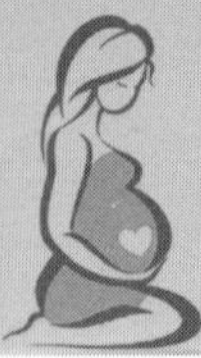

Antenatal Assessment (Case No. 5)

Client's Profile

Name	:	Education	: ....
Age	:	Occupation	: ....
Hospital name	:	Income per month	: ....
Date of booking	:	Marriage duration	: ....
Reg. No.	:	W/o	: ....
Religion	:	LMP	: ....
Parity	:	EDD	:..

Address : ....

Period of gestation : ....

Menstrual History

Age at menarche	:..............................	year of age	Blood flow :	average/scanty/heavy ....
Cycle of	:..............................	days	Dysmenorrhea :	....
Period duration of	:..............................	days		

History of Present Pregnancy

No. of antenatal visits : .... Immunization Status : ....

Tick mark (√), if present

Nausea/Vomiting/Back ache/Constipation/Frequency of Micturition/Leaking of watery fluid through vagina/Vaginal bleeding/Severe headache/Blurred vision/Difficulty in breathing/Palpitation/Decrease or absent fetal movement/ Acidity/generalized swelling of body or face/Fever

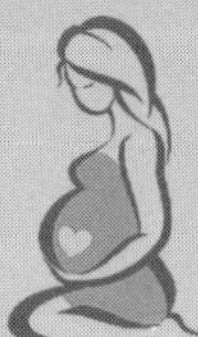

Obstetric History

S. No	Year	Term/ preterm	Abortion/ stillbirth	Nature of delivery	Child		Immunization	Growth and development	Nature of puerperium	Remark
					Alive	Sex/ weight				

Personal History

Allergies to drug : .... Body built : ....
Habit : Smoking/alcohol/betel chewing/any drug addiction : ....
Dietary habits : Vegetarian/nonvegetarian : ....
Hobbies : .... Diet per day - 2/3/4/5/6 : ....

Present and Past Medical History

Hypertension/diabetes/breathlessness on exertion/palpitation/tuberculosis/asthma/renal disease/convulsion/jaundice/malaria/RTI/STI/HIV/AIDS/no any/if any other specify ....

Family History

Family history of systemic illness: Hypertension/Diabetes/Tuberculosis/No any ....
Blood disorder: Thalassemia/Repeated blood transfusion
Delivery of: Twins/Congenital abnormalities

Examinations of Client

General Examinations

Height : ....cm Temperature : ......F Respiration : ....breath/mint
Weight : ....kg Pulse : ....beats/mint BP : ....mm Hg

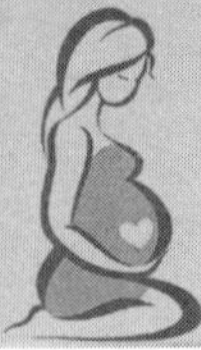

Physical Examinations

General appearance : Sick/active/anemic/pallor
Body built : Moderate/thin/obsess
Head : Dandruff/pediculosis/flakes/dryness/itching/normal
Eye : Pupil—normal/dilated/constricted, Conjunctiva—pink/white
Ear : Normal/wax impaction/abnormal auricle development
Nose : Normal/nasal septum deviation/polyps/rhinitis
Lips : Normal/cheilosis/dry/pale lips
Tongue : White and smooth/pallor
Nail : Pink/pallor
Breast examination : Breast—normal/lump/tenderness
Nipple : Normal/inverted or flat nipples/crust or sore nipple
Micturition : Scanty/retention/incontinence/painful/frequent/normal
Digestion : Heart burn/constipation/diarrhea/hemorrhoids/normal

Abdominal Examinations

Inspection

Abdomen : Size :.. Shape :..
Counter : Fundal notching/convex/flattened anterior wall/cylindrical/spherical ....
Umbilicus : Striae gravidarum: ....
Linea nigra : ....

Palpation

Abdominal girth : ....cm
Fundal height of uterus : ....cm ....weeks
Fetal lie and presentation :

- Fundal palpation/grip
  Presentation—hard and globular (head)/soft and irregular (breech)
- Lateral palpation/grip
  Left—continuous hard/irregular small knobs
  Right—continuous hard/irregular small knobs
- Superficial pelvic grip
  Head (hard and globular)/breech (soft and irregular)/empty
- Deep pelvic grip (only in 3rd trimester)
  Head engagement—head engaged/not engaged

Auscultation

Fetal heart rate (FHR) :.. Beats/Mint : ....

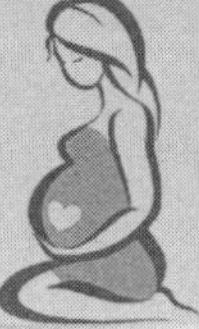

Laboratory Investigations

Date: .... Blood: Hb .... Group .... Sugar .... Urine: Albumin ....
HIV: .... HbsAg :..................... Malaria: VDRL .... Any other specify ....

Treatment

Drugs: .... Dose/Route: ....

Health Education

....

....

....

....

Remark

....

....

....

....

....

....

Signature of Sister in Charge

Signature of Supervisor

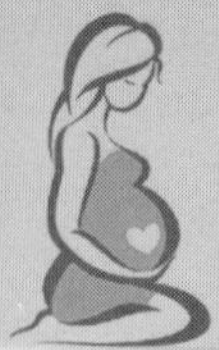

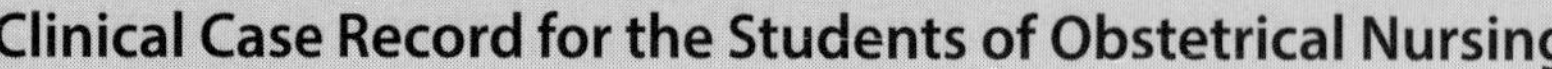

Antenatal Assessment (Case No. 6)

Client's Profile

Name : .... Education : ....

Age : .... Occupation : ....

Hospital name : .... Income per month : ....

Date of booking : .... Marriage duration : ....

Reg. No. : .... W/o : ....

Religion : .... LMP : ....

Parity : .... EDD :..

Address : ....

Period of gestation : ....

Menstrual History

Age at menarche :.............................. year of age Blood flow : average/scanty/heavy ....

Cycle of :.............................. days Dysmenorrhea : ....

Period duration of :.............................. days

History of Present Pregnancy

No. of antenatal visits : .... Immunization Status : ....

Tick mark (√), if present

Nausea/Vomiting/Back ache/Constipation/Frequency of Micturition/Leaking of watery fluid through vagina/Vaginal bleeding/Severe headache/Blurred vision/Difficulty in breathing/Palpitation/Decrease or absent fetal movement/ Acidity/generalized swelling of body or face/Fever

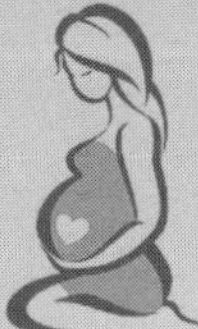

Obstetric History

S. No	Year	Term/ preterm	Abortion/ stillbirth	Nature of delivery	Child		Immunization	Growth and development	Nature of puerperium	Remark
					Alive	Sex/ weight				

Personal History

Allergies to drug : .... Body built : ....

Habit : Smoking/alcohol/betel chewing/any drug addiction : ....

Dietary habits : Vegetarian/nonvegetarian : ....

Hobbies : .... Diet per day - 2/3/4/5/6 : ....

Present and Past Medical History

Hypertension/diabetes/breathlessness on exertion/palpitation/tuberculosis/asthma/renal disease/convulsion/jaundice/malaria/RTI/STI/HIV/AIDS/no any/if any other specify ....

Family History

Family history of systemic illness: Hypertension/Diabetes/Tuberculosis/No any ....

Blood disorder: Thalassemia/Repeated blood transfusion

Delivery of: Twins/Congenital abnormalities

Examinations of Client

General Examinations

Height : ....cm Temperature : ......F Respiration : ....breath/mint

Weight : ....kg Pulse : ....beats/mint BP : ....mm Hg

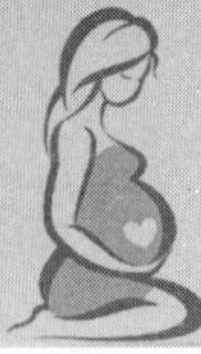

Physical Examinations

General appearance	:	Sick/active/anemic/pallor
Body built	:	Moderate/thin/obsess
Head	:	Dandruff/pediculosis/flakes/dryness/itching/normal
Eye	:	Pupil—normal/dilated/constricted, Conjunctiva—pink/white
Ear	:	Normal/wax impaction/abnormal auricle development
Nose	:	Normal/nasal septum deviation/polyps/rhinitis
Lips	:	Normal/cheilosis/dry/pale lips
Tongue	:	White and smooth/pallor
Nail	:	Pink/pallor
Breast examination	:	Breast—normal/lump/tenderness
Nipple	:	Normal/inverted or flat nipples/crust or sore nipple
Micturition	:	Scanty/retention/incontinence/painful/frequent/normal
Digestion	:	Heart burn/constipation/diarrhea/hemorrhoids/normal

Abdominal Examinations

Inspection

Abdomen : Size : .... Shape : ....

Counter : Fundal notching/convex/flattened anterior wall/cylindrical/spherical ....

Umbilicus : Striae gravidarum: ....

Linea nigra : ....

Palpation

Abdominal girth : ....cm

Fundal height of uterus : ....cm ....weeks

Fetal lie and presentation :

- Fundal palpation/grip
  Presentation—hard and globular (head)/soft and irregular (breech)
- Lateral palpation/grip
  Left—continuous hard/irregular small knobs
  Right—continuous hard/irregular small knobs
- Superficial pelvic grip
  Head (hard and globular)/breech (soft and irregular)/empty
- Deep pelvic grip (only in 3rd trimester)
  Head engagement—head engaged/not engaged

Auscultation

Fetal heart rate (FHR) :.. Beats/Mint : ....

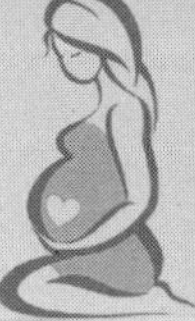

Laboratory Investigations

Date: .... Blood: Hb .... Group .... Sugar .... Urine: Albumin ....
HIV: .... HbsAg :..................... Malaria: VDRL .... Any other specify ....

Treatment

Drugs: .... Dose/Route: ....

Health Education

....

....

....

....

Remark

....

....

....

....

....

....

Signature of Sister in Charge

____

Signature of Supervisor

____

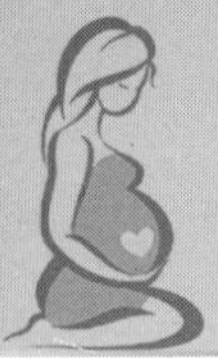

Antenatal Assessment (Case No. 7)

Client's Profile

Name	:	Education	: ....
Age	:	Occupation	: ....
Hospital name	:	Income per month	: ....
Date of booking	:	Marriage duration	: ....
Reg. No.	:	W/o	: ....
Religion	:	LMP	: ....
Parity	:	EDD	: ....

Address : ....

Period of gestation : ....

Menstrual History

Age at menarche	:............................	year of age	Blood flow :	average/scanty/heavy ....
Cycle of	:............................	days	Dysmenorrhea :	....
Period duration of	:............................	days		

History of Present Pregnancy

No. of antenatal visits : .... Immunization Status : ....

Tick mark (√), if present

Nausea/Vomiting/Back ache/Constipation/Frequency of Micturition/Leaking of watery fluid through vagina/Vaginal bleeding/Severe headache/Blurred vision/Difficulty in breathing/Palpitation/Decrease or absent fetal movement/Acidity/generalized swelling of body or face/Fever

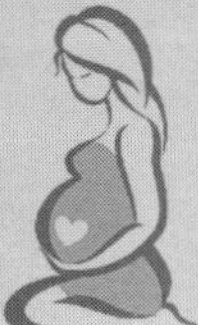

Obstetric History

S. No	Year	Term/ preterm	Abortion/ stillbirth	Nature of delivery	Child		Immunization	Growth and development	Nature of puerperium	Remark
					Alive	Sex/ weight				

Personal History

Allergies to drug : .... Body built : ....

Habit : Smoking/alcohol/betel chewing/any drug addiction : ....

Dietary habits : Vegetarian/nonvegetarian : ....

Hobbies : .... Diet per day - 2/3/4/5/6 : ....

Present and Past Medical History

Hypertension/diabetes/breathlessness on exertion/palpitation/tuberculosis/asthma/renal disease/convulsion/jaundice/malaria/RTI/STI/HIV/AIDS/no any/if any other specify ....

Family History

Family history of systemic illness: Hypertension/Diabetes/Tuberculosis/No any ....

Blood disorder: Thalassemia/Repeated blood transfusion

Delivery of: Twins/Congenital abnormalities

Examinations of Client

General Examinations

Height : ....cm Temperature : ......F Respiration : ....breath/mint

Weight : ....kg Pulse : ....beats/mint BP : ....mm Hg

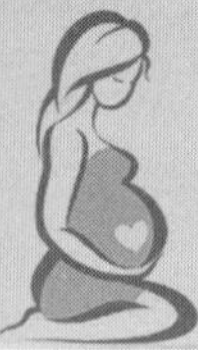

Physical Examinations

General appearance : Sick/active/anemic/pallor
Body built : Moderate/thin/obsess
Head : Dandruff/pediculosis/flakes/dryness/itching/normal
Eye : Pupil—normal/dilated/constricted, Conjunctiva—pink/white
Ear : Normal/wax impaction/abnormal auricle development
Nose : Normal/nasal septum deviation/polyps/rhinitis
Lips : Normal/cheilosis/dry/pale lips
Tongue : White and smooth/pallor
Nail : Pink/pallor
Breast examination : Breast—normal/lump/tenderness
Nipple : Normal/inverted or flat nipples/crust or sore nipple
Micturition : Scanty/retention/incontinence/painful/frequent/normal
Digestion : Heart burn/constipation/diarrhea/hemorrhoids/normal

Abdominal Examinations

Inspection

Abdomen : Size :.. Shape :..
Counter : Fundal notching/convex/flattened anterior wall/cylindrical/spherical ....
Umbilicus : Striae gravidarum: ....
Linea nigra : ....

Palpation

Abdominal girth : ....cm
Fundal height of uterus : ....cm ....weeks
Fetal lie and presentation :

- Fundal palpation/grip
  Presentation—hard and globular (head)/soft and irregular (breech)
- Lateral palpation/grip
  Left—continuous hard/irregular small knobs
  Right—continuous hard/irregular small knobs
- Superficial pelvic grip
  Head (hard and globular)/breech (soft and irregular)/empty
- Deep pelvic grip (only in 3rd trimester)
  Head engagement—head engaged/not engaged

Auscultation

Fetal heart rate (FHR) :.. Beats/Mint : ....

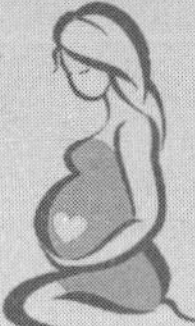

Laboratory Investigations

Date: .... Blood: Hb .... Group .... Sugar .... Urine: Albumin ....
HIV: .... HbsAg :..................... Malaria: VDRL .... Any other specify ....

Treatment

Drugs: .... Dose/Route: ....

Health Education

....

....

....

....

Remark

....

....

....

....

....

....

Signature of Sister in Charge **Signature of Supervisor**

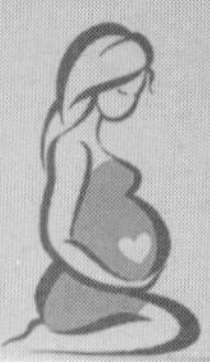

Antenatal Assessment (Case No. 8)

Client's Profile

Name	:	Education	: ....
Age	:	Occupation	: ....
Hospital name	:	Income per month	: ....
Date of booking	:	Marriage duration	: ....
Reg. No.	:	W/o	: ....
Religion	:	LMP	: ....
Parity	:	EDD	: ....

Address : ....

Period of gestation : ....

Menstrual History

Age at menarche	:....................	year of age	Blood flow :	average/scanty/heavy ....
Cycle of	:....................	days	Dysmenorrhea :	....
Period duration of	:....................	days		

History of Present Pregnancy

No. of antenatal visits : .... Immunization Status : ....

Tick mark (√), if present

Nausea/Vomiting/Back ache/Constipation/Frequency of Micturition/Leaking of watery fluid through vagina/Vaginal bleeding/Severe headache/Blurred vision/Difficulty in breathing/Palpitation/Decrease or absent fetal movement/Acidity/generalized swelling of body or face/Fever

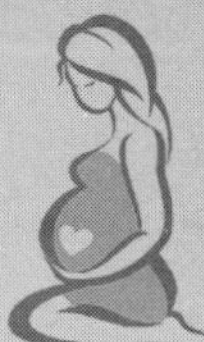

Obstetric History

S. No	Year	Term/ preterm	Abortion/ stillbirth	Nature of delivery	Child		Immunization	Growth and development	Nature of puerperium	Remark
					Alive	Sex/ weight				

Personal History

Allergies to drug : .... Body built : ....

Habit : Smoking/alcohol/betel chewing/any drug addiction : ....

Dietary habits : Vegetarian/nonvegetarian : ....

Hobbies : .... Diet per day - 2/3/4/5/6 : ....

Present and Past Medical History

Hypertension/diabetes/breathlessness on exertion/palpitation/tuberculosis/asthma/renal disease/convulsion/jaundice/malaria/RTI/STI/HIV/AIDS/no any/if any other specify ....

Family History

Family history of systemic illness: Hypertension/Diabetes/Tuberculosis/No any ....

Blood disorder: Thalassemia/Repeated blood transfusion

Delivery of: Twins/Congenital abnormalities

Examinations of Client

General Examinations

Height : ....cm Temperature : ......F Respiration : ....breath/mint

Weight : ....kg Pulse : ....beats/mint BP : ....mm Hg

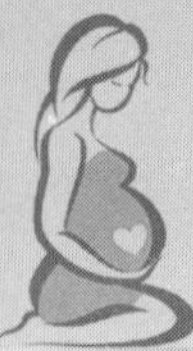

Physical Examinations

General appearance : Sick/active/anemic/pallor
Body built : Moderate/thin/obsess
Head : Dandruff/pediculosis/flakes/dryness/itching/normal
Eye : Pupil—normal/dilated/constricted, Conjunctiva—pink/white
Ear : Normal/wax impaction/abnormal auricle development
Nose : Normal/nasal septum deviation/polyps/rhinitis
Lips : Normal/cheilosis/dry/pale lips
Tongue : White and smooth/pallor
Nail : Pink/pallor
Breast examination : Breast—normal/lump/tenderness
Nipple : Normal/inverted or flat nipples/crust or sore nipple
Micturition : Scanty/retention/incontinence/painful/frequent/normal
Digestion : Heart burn/constipation/diarrhea/hemorrhoids/normal

Abdominal Examinations

Inspection

Abdomen : Size : .... Shape : ....
Counter : Fundal notching/convex/flattened anterior wall/cylindrical/spherical ....
Umbilicus : Striae gravidarum: ....
Linea nigra : ....

Palpation

Abdominal girth : ....cm
Fundal height of uterus : ....cm ....weeks
Fetal lie and presentation :

- Fundal palpation/grip
  Presentation—hard and globular (head)/soft and irregular (breech)
- Lateral palpation/grip
  Left—continuous hard/irregular small knobs
  Right—continuous hard/irregular small knobs
- Superficial pelvic grip
  Head (hard and globular)/breech (soft and irregular)/empty
- Deep pelvic grip (only in 3rd trimester)
  Head engagement—head engaged/not engaged

Auscultation

Fetal heart rate (FHR) :.. Beats/Mint : ....

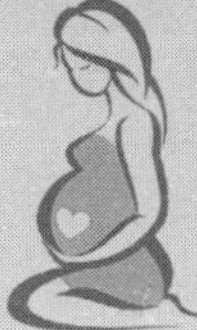

Laboratory Investigations

Date: .... Blood: Hb .... Group .... Sugar .... Urine: Albumin ....
HIV: .... HbsAg :..................... Malaria: VDRL .... Any other specify ....

Treatment

Drugs: .... Dose/Route: ....

Health Education

....

....

....

....

Remark

....

....

....

....

....

....

Signature of Sister in Charge **Signature of Supervisor**

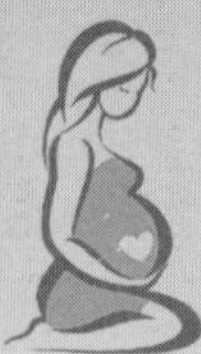

Antenatal Assessment (Case No. 9)

Client's Profile

Name	:	Education	: ....
Age	:	Occupation	: ....
Hospital name	:	Income per month	: ....
Date of booking	:	Marriage duration	: ....
Reg. No.	:	W/o	: ....
Religion	:	LMP	: ....
Parity	:	EDD	: ....

Address : ....

Period of gestation : ....

Menstrual History

Age at menarche	:..............................	year of age	Blood flow :	average/scanty/heavy ....
Cycle of	:..............................	days	Dysmenorrhea :	....
Period duration of	:..............................	days		

History of Present Pregnancy

No. of antenatal visits : .... Immunization Status : ....

Tick mark (√), if present

Nausea/Vomiting/Back ache/Constipation/Frequency of Micturition/Leaking of watery fluid through vagina/Vaginal bleeding/Severe headache/Blurred vision/Difficulty in breathing/Palpitation/Decrease or absent fetal movement/Acidity/generalized swelling of body or face/Fever

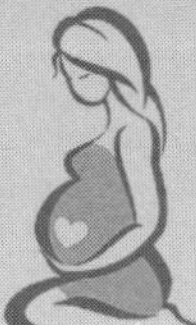

Obstetric History

S. No	Year	Term/ preterm	Abortion/ stillbirth	Nature of delivery	Child		Immunization	Growth and development	Nature of puerperium	Remark
					Alive	Sex/ weight				

Personal History

Allergies to drug : .... Body built : ....
Habit : Smoking/alcohol/betel chewing/any drug addiction : ....
Dietary habits : Vegetarian/nonvegetarian : ....
Hobbies : .... Diet per day - 2/3/4/5/6 : ....

Present and Past Medical History

Hypertension/diabetes/breathlessness on exertion/palpitation/tuberculosis/asthma/renal disease/convulsion/jaundice/malaria/RTI/STI/HIV/AIDS/no any/if any other specify ....

Family History

Family history of systemic illness: Hypertension/Diabetes/Tuberculosis/No any ....
Blood disorder: Thalassemia/Repeated blood transfusion
Delivery of: Twins/Congenital abnormalities

Examinations of Client

General Examinations

Height : ....cm Temperature : ......F Respiration : ....breath/mint
Weight : ....kg Pulse : ....beats/mint BP : ....mm Hg

Physical Examinations

General appearance	:	Sick/active/anemic/pallor
Body built	:	Moderate/thin/obsess
Head	:	Dandruff/pediculosis/flakes/dryness/itching/normal
Eye	:	Pupil—normal/dilated/constricted, Conjunctiva—pink/white
Ear	:	Normal/wax impaction/abnormal auricle development
Nose	:	Normal/nasal septum deviation/polyps/rhinitis
Lips	:	Normal/cheilosis/dry/pale lips
Tongue	:	White and smooth/pallor
Nail	:	Pink/pallor
Breast examination	:	Breast—normal/lump/tenderness
Nipple	:	Normal/inverted or flat nipples/crust or sore nipple
Micturition	:	Scanty/retention/incontinence/painful/frequent/normal
Digestion	:	Heart burn/constipation/diarrhea/hemorrhoids/normal

Abdominal Examinations

Inspection

Abdomen	:	Size :	Shape : ....
Counter	:	Fundal notching/convex/flattened anterior wall/cylindrical/spherical	
Umbilicus	:	Striae gravidarum:	
Linea nigra	:	....	

Palpation

Abdominal girth : ....cm

Fundal height of uterus : ....cm ....weeks

Fetal lie and presentation :

- Fundal palpation/grip
  Presentation—hard and globular (head)/soft and irregular (breech)
- Lateral palpation/grip
  Left—continuous hard/irregular small knobs
  Right—continuous hard/irregular small knobs
- Superficial pelvic grip
  Head (hard and globular)/breech (soft and irregular)/empty
- Deep pelvic grip (only in 3rd trimester)
  Head engagement—head engaged/not engaged

Auscultation

Fetal heart rate (FHR) :.. Beats/Mint : ....

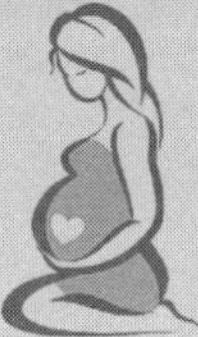

Laboratory Investigations

Date: .... Blood: Hb .... Group .... Sugar .... Urine: Albumin ....
HIV: .... HbsAg :..................... Malaria: VDRL .... Any other specify ....

Treatment

Drugs: .... Dose/Route: ....

Health Education

....

....

....

....

Remark

....

....

....

....

....

....

Signature of Sister in Charge **Signature of Supervisor**

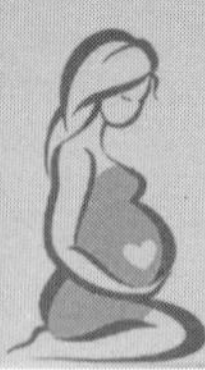

Antenatal Assessment (Case No. 10)

Client's Profile

Name	:	Education	: ....
Age	:	Occupation	: ....
Hospital name	:	Income per month	: ....
Date of booking	:	Marriage duration	: ....
Reg. No.	:	W/o	: ....
Religion	:	LMP	: ....
Parity	:	EDD	: ....

Address : ....

Period of gestation : ....

Menstrual History

Age at menarche	:..............................	year of age	Blood flow :	average/scanty/heavy ....
Cycle of	:..............................	days	Dysmenorrhea :	....
Period duration of	:..............................	days		

History of Present Pregnancy

No. of antenatal visits : .... Immunization Status : ....

Tick mark (√), if present

Nausea/Vomiting/Back ache/Constipation/Frequency of Micturition/Leaking of watery fluid through vagina/Vaginal bleeding/Severe headache/Blurred vision/Difficulty in breathing/Palpitation/Decrease or absent fetal movement/ Acidity/generalized swelling of body or face/Fever

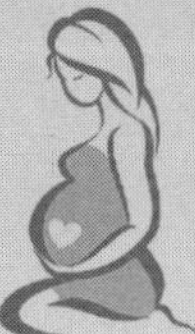

Obstetric History

S. No	Year	Term/ preterm	Abortion/ stillbirth	Nature of delivery	Child		Immunization	Growth and development	Nature of puerperium	Remark
					Alive	Sex/ weight				

Personal History

Allergies to drug : .... Body built : ....
Habit : Smoking/alcohol/betel chewing/any drug addiction : ....
Dietary habits : Vegetarian/nonvegetarian : ....
Hobbies : .... Diet per day - 2/3/4/5/6 : ....

Present and Past Medical History

Hypertension/diabetes/breathlessness on exertion/palpitation/tuberculosis/asthma/renal disease/convulsion/jaundice/malaria/RTI/STI/HIV/AIDS/no any/if any other specify ....

Family History

Family history of systemic illness: Hypertension/Diabetes/Tuberculosis/No any ....
Blood disorder: Thalassemia/Repeated blood transfusion
Delivery of: Twins/Congenital abnormalities

Examinations of Client

General Examinations

Height : ....cm Temperature : ......F Respiration : ....breath/mint
Weight : ....kg Pulse : ....beats/mint BP : ....mm Hg

Physical Examinations

General appearance	:	Sick/active/anemic/pallor
Body built	:	Moderate/thin/obsess
Head	:	Dandruff/pediculosis/flakes/dryness/itching/normal
Eye	:	Pupil—normal/dilated/constricted, Conjunctiva—pink/white
Ear	:	Normal/wax impaction/abnormal auricle development
Nose	:	Normal/nasal septum deviation/polyps/rhinitis
Lips	:	Normal/cheilosis/dry/pale lips
Tongue	:	White and smooth/pallor
Nail	:	Pink/pallor
Breast examination	:	Breast—normal/lump/tenderness
Nipple	:	Normal/inverted or flat nipples/crust or sore nipple
Micturition	:	Scanty/retention/incontinence/painful/frequent/normal
Digestion	:	Heart burn/constipation/diarrhea/hemorrhoids/normal

Abdominal Examinations

Inspection

Abdomen	:	Size : .... Shape : ....
Counter	:	Fundal notching/convex/flattened anterior wall/cylindrical/spherical ....
Umbilicus	:	Striae gravidarum: ....
Linea nigra	:	....

Palpation

Abdominal girth	:	....................cm
Fundal height of uterus	:	....................cm ....weeks
Fetal lie and presentation	:	

- Fundal palpation/grip
  Presentation—hard and globular (head)/soft and irregular (breech)
- Lateral palpation/grip
  Left—continuous hard/irregular small knobs
  Right—continuous hard/irregular small knobs
- Superficial pelvic grip
  Head (hard and globular)/breech (soft and irregular)/empty
- Deep pelvic grip (only in 3rd trimester)
  Head engagement—head engaged/not engaged

Auscultation

Fetal heart rate (FHR) :.. Beats/Mint : ....

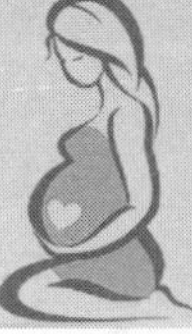

Laboratory Investigations

Date: .... Blood: Hb .... Group .... Sugar .... Urine: Albumin ....
HIV: .... HbsAg :.................... Malaria: VDRL .... Any other specify ....

Treatment

Drugs: .... Dose/Route: ....

Health Education

....

....

....

....

Remark

....

....

....

....

....

....

Signature of Sister in Charge **Signature of Supervisor**

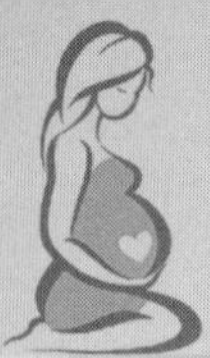

Antenatal Assessment (Case No. 11)

Client's Profile

Name	:	Education	: ....
Age	:	Occupation	: ....
Hospital name	:	Income per month	: ....
Date of booking	:	Marriage duration	: ....
Reg. No.	:	W/o	: ....
Religion	:	LMP	: ....
Parity	:	EDD	: ....

Address : ....

Period of gestation : ....

Menstrual History

Age at menarche	:............................	year of age	Blood flow :	average/scanty/heavy ....
Cycle of	:............................	days	Dysmenorrhea :	....
Period duration of	:............................	days		

History of Present Pregnancy

No. of antenatal visits : .... Immunization Status : ....

Tick mark (√), if present

Nausea/Vomiting/Back ache/Constipation/Frequency of Micturition/Leaking of watery fluid through vagina/Vaginal bleeding/Severe headache/Blurred vision/Difficulty in breathing/Palpitation/Decrease or absent fetal movement/Acidity/generalized swelling of body or face/Fever

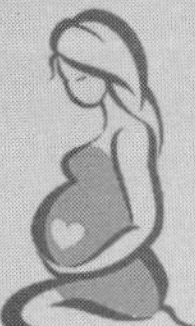

Obstetric History

S. No	Year	Term/ preterm	Abortion/ stillbirth	Nature of delivery	Child		Immunization	Growth and development	Nature of puerperium	Remark
					Alive	Sex/ weight				

Personal History

Allergies to drug : .... Body built : ....

Habit : Smoking/alcohol/betel chewing/any drug addiction : ....

Dietary habits : Vegetarian/nonvegetarian : ....

Hobbies : .... Diet per day - 2/3/4/5/6 : ....

Present and Past Medical History

Hypertension/diabetes/breathlessness on exertion/palpitation/tuberculosis/asthma/renal disease/convulsion/jaundice/malaria/RTI/STI/HIV/AIDS/no any/if any other specify ....

Family History

Family history of systemic illness: Hypertension/Diabetes/Tuberculosis/No any ....

Blood disorder: Thalassemia/Repeated blood transfusion

Delivery of: Twins/Congenital abnormalities

Examinations of Client

General Examinations

Height : ....cm Temperature : ......F Respiration : ....breath/mint

Weight : ....kg Pulse : ....beats/mint BP : ....mm Hg

Physical Examinations

General appearance	:	Sick/active/anemic/pallor
Body built	:	Moderate/thin/obsess
Head	:	Dandruff/pediculosis/flakes/dryness/itching/normal
Eye	:	Pupil—normal/dilated/constricted, Conjunctiva—pink/white
Ear	:	Normal/wax impaction/abnormal auricle development
Nose	:	Normal/nasal septum deviation/polyps/rhinitis
Lips	:	Normal/cheilosis/dry/pale lips
Tongue	:	White and smooth/pallor
Nail	:	Pink/pallor
Breast examination	:	Breast—normal/lump/tenderness
Nipple	:	Normal/inverted or flat nipples/crust or sore nipple
Micturition	:	Scanty/retention/incontinence/painful/frequent/normal
Digestion	:	Heart burn/constipation/diarrhea/hemorrhoids/normal

Abdominal Examinations

Inspection

Abdomen : Size :.. Shape :...

Counter : Fundal notching/convex/flattened anterior wall/cylindrical/spherical ....

Umbilicus : Striae gravidarum: ....

Linea nigra : ....

Palpation

Abdominal girth : ....cm

Fundal height of uterus : ....cm ....weeks

Fetal lie and presentation :

- Fundal palpation/grip
  Presentation—hard and globular (head)/soft and irregular (breech)
- Lateral palpation/grip
  Left—continuous hard/irregular small knobs
  Right—continuous hard/irregular small knobs
- Superficial pelvic grip
  Head (hard and globular)/breech (soft and irregular)/empty
- Deep pelvic grip (only in 3rd trimester)
  Head engagement—head engaged/not engaged

Auscultation

Fetal heart rate (FHR) :.. Beats/Mint : ....

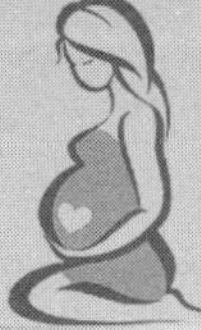

Laboratory Investigations

Date: .... Blood: Hb .... Group .... Sugar .... Urine: Albumin ....
HIV: .... HbsAg :..................... Malaria: VDRL .... Any other specify ....

Treatment

Drugs: .... Dose/Route: ....

Health Education

....

....

....

....

Remark

....

....

....

....

....

....

Signature of Sister in Charge **Signature of Supervisor**

Antenatal Assessment (Case No. 12)

Client's Profile

Name	:	Education	: ....
Age	:	Occupation	: ....
Hospital name	:	Income per month	: ....
Date of booking	:	Marriage duration	: ....
Reg. No.	:	W/o	: ....
Religion	:	LMP	: ....
Parity	:	EDD	:..

Address : ....

Period of gestation : ....

Menstrual History

Age at menarche	:..............................	year of age	Blood flow :	average/scanty/heavy ....
Cycle of	:..............................	days	Dysmenorrhea :	....
Period duration of	:..............................	days		

History of Present Pregnancy

No. of antenatal visits : .... Immunization Status : ....

Tick mark (√), if present

Nausea/Vomiting/Back ache/Constipation/Frequency of Micturition/Leaking of watery fluid through vagina/Vaginal bleeding/Severe headache/Blurred vision/Difficulty in breathing/Palpitation/Decrease or absent fetal movement/ Acidity/generalized swelling of body or face/Fever

Obstetric History

S. No	Year	Term/ preterm	Abortion/ stillbirth	Nature of delivery	Child		Immunization	Growth and development	Nature of puerperium	Remark
					Alive	Sex/ weight				

Personal History

Allergies to drug : .... Body built : ....

Habit : Smoking/alcohol/betel chewing/any drug addiction : ....

Dietary habits : Vegetarian/nonvegetarian : ....

Hobbies : .... Diet per day - 2/3/4/5/6 : ....

Present and Past Medical History

Hypertension/diabetes/breathlessness on exertion/palpitation/tuberculosis/asthma/renal disease/convulsion/jaundice/malaria/RTI/STI/HIV/AIDS/no any/if any other specify ....

Family History

Family history of systemic illness: Hypertension/Diabetes/Tuberculosis/No any ....
Blood disorder: Thalassemia/Repeated blood transfusion
Delivery of: Twins/Congenital abnormalities

Examinations of Client

General Examinations

Height : ....cm Temperature : ......F Respiration : ....breath/mint
Weight : ....kg Pulse : ....beats/mint BP : ....mm Hg

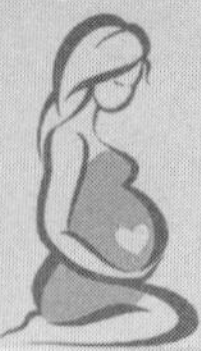

Physical Examinations

General appearance	:	Sick/active/anemic/pallor
Body built	:	Moderate/thin/obsess
Head	:	Dandruff/pediculosis/flakes/dryness/itching/normal
Eye	:	Pupil—normal/dilated/constricted, Conjunctiva—pink/white
Ear	:	Normal/wax impaction/abnormal auricle development
Nose	:	Normal/nasal septum deviation/polyps/rhinitis
Lips	:	Normal/cheilosis/dry/pale lips
Tongue	:	White and smooth/pallor
Nail	:	Pink/pallor
Breast examination	:	Breast—normal/lump/tenderness
Nipple	:	Normal/inverted or flat nipples/crust or sore nipple
Micturition	:	Scanty/retention/incontinence/painful/frequent/normal
Digestion	:	Heart burn/constipation/diarrhea/hemorrhoids/normal

Abdominal Examinations

Inspection

Abdomen : Size : .... Shape : ....

Counter : Fundal notching/convex/flattened anterior wall/cylindrical/spherical ....

Umbilicus : Striae gravidarum: ....

Linea nigra : ....

Palpation

Abdominal girth : ....cm

Fundal height of uterus : ....cm ....weeks

Fetal lie and presentation :

- Fundal palpation/grip
  Presentation—hard and globular (head)/soft and irregular (breech)
- Lateral palpation/grip
  Left—continuous hard/irregular small knobs
  Right—continuous hard/irregular small knobs
- Superficial pelvic grip
  Head (hard and globular)/breech (soft and irregular)/empty
- Deep pelvic grip (only in 3rd trimester)
  Head engagement—head engaged/not engaged

Auscultation

Fetal heart rate (FHR) :.. Beats/Mint : ....

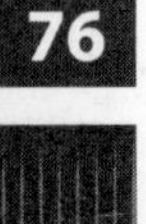

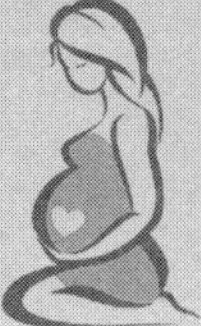

Laboratory Investigations

Date: .... Blood: Hb .... Group .... Sugar .... Urine: Albumin ....
HIV: .... HbsAg :..................... Malaria: VDRL .... Any other specify ....

Treatment

Drugs: .... Dose/Route: ....

Health Education

....

....

....

....

Remark

....

....

....

....

....

....

Signature of Sister in Charge

Signature of Supervisor

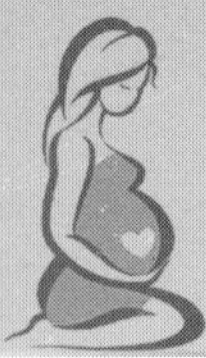

Antenatal Assessment (Case No. 13)

Client's Profile

Name : .... Education : ....

Age : .... Occupation : ....

Hospital name : .... Income per month : ....

Date of booking : .... Marriage duration : ....

Reg. No. : .... W/o : ....

Religion : .... LMP : ....

Parity : .... EDD : ....

Address : ....

Period of gestation : ....

Menstrual History

Age at menarche :............................ year of age Blood flow : average/scanty/heavy ....

Cycle of :............................ days Dysmenorrhea : ....

Period duration of :............................ days

History of Present Pregnancy

No. of antenatal visits : .... Immunization Status : ....

Tick mark (√), if present

Nausea/Vomiting/Back ache/Constipation/Frequency of Micturition/Leaking of watery fluid through vagina/Vaginal bleeding/Severe headache/Blurred vision/Difficulty in breathing/Palpitation/Decrease or absent fetal movement/Acidity/generalized swelling of body or face/Fever

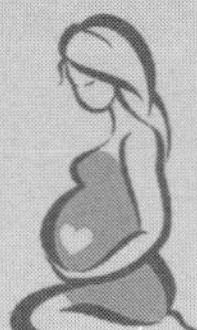

Obstetric History

S. No	Year	Term/ preterm	Abortion/ stillbirth	Nature of delivery	Child		Immunization	Growth and development	Nature of puerperium	Remark
					Alive	Sex/ weight				

Personal History

Allergies to drug : .... Body built : ....

Habit : Smoking/alcohol/betel chewing/any drug addiction : ....

Dietary habits : Vegetarian/nonvegetarian : ....

Hobbies : .... Diet per day - 2/3/4/5/6 : ....

Present and Past Medical History

Hypertension/diabetes/breathlessness on exertion/palpitation/tuberculosis/asthma/renal disease/convulsion/jaundice/malaria/RTI/STI/HIV/AIDS/no any/if any other specify ....

Family History

Family history of systemic illness: Hypertension/Diabetes/Tuberculosis/No any ....

Blood disorder: Thalassemia/Repeated blood transfusion

Delivery of: Twins/Congenital abnormalities

Examinations of Client

General Examinations

Height : ....cm Temperature : ......F Respiration : ....breath/mint

Weight : ....kg Pulse : ....beats/mint BP : ....mm Hg

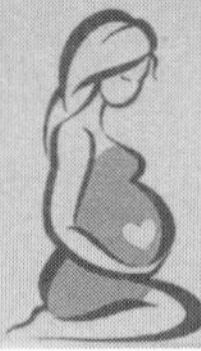

Physical Examinations

General appearance	:	Sick/active/anemic/pallor
Body built	:	Moderate/thin/obsess
Head	:	Dandruff/pediculosis/flakes/dryness/itching/normal
Eye	:	Pupil—normal/dilated/constricted, Conjunctiva—pink/white
Ear	:	Normal/wax impaction/abnormal auricle development
Nose	:	Normal/nasal septum deviation/polyps/rhinitis
Lips	:	Normal/cheilosis/dry/pale lips
Tongue	:	White and smooth/pallor
Nail	:	Pink/pallor
Breast examination	:	Breast—normal/lump/tenderness
Nipple	:	Normal/inverted or flat nipples/crust or sore nipple
Micturition	:	Scanty/retention/incontinence/painful/frequent/normal
Digestion	:	Heart burn/constipation/diarrhea/hemorrhoids/normal

Abdominal Examinations

Inspection

Abdomen : Size : .... Shape : ....

Counter : Fundal notching/convex/flattened anterior wall/cylindrical/spherical ....

Umbilicus : Striae gravidarum: ....

Linea nigra : ....

Palpation

Abdominal girth : ....cm

Fundal height of uterus : ....cm ....weeks

Fetal lie and presentation :

- Fundal palpation/grip
  Presentation—hard and globular (head)/soft and irregular (breech)
- Lateral palpation/grip
  Left—continuous hard/irregular small knobs
  Right—continuous hard/irregular small knobs
- Superficial pelvic grip
  Head (hard and globular)/breech (soft and irregular)/empty
- Deep pelvic grip (only in 3rd trimester)
  Head engagement—head engaged/not engaged

Auscultation

Fetal heart rate (FHR) :.. Beats/Mint : ....

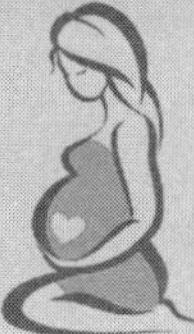

Laboratory Investigations

Date: .... Blood: Hb .... Group .... Sugar .... Urine: Albumin ....
HIV: .... HbsAg :..................... Malaria: VDRL .... Any other specify ....

Treatment

Drugs: .... Dose/Route: ....

Health Education

....

....

....

....

Remark

....

....

....

....

....

....

Signature of Sister in Charge

Signature of Supervisor

Antenatal Assessment (Case No. 14)

Client's Profile

Name	:	Education	: ....
Age	:	Occupation	: ....
Hospital name	:	Income per month	: ....
Date of booking	:	Marriage duration	: ....
Reg. No.	:	W/o	: ....
Religion	:	LMP	: ....
Parity	:	EDD	: ....

Address : ....

Period of gestation : ....

Menstrual History

Age at menarche	:..............................	year of age	Blood flow :	average/scanty/heavy ....
Cycle of	:..............................	days	Dysmenorrhea :	....
Period duration of	:..............................	days		

History of Present Pregnancy

No. of antenatal visits : .... Immunization Status : ....

Tick mark (√), if present

Nausea/Vomiting/Back ache/Constipation/Frequency of Micturition/Leaking of watery fluid through vagina/Vaginal bleeding/Severe headache/Blurred vision/Difficulty in breathing/Palpitation/Decrease or absent fetal movement/Acidity/generalized swelling of body or face/Fever

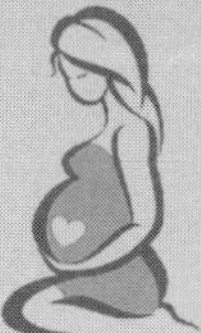

Obstetric History

S. No	Year	Term/ preterm	Abortion/ stillbirth	Nature of delivery	Child		Immunization	Growth and development	Nature of puerperium	Remark
					Alive	Sex/ weight				

Personal History

Allergies to drug : .... Body built : ....

Habit : Smoking/alcohol/betel chewing/any drug addiction : ....

Dietary habits : Vegetarian/nonvegetarian : ....

Hobbies : .... Diet per day - 2/3/4/5/6 : ....

Present and Past Medical History

Hypertension/diabetes/breathlessness on exertion/palpitation/tuberculosis/asthma/renal disease/convulsion/jaundice/malaria/RTI/STI/HIV/AIDS/no any/if any other specify ....

Family History

Family history of systemic illness: Hypertension/Diabetes/Tuberculosis/No any ....

Blood disorder: Thalassemia/Repeated blood transfusion

Delivery of: Twins/Congenital abnormalities

Examinations of Client

General Examinations

Height : ....cm Temperature : ......F Respiration : ....breath/mint

Weight : ....kg Pulse : ....beats/mint BP : ....mm Hg

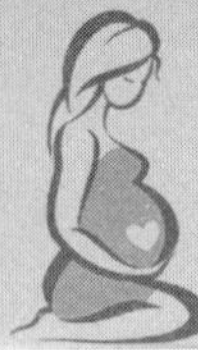

Physical Examinations

General appearance : Sick/active/anemic/pallor
Body built : Moderate/thin/obsess
Head : Dandruff/pediculosis/flakes/dryness/itching/normal
Eye : Pupil—normal/dilated/constricted, Conjunctiva—pink/white
Ear : Normal/wax impaction/abnormal auricle development
Nose : Normal/nasal septum deviation/polyps/rhinitis
Lips : Normal/cheilosis/dry/pale lips
Tongue : White and smooth/pallor
Nail : Pink/pallor
Breast examination : Breast—normal/lump/tenderness
Nipple : Normal/inverted or flat nipples/crust or sore nipple
Micturition : Scanty/retention/incontinence/painful/frequent/normal
Digestion : Heart burn/constipation/diarrhea/hemorrhoids/normal

Abdominal Examinations

Inspection

Abdomen : Size : .... Shape : ....
Counter : Fundal notching/convex/flattened anterior wall/cylindrical/spherical ....
Umbilicus : Striae gravidarum: ....
Linea nigra : ....

Palpation

Abdominal girth : ....cm
Fundal height of uterus : ....cm ....weeks
Fetal lie and presentation :

- Fundal palpation/grip
  Presentation—hard and globular (head)/soft and irregular (breech)
- Lateral palpation/grip
  Left—continuous hard/irregular small knobs
  Right—continuous hard/irregular small knobs
- Superficial pelvic grip
  Head (hard and globular)/breech (soft and irregular)/empty
- Deep pelvic grip (only in 3rd trimester)
  Head engagement—head engaged/not engaged

Auscultation

Fetal heart rate (FHR) :.. Beats/Mint : ....

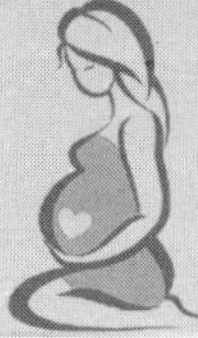

Laboratory Investigations

Date: .... Blood: Hb .... Group .... Sugar .... Urine: Albumin ....
HIV: .... HbsAg :.................... Malaria: VDRL .... Any other specify ....

Treatment

Drugs: .... Dose/Route: ....

Health Education

....

....

....

....

Remark

....

....

....

....

....

....

Signature of Sister in Charge **Signature of Supervisor**

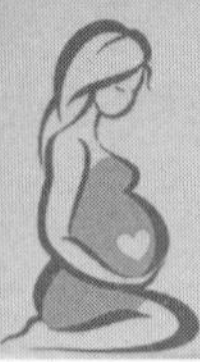

Antenatal Assessment (Case No. 15)

Client's Profile

Name	:	Education	: ....
Age	:	Occupation	: ....
Hospital name	:	Income per month	: ....
Date of booking	:	Marriage duration	: ....
Reg. No.	:	W/o	: ....
Religion	:	LMP	: ....
Parity	:	EDD	: ....

Address : ....

Period of gestation : ....

Menstrual History

Age at menarche	:..............................	year of age	Blood flow :	average/scanty/heavy ....
Cycle of	:..............................	days	Dysmenorrhea :	....
Period duration of	:..............................	days		

History of Present Pregnancy

No. of antenatal visits : .... Immunization Status : ....

Tick mark (√), if present

Nausea/Vomiting/Back ache/Constipation/Frequency of Micturition/Leaking of watery fluid through vagina/Vaginal bleeding/Severe headache/Blurred vision/Difficulty in breathing/Palpitation/Decrease or absent fetal movement/Acidity/generalized swelling of body or face/Fever

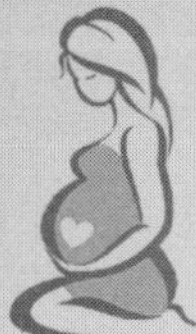

Obstetric History

S. No	Year	Term/ preterm	Abortion/ stillbirth	Nature of delivery	Child		Immunization	Growth and development	Nature of puerperium	Remark
					Alive	Sex/ weight				

Personal History

Allergies to drug : .... Body built : ....

Habit : Smoking/alcohol/betel chewing/any drug addiction : ....

Dietary habits : Vegetarian/nonvegetarian : ....

Hobbies : .... Diet per day - 2/3/4/5/6 : ....

Present and Past Medical History

Hypertension/diabetes/breathlessness on exertion/palpitation/tuberculosis/asthma/renal disease/convulsion/jaundice/malaria/RTI/STI/HIV/AIDS/no any/if any other specify ....

Family History

Family history of systemic illness: Hypertension/Diabetes/Tuberculosis/No any ....

Blood disorder: Thalassemia/Repeated blood transfusion

Delivery of: Twins/Congenital abnormalities

Examinations of Client

General Examinations

Height : ....cm Temperature : ......F Respiration : ....breath/mint

Weight : ....kg Pulse : ....beats/mint BP : ....mm Hg

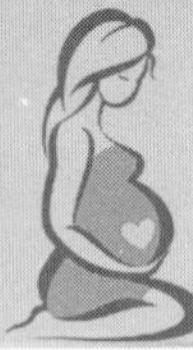

Physical Examinations

General appearance : Sick/active/anemic/pallor
Body built : Moderate/thin/obsess
Head : Dandruff/pediculosis/flakes/dryness/itching/normal
Eye : Pupil—normal/dilated/constricted, Conjunctiva—pink/white
Ear : Normal/wax impaction/abnormal auricle development
Nose : Normal/nasal septum deviation/polyps/rhinitis
Lips : Normal/cheilosis/dry/pale lips
Tongue : White and smooth/pallor
Nail : Pink/pallor
Breast examination : Breast—normal/lump/tenderness
Nipple : Normal/inverted or flat nipples/crust or sore nipple
Micturition : Scanty/retention/incontinence/painful/frequent/normal
Digestion : Heart burn/constipation/diarrhea/hemorrhoids/normal

Abdominal Examinations

Inspection

Abdomen : Size : .... Shape : ....
Counter : Fundal notching/convex/flattened anterior wall/cylindrical/spherical ....
Umbilicus : Striae gravidarum: ....
Linea nigra : ....

Palpation

Abdominal girth : ....cm
Fundal height of uterus : ....cm ....weeks
Fetal lie and presentation :

- Fundal palpation/grip
  Presentation—hard and globular (head)/soft and irregular (breech)
- Lateral palpation/grip
  Left—continuous hard/irregular small knobs
  Right—continuous hard/irregular small knobs
- Superficial pelvic grip
  Head (hard and globular)/breech (soft and irregular)/empty
- Deep pelvic grip (only in 3rd trimester)
  Head engagement—head engaged/not engaged

Auscultation

Fetal heart rate (FHR) :... Beats/Mint : ....

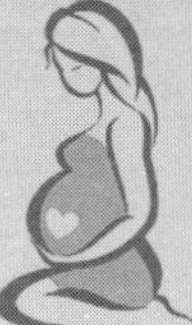

Laboratory Investigations

Date: .... Blood: Hb .... Group .... Sugar .... Urine: Albumin ....
HIV: .... HbsAg :..................... Malaria: VDRL .... Any other specify ....

Treatment

Drugs: .... Dose/Route: ....

Health Education

....

....

....

....

Remark

....

....

....

....

....

....

Signature of Sister in Charge

Signature of Supervisor

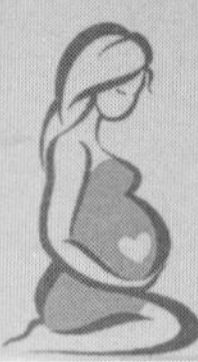

Antenatal Assessment (Case No. 16)

Client's Profile

Name : .... Education : ....

Age : .... Occupation : ....

Hospital name : .... Income per month : ....

Date of booking : .... Marriage duration : ....

Reg. No. : .... W/o : ....

Religion : .... LMP : ....

Parity : .... EDD : ....

Address : ....

Period of gestation : ....

Menstrual History

Age at menarche :.............................. year of age Blood flow : average/scanty/heavy ....

Cycle of :.............................. days Dysmenorrhea : ....

Period duration of :.............................. days

History of Present Pregnancy

No. of antenatal visits : .... Immunization Status : ....

Tick mark (√), if present

Nausea/Vomiting/Back ache/Constipation/Frequency of Micturition/Leaking of watery fluid through vagina/Vaginal bleeding/Severe headache/Blurred vision/Difficulty in breathing/Palpitation/Decrease or absent fetal movement/Acidity/generalized swelling of body or face/Fever

Obstetric History

S. No	Year	Term/ preterm	Abortion/ stillbirth	Nature of delivery	Child		Immunization	Growth and development	Nature of puerperium	Remark
					Alive	Sex/ weight				

Personal History

Allergies to drug : .... Body built : ....
Habit : Smoking/alcohol/betel chewing/any drug addiction : ....
Dietary habits : Vegetarian/nonvegetarian : ....
Hobbies : .... Diet per day - 2/3/4/5/6 : ....

Present and Past Medical History

Hypertension/diabetes/breathlessness on exertion/palpitation/tuberculosis/asthma/renal disease/convulsion/jaundice/malaria/RTI/STI/HIV/AIDS/no any/if any other specify ....

Family History

Family history of systemic illness: Hypertension/Diabetes/Tuberculosis/No any ....
Blood disorder: Thalassemia/Repeated blood transfusion
Delivery of: Twins/Congenital abnormalities

Examinations of Client

General Examinations

Height : ....cm Temperature : ......F Respiration : ....breath/mint
Weight : ....kg Pulse : ....beats/mint BP : ....mm Hg

Physical Examinations

General appearance	:	Sick/active/anemic/pallor
Body built	:	Moderate/thin/obsess
Head	:	Dandruff/pediculosis/flakes/dryness/itching/normal
Eye	:	Pupil—normal/dilated/constricted, Conjunctiva—pink/white
Ear	:	Normal/wax impaction/abnormal auricle development
Nose	:	Normal/nasal septum deviation/polyps/rhinitis
Lips	:	Normal/cheilosis/dry/pale lips
Tongue	:	White and smooth/pallor
Nail	:	Pink/pallor
Breast examination	:	Breast—normal/lump/tenderness
Nipple	:	Normal/inverted or flat nipples/crust or sore nipple
Micturition	:	Scanty/retention/incontinence/painful/frequent/normal
Digestion	:	Heart burn/constipation/diarrhea/hemorrhoids/normal

Abdominal Examinations

Inspection

Abdomen : Size : .... Shape : ....

Counter : Fundal notching/convex/flattened anterior wall/cylindrical/spherical ....

Umbilicus : Striae gravidarum: ....

Linea nigra : ....

Palpation

Abdominal girth : ....cm

Fundal height of uterus : ....cm ....weeks

Fetal lie and presentation :

- Fundal palpation/grip
  Presentation—hard and globular (head)/soft and irregular (breech)
- Lateral palpation/grip
  Left—continuous hard/irregular small knobs
  Right—continuous hard/irregular small knobs
- Superficial pelvic grip
  Head (hard and globular)/breech (soft and irregular)/empty
- Deep pelvic grip (only in 3rd trimester)
  Head engagement—head engaged/not engaged

Auscultation

Fetal heart rate (FHR) :.. Beats/Mint : ....

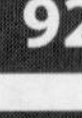

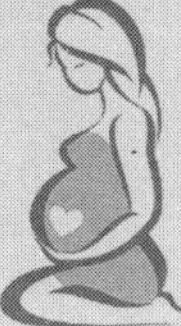

Laboratory Investigations

Date: .... Blood: Hb .... Group .... Sugar .... Urine: Albumin ....
HIV: .... HbsAg :.................... Malaria: VDRL .... Any other specify ....

Treatment

Drugs: .... Dose/Route: ....

Health Education

....

....

....

....

Remark

....

....

....

....

....

....

Signature of Sister in Charge **Signature of Supervisor**

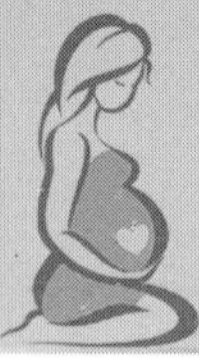

Antenatal Assessment (Case No. 17)

Client's Profile

Name : .... Education : ....

Age : .... Occupation : ....

Hospital name : .... Income per month : ....

Date of booking : .... Marriage duration : ....

Reg. No. : .... W/o : ....

Religion : .... LMP : ....

Parity : .... EDD : ....

Address : ....

Period of gestation : ....

Menstrual History

Age at menarche :............................... year of age Blood flow : average/scanty/heavy ....

Cycle of :............................... days Dysmenorrhea : ....

Period duration of :............................... days

History of Present Pregnancy

No. of antenatal visits : .... Immunization Status : ....

Tick mark (√), if present

Nausea/Vomiting/Back ache/Constipation/Frequency of Micturition/Leaking of watery fluid through vagina/Vaginal bleeding/Severe headache/Blurred vision/Difficulty in breathing/Palpitation/Decrease or absent fetal movement/Acidity/generalized swelling of body or face/Fever

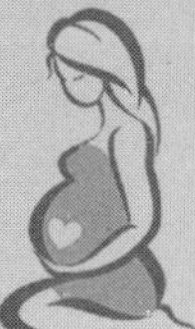

Obstetric History

S. No	Year	Term/ preterm	Abortion/ stillbirth	Nature of delivery	Child		Immunization	Growth and development	Nature of puerperium	Remark
					Alive	Sex/ weight				

Personal History

Allergies to drug : .... Body built : ....
Habit : Smoking/alcohol/betel chewing/any drug addiction : ....
Dietary habits : Vegetarian/nonvegetarian : ....
Hobbies : .... Diet per day - 2/3/4/5/6 : ....

Present and Past Medical History

Hypertension/diabetes/breathlessness on exertion/palpitation/tuberculosis/asthma/renal disease/convulsion/jaundice/malaria/RTI/STI/HIV/AIDS/no any/if any other specify ....

Family History

Family history of systemic illness: Hypertension/Diabetes/Tuberculosis/No any ....
Blood disorder: Thalassemia/Repeated blood transfusion
Delivery of: Twins/Congenital abnormalities

Examinations of Client

General Examinations

Height : ....cm Temperature : ......F Respiration : ....breath/mint
Weight : ....kg Pulse : ....beats/mint BP : ....mm Hg

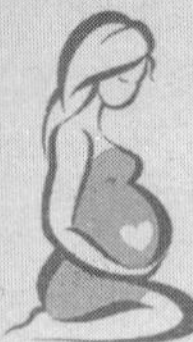

Physical Examinations

General appearance : Sick/active/anemic/pallor
Body built : Moderate/thin/obsess
Head : Dandruff/pediculosis/flakes/dryness/itching/normal
Eye : Pupil—normal/dilated/constricted, Conjunctiva—pink/white
Ear : Normal/wax impaction/abnormal auricle development
Nose : Normal/nasal septum deviation/polyps/rhinitis
Lips : Normal/cheilosis/dry/pale lips
Tongue : White and smooth/pallor
Nail : Pink/pallor
Breast examination : Breast—normal/lump/tenderness
Nipple : Normal/inverted or flat nipples/crust or sore nipple
Micturition : Scanty/retention/incontinence/painful/frequent/normal
Digestion : Heart burn/constipation/diarrhea/hemorrhoids/normal

Abdominal Examinations

Inspection

Abdomen : Size : .... Shape : ....
Counter : Fundal notching/convex/flattened anterior wall/cylindrical/spherical ....
Umbilicus : Striae gravidarum: ....
Linea nigra : ....

Palpation

Abdominal girth : ....cm
Fundal height of uterus : ....cm ....weeks
Fetal lie and presentation :

- Fundal palpation/grip
  Presentation—hard and globular (head)/soft and irregular (breech)
- Lateral palpation/grip
  Left—continuous hard/irregular small knobs
  Right—continuous hard/irregular small knobs
- Superficial pelvic grip
  Head (hard and globular)/breech (soft and irregular)/empty
- Deep pelvic grip (only in 3rd trimester)
  Head engagement—head engaged/not engaged

Auscultation

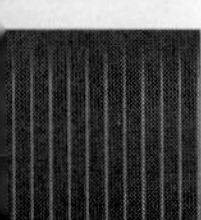

Fetal heart rate (FHR) :... Beats/Mint : ....

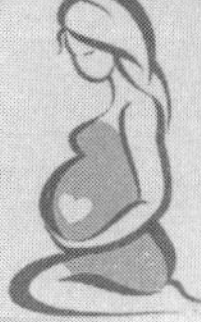

Laboratory Investigations

Date: .... Blood: Hb .... Group .... Sugar .... Urine: Albumin ....
HIV: .... HbsAg :..................... Malaria: VDRL .... Any other specify ....

Treatment

Drugs: .... Dose/Route: ....

Health Education

....

....

....

....

Remark

....

....

....

....

....

....

Signature of Sister in Charge **Signature of Supervisor**

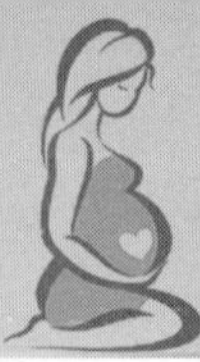

Antenatal Assessment (Case No. 18)

Client's Profile

Name	:	Education	: ....
Age	:	Occupation	: ....
Hospital name	:	Income per month	: ....
Date of booking	:	Marriage duration	: ....
Reg. No.	:	W/o	: ....
Religion	:	LMP	: ....
Parity	:	EDD	: ....

Address : ....

Period of gestation : ....

Menstrual History

Age at menarche	:..........................	year of age	Blood flow :	average/scanty/heavy ....
Cycle of	:..........................	days	Dysmenorrhea :	....
Period duration of	:..........................	days		

History of Present Pregnancy

No. of antenatal visits : .... Immunization Status : ....

Tick mark (√), if present

Nausea/Vomiting/Back ache/Constipation/Frequency of Micturition/Leaking of watery fluid through vagina/Vaginal bleeding/Severe headache/Blurred vision/Difficulty in breathing/Palpitation/Decrease or absent fetal movement/Acidity/generalized swelling of body or face/Fever

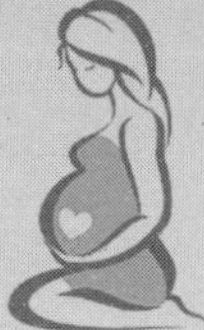

Obstetric History

S. No	Year	Term/ preterm	Abortion/ stillbirth	Nature of delivery	Child		Immunization	Growth and development	Nature of puerperium	Remark
					Alive	Sex/ weight				

Personal History

Allergies to drug : .... Body built : ....

Habit : Smoking/alcohol/betel chewing/any drug addiction : ....

Dietary habits : Vegetarian/nonvegetarian : ....

Hobbies : .... Diet per day - 2/3/4/5/6 : ....

Present and Past Medical History

Hypertension/diabetes/breathlessness on exertion/palpitation/tuberculosis/asthma/renal disease/convulsion/jaundice/malaria/RTI/STI/HIV/AIDS/no any/if any other specify ....

Family History

Family history of systemic illness: Hypertension/Diabetes/Tuberculosis/No any ....

Blood disorder: Thalassemia/Repeated blood transfusion

Delivery of: Twins/Congenital abnormalities

Examinations of Client

General Examinations

Height : ....cm Temperature : ......F Respiration : ....breath/mint

Weight : .... kg Pulse : ....beats/mint BP : ....mm Hg

Physical Examinations

General appearance : Sick/active/anemic/pallor
Body built : Moderate/thin/obsess
Head : Dandruff/pediculosis/flakes/dryness/itching/normal
Eye : Pupil—normal/dilated/constricted, Conjunctiva—pink/white
Ear : Normal/wax impaction/abnormal auricle development
Nose : Normal/nasal septum deviation/polyps/rhinitis
Lips : Normal/cheilosis/dry/pale lips
Tongue : White and smooth/pallor
Nail : Pink/pallor
Breast examination : Breast—normal/lump/tenderness
Nipple : Normal/inverted or flat nipples/crust or sore nipple
Micturition : Scanty/retention/incontinence/painful/frequent/normal
Digestion : Heart burn/constipation/diarrhea/hemorrhoids/normal

Abdominal Examinations

Inspection

Abdomen : Size :.. Shape :..
Counter : Fundal notching/convex/flattened anterior wall/cylindrical/spherical ....
Umbilicus : Striae gravidarum: ....
Linea nigra : ....

Palpation

Abdominal girth : ....cm
Fundal height of uterus : ....cm ....weeks
Fetal lie and presentation :

- Fundal palpation/grip
  Presentation—hard and globular (head)/soft and irregular (breech)
- Lateral palpation/grip
  Left—continuous hard/irregular small knobs
  Right—continuous hard/irregular small knobs
- Superficial pelvic grip
  Head (hard and globular)/breech (soft and irregular)/empty
- Deep pelvic grip (only in 3rd trimester)
  Head engagement—head engaged/not engaged

Auscultation

Fetal heart rate (FHR) :.. Beats/Mint : ....

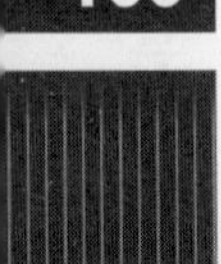

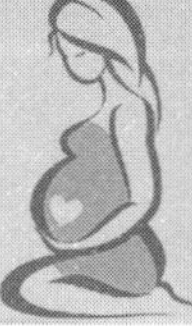

Laboratory Investigations

Date: .... Blood: Hb .... Group .... Sugar .... Urine: Albumin ....
HIV: .... HbsAg :..................... Malaria: VDRL .... Any other specify ....

Treatment

Drugs: .... Dose/Route: ....

Health Education

....

....

....

....

Remark

....

....

....

....

....

....

Signature of Sister in Charge

____

Signature of Supervisor

____

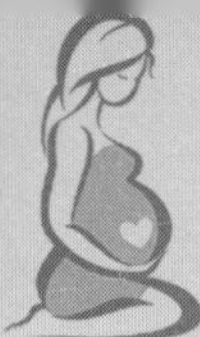

Antenatal Assessment (Case No. 19)

Client's Profile

Name	:	Education	: ....
Age	:	Occupation	: ....
Hospital name	:	Income per month	: ....
Date of booking	:	Marriage duration	: ....
Reg. No.	:	W/o	: ....
Religion	:	LMP	: ....
Parity	:	EDD	: ....

Address : ....

Period of gestation : ....

Menstrual History

Age at menarche	:..............................	year of age	Blood flow :	average/scanty/heavy ....
Cycle of	:..............................	days	Dysmenorrhea :	....
Period duration of	:..............................	days		

History of Present Pregnancy

No. of antenatal visits : .... Immunization Status : ....

Tick mark (√), if present

Nausea/Vomiting/Back ache/Constipation/Frequency of Micturition/Leaking of watery fluid through vagina/Vaginal bleeding/Severe headache/Blurred vision/Difficulty in breathing/Palpitation/Decrease or absent fetal movement/Acidity/generalized swelling of body or face/Fever

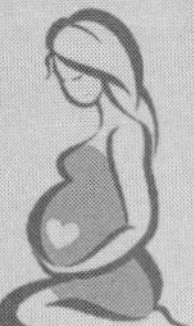

Obstetric History

S. No	Year	Term/ preterm	Abortion/ stillbirth	Nature of delivery	Child		Immunization	Growth and development	Nature of puerperium	Remark
					Alive	Sex/ weight				

Personal History

Allergies to drug : .... Body built : ....
Habit : Smoking/alcohol/betel chewing/any drug addiction : ....
Dietary habits : Vegetarian/nonvegetarian : ....
Hobbies : .... Diet per day - 2/3/4/5/6 : ....

Present and Past Medical History

Hypertension/diabetes/breathlessness on exertion/palpitation/tuberculosis/asthma/renal disease/convulsion/jaundice/malaria/RTI/STI/HIV/AIDS/no any/if any other specify ....

Family History

Family history of systemic illness: Hypertension/Diabetes/Tuberculosis/No any ....
Blood disorder: Thalassemia/Repeated blood transfusion
Delivery of: Twins/Congenital abnormalities

Examinations of Client

General Examinations

Height : ....cm Temperature : ......F Respiration : ....breath/mint
Weight : ....kg Pulse : ....beats/mint BP : ....mm Hg

Physical Examinations

General appearance : Sick/active/anemic/pallor
Body built : Moderate/thin/obsess
Head : Dandruff/pediculosis/flakes/dryness/itching/normal
Eye : Pupil—normal/dilated/constricted, Conjunctiva—pink/white
Ear : Normal/wax impaction/abnormal auricle development
Nose : Normal/nasal septum deviation/polyps/rhinitis
Lips : Normal/cheilosis/dry/pale lips
Tongue : White and smooth/pallor
Nail : Pink/pallor
Breast examination : Breast—normal/lump/tenderness
Nipple : Normal/inverted or flat nipples/crust or sore nipple
Micturition : Scanty/retention/incontinence/painful/frequent/normal
Digestion : Heart burn/constipation/diarrhea/hemorrhoids/normal

Abdominal Examinations

Inspection

Abdomen : Size : .... Shape : ....
Counter : Fundal notching/convex/flattened anterior wall/cylindrical/spherical ....
Umbilicus : Striae gravidarum: ....
Linea nigra : ....

Palpation

Abdominal girth : ....cm
Fundal height of uterus : ....cm ....weeks
Fetal lie and presentation :

- Fundal palpation/grip
  Presentation—hard and globular (head)/soft and irregular (breech)
- Lateral palpation/grip
  Left—continuous hard/irregular small knobs
  Right—continuous hard/irregular small knobs
- Superficial pelvic grip
  Head (hard and globular)/breech (soft and irregular)/empty
- Deep pelvic grip (only in 3rd trimester)
  Head engagement—head engaged/not engaged

Auscultation

Fetal heart rate (FHR) :... Beats/Mint : ....

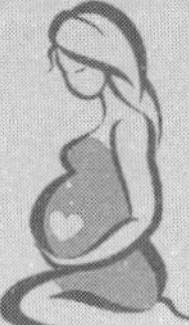

Laboratory Investigations

Date: .... Blood: Hb .... Group .... Sugar .... Urine: Albumin ....
HIV: .... HbsAg :..................... Malaria: VDRL .... Any other specify ....

Treatment

Drugs: .... Dose/Route: ....

Health Education

....

....

....

....

Remark

....

....

....

....

....

....

Signature of Sister in Charge **Signature of Supervisor**

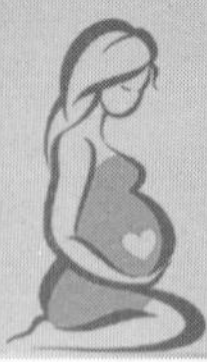

Antenatal Assessment (Case No. 20)

Client's Profile

Name	:	Education	: ....
Age	:	Occupation	: ....
Hospital name	:	Income per month	: ....
Date of booking	:	Marriage duration	: ....
Reg. No.	:	W/o	: ....
Religion	:	LMP	: ....
Parity	:	EDD	:..

Address : ....

Period of gestation : ....

Menstrual History

Age at menarche	:..........................	year of age	Blood flow :	average/scanty/heavy ....
Cycle of	:..........................	days	Dysmenorrhea :	....
Period duration of	:..........................	days		

History of Present Pregnancy

No. of antenatal visits : .... Immunization Status : ....

Tick mark (√), if present

Nausea/Vomiting/Back ache/Constipation/Frequency of Micturition/Leaking of watery fluid through vagina/Vaginal bleeding/Severe headache/Blurred vision/Difficulty in breathing/Palpitation/Decrease or absent fetal movement/Acidity/generalized swelling of body or face/Fever

Obstetric History

S. No	Year	Term/ preterm	Abortion/ stillbirth	Nature of delivery	Child		Immunization	Growth and development	Nature of puerperium	Remark
					Alive	Sex/ weight				

Personal History

Allergies to drug : .... Body built : ....

Habit : Smoking/alcohol/betel chewing/any drug addiction : ....

Dietary habits : Vegetarian/nonvegetarian : ....

Hobbies : .... Diet per day - 2/3/4/5/6 : ....

Present and Past Medical History

Hypertension/diabetes/breathlessness on exertion/palpitation/tuberculosis/asthma/renal disease/convulsion/jaundice/malaria/RTI/STI/HIV/AIDS/no any/if any other specify ....

Family History

Family history of systemic illness: Hypertension/Diabetes/Tuberculosis/No any ....

Blood disorder: Thalassemia/Repeated blood transfusion

Delivery of: Twins/Congenital abnormalities

Examinations of Client

General Examinations

Height : ....cm Temperature : ......F Respiration : ....breath/mint

Weight : ....kg Pulse : ....beats/mint BP : ....mm Hg

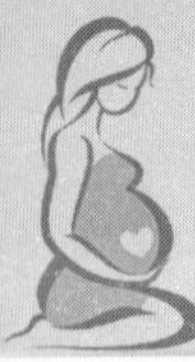

Physical Examinations

General appearance	:	Sick/active/anemic/pallor
Body built	:	Moderate/thin/obsess
Head	:	Dandruff/pediculosis/flakes/dryness/itching/normal
Eye	:	Pupil—normal/dilated/constricted, Conjunctiva—pink/white
Ear	:	Normal/wax impaction/abnormal auricle development
Nose	:	Normal/nasal septum deviation/polyps/rhinitis
Lips	:	Normal/cheilosis/dry/pale lips
Tongue	:	White and smooth/pallor
Nail	:	Pink/pallor
Breast examination	:	Breast—normal/lump/tenderness
Nipple	:	Normal/inverted or flat nipples/crust or sore nipple
Micturition	:	Scanty/retention/incontinence/painful/frequent/normal
Digestion	:	Heart burn/constipation/diarrhea/hemorrhoids/normal

Abdominal Examinations

Inspection

Abdomen : Size : .... Shape : ....

Counter : Fundal notching/convex/flattened anterior wall/cylindrical/spherical ....

Umbilicus : Striae gravidarum: ....

Linea nigra : ....

Palpation

Abdominal girth : ....cm

Fundal height of uterus : ....cm ....weeks

Fetal lie and presentation :

- Fundal palpation/grip
  Presentation—hard and globular (head)/soft and irregular (breech)
- Lateral palpation/grip
  Left—continuous hard/irregular small knobs
  Right—continuous hard/irregular small knobs
- Superficial pelvic grip
  Head (hard and globular)/breech (soft and irregular)/empty
- Deep pelvic grip (only in 3rd trimester)
  Head engagement—head engaged/not engaged

Auscultation

Fetal heart rate (FHR) :... Beats/Mint : ....

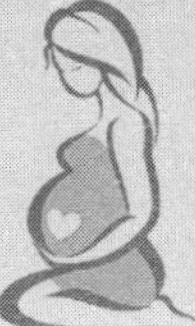

Laboratory Investigations

Date: .... Blood: Hb .... Group .... Sugar .... Urine: Albumin ....

HIV: .... HbsAg :..................... Malaria: VDRL .... Any other specify ....

Treatment

Drugs: .... Dose/Route: ....

Health Education

....

....

....

....

Remark

....

....

....

....

....

....

Signature of Sister in Charge **Signature of Supervisor**

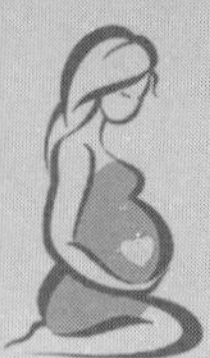

Antenatal Assessment (Case No. 21)

Client's Profile

Name : .... Education : ....

Age : .... Occupation : ....

Hospital name : .... Income per month : ....

Date of booking : .... Marriage duration : ....

Reg. No. : .... W/o : ....

Religion : .... LMP : ....

Parity : .... EDD :..

Address : ....

Period of gestation : ....

Menstrual History

Age at menarche :.............................. year of age Blood flow : average/scanty/heavy ....

Cycle of :.............................. days Dysmenorrhea : ....

Period duration of :.............................. days

History of Present Pregnancy

No. of antenatal visits : .... Immunization Status : ....

Tick mark (√), if present

Nausea/Vomiting/Back ache/Constipation/Frequency of Micturition/Leaking of watery fluid through vagina/Vaginal bleeding/Severe headache/Blurred vision/Difficulty in breathing/Palpitation/Decrease or absent fetal movement/Acidity/generalized swelling of body or face/Fever

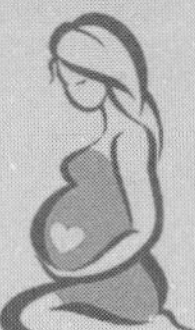

Obstetric History

S. No	Year	Term/ preterm	Abortion/ stillbirth	Nature of delivery	Child		Immunization	Growth and development	Nature of puerperium	Remark
					Alive	Sex/ weight				

Personal History

Allergies to drug : .... Body built : ....
Habit : Smoking/alcohol/betel chewing/any drug addiction : ....
Dietary habits : Vegetarian/nonvegetarian : ....
Hobbies : .... Diet per day - 2/3/4/5/6 : ....

Present and Past Medical History

Hypertension/diabetes/breathlessness on exertion/palpitation/tuberculosis/asthma/renal disease/convulsion/jaundice/malaria/RTI/STI/HIV/AIDS/no any/if any other specify ....

Family History

Family history of systemic illness: Hypertension/Diabetes/Tuberculosis/No any ....
Blood disorder: Thalassemia/Repeated blood transfusion
Delivery of: Twins/Congenital abnormalities

Examinations of Client

General Examinations

Height : ....cm Temperature : ......F Respiration : ....breath/mint
Weight : ....kg Pulse : ....beats/mint BP : ....mm Hg

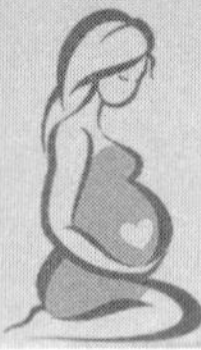

Physical Examinations

General appearance : Sick/active/anemic/pallor
Body built : Moderate/thin/obsess
Head : Dandruff/pediculosis/flakes/dryness/itching/normal
Eye : Pupil—normal/dilated/constricted, Conjunctiva—pink/white
Ear : Normal/wax impaction/abnormal auricle development
Nose : Normal/nasal septum deviation/polyps/rhinitis
Lips : Normal/cheilosis/dry/pale lips
Tongue : White and smooth/pallor
Nail : Pink/pallor
Breast examination : Breast—normal/lump/tenderness
Nipple : Normal/inverted or flat nipples/crust or sore nipple
Micturition : Scanty/retention/incontinence/painful/frequent/normal
Digestion : Heart burn/constipation/diarrhea/hemorrhoids/normal

Abdominal Examinations

Inspection

Abdomen : Size :.. Shape :..
Counter : Fundal notching/convex/flattened anterior wall/cylindrical/spherical ....
Umbilicus : Striae gravidarum: ....
Linea nigra : ....

Palpation

Abdominal girth : ....cm
Fundal height of uterus : ....cm ....weeks
Fetal lie and presentation :

- Fundal palpation/grip
  Presentation—hard and globular (head)/soft and irregular (breech)
- Lateral palpation/grip
  Left—continuous hard/irregular small knobs
  Right—continuous hard/irregular small knobs
- Superficial pelvic grip
  Head (hard and globular)/breech (soft and irregular)/empty
- Deep pelvic grip (only in 3rd trimester)
  Head engagement—head engaged/not engaged

Auscultation

Fetal heart rate (FHR) :... Beats/Mint : ....

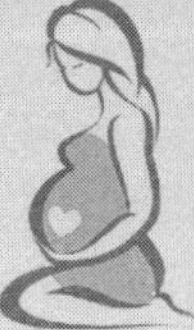

Laboratory Investigations

Date: .... Blood: Hb .... Group .... Sugar .... Urine: Albumin ....
HIV: .... HbsAg :..................... Malaria: VDRL .... Any other specify ....

Treatment

Drugs: .... Dose/Route: ....

Health Education

....

....

....

....

Remark

....

....

....

....

....

....

Signature of Sister in Charge **Signature of Supervisor**

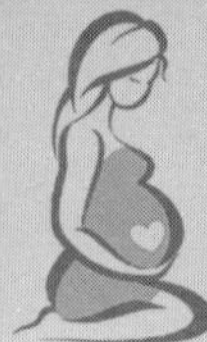

Antenatal Assessment (Case No. 22)

Client's Profile

Name	:	Education	: ....
Age	:	Occupation	: ....
Hospital name	:	Income per month	: ....
Date of booking	:	Marriage duration	: ....
Reg. No.	:	W/o	: ....
Religion	:	LMP	: ....
Parity	:	EDD	: ....

Address : ....

Period of gestation : ....

Menstrual History

Age at menarche	:............................	year of age	Blood flow :	average/scanty/heavy ....
Cycle of	:............................	days	Dysmenorrhea :	....
Period duration of	:............................	days		

History of Present Pregnancy

No. of antenatal visits : .... Immunization Status : ....

Tick mark (√), if present

Nausea/Vomiting/Back ache/Constipation/Frequency of Micturition/Leaking of watery fluid through vagina/Vaginal bleeding/Severe headache/Blurred vision/Difficulty in breathing/Palpitation/Decrease or absent fetal movement/Acidity/generalized swelling of body or face/Fever

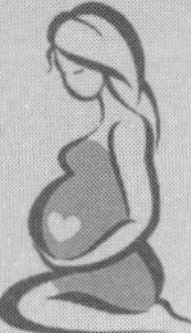

Obstetric History

S. No	Year	Term/ preterm	Abortion/ stillbirth	Nature of delivery	Child		Immunization	Growth and development	Nature of puerperium	Remark
					Alive	Sex/ weight				

Personal History

Allergies to drug : .... Body built : ....
Habit : Smoking/alcohol/betel chewing/any drug addiction : ....
Dietary habits : Vegetarian/nonvegetarian : ....
Hobbies : .... Diet per day - 2/3/4/5/6 : ....

Present and Past Medical History

Hypertension/diabetes/breathlessness on exertion/palpitation/tuberculosis/asthma/renal disease/convulsion/jaundice/malaria/RTI/STI/HIV/AIDS/no any/if any other specify ....

Family History

Family history of systemic illness: Hypertension/Diabetes/Tuberculosis/No any ....
Blood disorder: Thalassemia/Repeated blood transfusion
Delivery of: Twins/Congenital abnormalities

Examinations of Client

General Examinations

Height : ....cm Temperature : ......F Respiration : ....breath/mint
Weight : ....kg Pulse : ....beats/mint BP : ....mm Hg

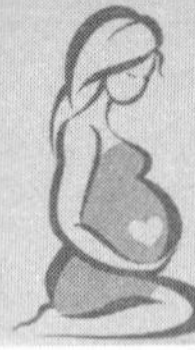

Physical Examinations

General appearance	:	Sick/active/anemic/pallor
Body built	:	Moderate/thin/obsess
Head	:	Dandruff/pediculosis/flakes/dryness/itching/normal
Eye	:	Pupil—normal/dilated/constricted, Conjunctiva—pink/white
Ear	:	Normal/wax impaction/abnormal auricle development
Nose	:	Normal/nasal septum deviation/polyps/rhinitis
Lips	:	Normal/cheilosis/dry/pale lips
Tongue	:	White and smooth/pallor
Nail	:	Pink/pallor
Breast examination	:	Breast—normal/lump/tenderness
Nipple	:	Normal/inverted or flat nipples/crust or sore nipple
Micturition	:	Scanty/retention/incontinence/painful/frequent/normal
Digestion	:	Heart burn/constipation/diarrhea/hemorrhoids/normal

Abdominal Examinations

Inspection

Abdomen : Size : .... Shape : ....

Counter : Fundal notching/convex/flattened anterior wall/cylindrical/spherical ....

Umbilicus : Striae gravidarum: ....

Linea nigra : ....

Palpation

Abdominal girth : ....cm

Fundal height of uterus : ....cm ....weeks

Fetal lie and presentation :

- Fundal palpation/grip
  Presentation—hard and globular (head)/soft and irregular (breech)
- Lateral palpation/grip
  Left—continuous hard/irregular small knobs
  Right—continuous hard/irregular small knobs
- Superficial pelvic grip
  Head (hard and globular)/breech (soft and irregular)/empty
- Deep pelvic grip (only in 3rd trimester)
  Head engagement—head engaged/not engaged

Auscultation

Fetal heart rate (FHR) :... Beats/Mint : ....

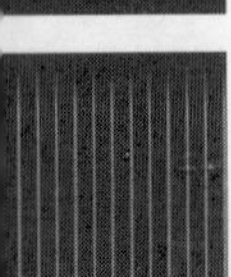

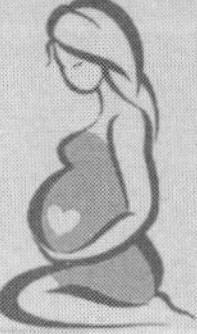

Laboratory Investigations

Date: .... Blood: Hb .... Group .... Sugar .... Urine: Albumin ....
HIV: .... HbsAg :..................... Malaria: VDRL .... Any other specify ....

Treatment

Drugs: .... Dose/Route: ....

Health Education

....

....

....

....

Remark

....

....

....

....

....

....

Signature of Sister in Charge

____

Signature of Supervisor

____

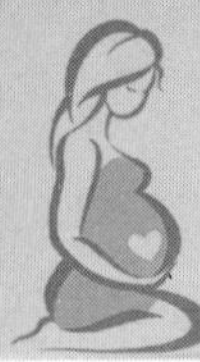

Antenatal Assessment (Case No. 23)

Client's Profile

Name	:	Education	: ....
Age	:	Occupation	: ....
Hospital name	:	Income per month	: ....
Date of booking	:	Marriage duration	: ....
Reg. No.	:	W/o	: ....
Religion	:	LMP	: ....
Parity	:	EDD	:..

Address : ....

Period of gestation : ....

Menstrual History

Age at menarche	:............................	year of age	Blood flow :	average/scanty/heavy ....
Cycle of	:............................	days	Dysmenorrhea :	....
Period duration of	:............................	days		

History of Present Pregnancy

No. of antenatal visits : .... Immunization Status : ....

Tick mark (√), if present

Nausea/Vomiting/Back ache/Constipation/Frequency of Micturition/Leaking of watery fluid through vagina/Vaginal bleeding/Severe headache/Blurred vision/Difficulty in breathing/Palpitation/Decrease or absent fetal movement/Acidity/generalized swelling of body or face/Fever

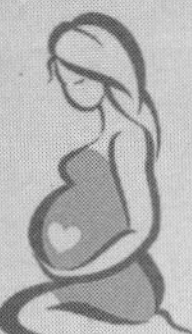

Obstetric History

S. No	Year	Term/ preterm	Abortion/ stillbirth	Nature of delivery	Child		Immunization	Growth and development	Nature of puerperium	Remark
					Alive	Sex/ weight				

Personal History

Allergies to drug : .... Body built : ....

Habit : Smoking/alcohol/betel chewing/any drug addiction : ....

Dietary habits : Vegetarian/nonvegetarian : ....

Hobbies : .... Diet per day - 2/3/4/5/6 : ....

Present and Past Medical History

Hypertension/diabetes/breathlessness on exertion/palpitation/tuberculosis/asthma/renal disease/convulsion/jaundice/malaria/RTI/STI/HIV/AIDS/no any/if any other specify ....

Family History

Family history of systemic illness: Hypertension/Diabetes/Tuberculosis/No any ....

Blood disorder: Thalassemia/Repeated blood transfusion

Delivery of: Twins/Congenital abnormalities

Examinations of Client

General Examinations

Height : ....cm Temperature : ......F Respiration : ....breath/mint

Weight : ....kg Pulse : ....beats/mint BP : ....mm Hg

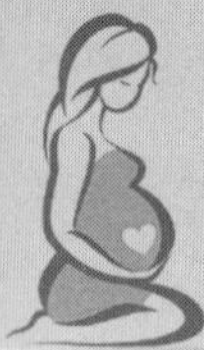

Physical Examinations

General appearance : Sick/active/anemic/pallor
Body built : Moderate/thin/obsess
Head : Dandruff/pediculosis/flakes/dryness/itching/normal
Eye : Pupil—normal/dilated/constricted, Conjunctiva—pink/white
Ear : Normal/wax impaction/abnormal auricle development
Nose : Normal/nasal septum deviation/polyps/rhinitis
Lips : Normal/cheilosis/dry/pale lips
Tongue : White and smooth/pallor
Nail : Pink/pallor
Breast examination : Breast—normal/lump/tenderness
Nipple : Normal/inverted or flat nipples/crust or sore nipple
Micturition : Scanty/retention/incontinence/painful/frequent/normal
Digestion : Heart burn/constipation/diarrhea/hemorrhoids/normal

Abdominal Examinations

Inspection

Abdomen : Size :.. Shape :...
Counter : Fundal notching/convex/flattened anterior wall/cylindrical/spherical ....
Umbilicus : Striae gravidarum: ....
Linea nigra : ....

Palpation

Abdominal girth : ....cm
Fundal height of uterus : ....cm ....weeks
Fetal lie and presentation :

- Fundal palpation/grip
  Presentation—hard and globular (head)/soft and irregular (breech)
- Lateral palpation/grip
  Left—continuous hard/irregular small knobs
  Right—continuous hard/irregular small knobs
- Superficial pelvic grip
  Head (hard and globular)/breech (soft and irregular)/empty
- Deep pelvic grip (only in 3rd trimester)
  Head engagement—head engaged/not engaged

Auscultation

Fetal heart rate (FHR) :.. Beats/Mint : ....

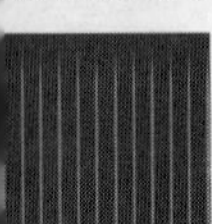

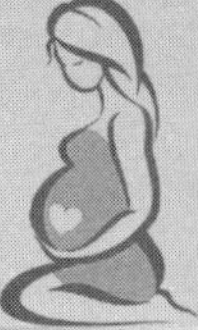

Laboratory Investigations

Date: .... Blood: Hb .... Group .... Sugar .... Urine: Albumin ....
HIV: .... HbsAg :..................... Malaria: VDRL .... Any other specify ....

Treatment

Drugs: .... Dose/Route: ....

Health Education

....

....

....

....

Remark

....

....

....

....

....

....

Signature of Sister in Charge **Signature of Supervisor**

Antenatal Assessment (Case No. 24)

Client's Profile

Name : .... Education : ....

Age : .... Occupation : ....

Hospital name : .... Income per month : ....

Date of booking : .... Marriage duration : ....

Reg. No. : .... W/o : ....

Religion : .... LMP : ....

Parity : .... EDD : ....

Address : ....

Period of gestation : ....

Menstrual History

Age at menarche :.............................. year of age Blood flow : average/scanty/heavy ....

Cycle of :.............................. days Dysmenorrhea : ....

Period duration of :.............................. days

History of Present Pregnancy

No. of antenatal visits : .... Immunization Status : ....

Tick mark (√), if present

Nausea/Vomiting/Back ache/Constipation/Frequency of Micturition/Leaking of watery fluid through vagina/Vaginal bleeding/Severe headache/Blurred vision/Difficulty in breathing/Palpitation/Decrease or absent fetal movement/Acidity/generalized swelling of body or face/Fever

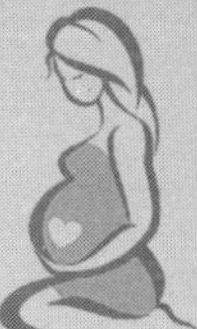

Obstetric History

S. No	Year	Term/ preterm	Abortion/ stillbirth	Nature of delivery	Child		Immunization	Growth and development	Nature of puerperium	Remark
					Alive	Sex/ weight				

Personal History

Allergies to drug : .... Body built : ....

Habit : Smoking/alcohol/betel chewing/any drug addiction : ....

Dietary habits : Vegetarian/nonvegetarian : ....

Hobbies : .... Diet per day - 2/3/4/5/6 : ....

Present and Past Medical History

Hypertension/diabetes/breathlessness on exertion/palpitation/tuberculosis/asthma/renal disease/convulsion/jaundice/malaria/RTI/STI/HIV/AIDS/no any/if any other specify ....

Family History

Family history of systemic illness: Hypertension/Diabetes/Tuberculosis/No any ....

Blood disorder: Thalassemia/Repeated blood transfusion

Delivery of: Twins/Congenital abnormalities

Examinations of Client

General Examinations

Height : ....cm Temperature : ......F Respiration : ....breath/mint

Weight : ....kg Pulse : ....beats/mint BP : ....mm Hg

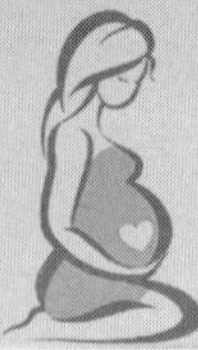

Physical Examinations

General appearance : Sick/active/anemic/pallor
Body built : Moderate/thin/obsess
Head : Dandruff/pediculosis/flakes/dryness/itching/normal
Eye : Pupil—normal/dilated/constricted, Conjunctiva—pink/white
Ear : Normal/wax impaction/abnormal auricle development
Nose : Normal/nasal septum deviation/polyps/rhinitis
Lips : Normal/cheilosis/dry/pale lips
Tongue : White and smooth/pallor
Nail : Pink/pallor
Breast examination : Breast—normal/lump/tenderness
Nipple : Normal/inverted or flat nipples/crust or sore nipple
Micturition : Scanty/retention/incontinence/painful/frequent/normal
Digestion : Heart burn/constipation/diarrhea/hemorrhoids/normal

Abdominal Examinations

Inspection

Abdomen : Size : .... Shape : ....
Counter : Fundal notching/convex/flattened anterior wall/cylindrical/spherical ....
Umbilicus : Striae gravidarum: ....
Linea nigra : ....

Palpation

Abdominal girth : ....cm
Fundal height of uterus : ....cm ....weeks
Fetal lie and presentation :

- Fundal palpation/grip
  Presentation—hard and globular (head)/soft and irregular (breech)
- Lateral palpation/grip
  Left—continuous hard/irregular small knobs
  Right—continuous hard/irregular small knobs
- Superficial pelvic grip
  Head (hard and globular)/breech (soft and irregular)/empty
- Deep pelvic grip (only in 3rd trimester)
  Head engagement—head engaged/not engaged

Auscultation

Fetal heart rate (FHR) :.. Beats/Mint : ....

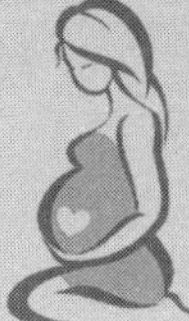

Laboratory Investigations

Date: .... Blood: Hb .... Group .... Sugar .... Urine: Albumin ....
HIV: .... HbsAg :.................... Malaria: VDRL .... Any other specify ....

Treatment

Drugs: .... Dose/Route: ....

Health Education

....

....

....

....

Remark

....

....

....

....

....

....

Signature of Sister in Charge **Signature of Supervisor**

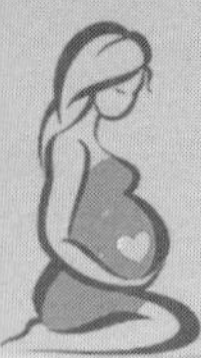

Antenatal Assessment (Case No. 25)

Client's Profile

Name	:	Education	: ....
Age	:	Occupation	: ....
Hospital name	:	Income per month	: ....
Date of booking	:	Marriage duration	: ....
Reg. No.	:	W/o	: ....
Religion	:	LMP	: ....
Parity	:	EDD	:..

Address : ....

Period of gestation : ....

Menstrual History

Age at menarche	:............................	year of age	Blood flow :	average/scanty/heavy ....
Cycle of	:............................	days	Dysmenorrhea :	....
Period duration of	:............................	days		

History of Present Pregnancy

No. of antenatal visits : .... Immunization Status : ....

Tick mark (√), if present

Nausea/Vomiting/Back ache/Constipation/Frequency of Micturition/Leaking of watery fluid through vagina/Vaginal bleeding/Severe headache/Blurred vision/Difficulty in breathing/Palpitation/Decrease or absent fetal movement/Acidity/generalized swelling of body or face/Fever

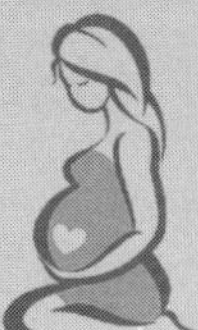

Obstetric History

S. No	Year	Term/ preterm	Abortion/ stillbirth	Nature of delivery	Child		Immunization	Growth and development	Nature of puerperium	Remark
					Alive	Sex/ weight				

Personal History

Allergies to drug : .... Body built : ....
Habit : Smoking/alcohol/betel chewing/any drug addiction : ....
Dietary habits : Vegetarian/nonvegetarian : ....
Hobbies : .... Diet per day - 2/3/4/5/6 : ....

Present and Past Medical History

Hypertension/diabetes/breathlessness on exertion/palpitation/tuberculosis/asthma/renal disease/convulsion/jaundice/malaria/RTI/STI/HIV/AIDS/no any/if any other specify ....

Family History

Family history of systemic illness: Hypertension/Diabetes/Tuberculosis/No any ....
Blood disorder: Thalassemia/Repeated blood transfusion
Delivery of: Twins/Congenital abnormalities

Examinations of Client

General Examinations

Height : ....cm Temperature : ......F Respiration : ....breath/mint
Weight : ....kg Pulse : ....beats/mint BP : ....mm Hg

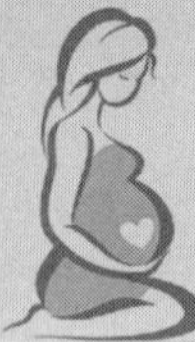

Physical Examinations

General appearance : Sick/active/anemic/pallor
Body built : Moderate/thin/obsess
Head : Dandruff/pediculosis/flakes/dryness/itching/normal
Eye : Pupil—normal/dilated/constricted, Conjunctiva—pink/white
Ear : Normal/wax impaction/abnormal auricle development
Nose : Normal/nasal septum deviation/polyps/rhinitis
Lips : Normal/cheilosis/dry/pale lips
Tongue : White and smooth/pallor
Nail : Pink/pallor
Breast examination : Breast—normal/lump/tenderness
Nipple : Normal/inverted or flat nipples/crust or sore nipple
Micturition : Scanty/retention/incontinence/painful/frequent/normal
Digestion : Heart burn/constipation/diarrhea/hemorrhoids/normal

Abdominal Examinations

Inspection

Abdomen : Size : .... Shape : ....
Counter : Fundal notching/convex/flattened anterior wall/cylindrical/spherical ....
Umbilicus : Striae gravidarum: ....
Linea nigra : ....

Palpation

Abdominal girth : ....cm
Fundal height of uterus : ....cm ....weeks
Fetal lie and presentation :

- Fundal palpation/grip
  Presentation—hard and globular (head)/soft and irregular (breech)
- Lateral palpation/grip
  Left—continuous hard/irregular small knobs
  Right—continuous hard/irregular small knobs
- Superficial pelvic grip
  Head (hard and globular)/breech (soft and irregular)/empty
- Deep pelvic grip (only in 3rd trimester)
  Head engagement—head engaged/not engaged

Auscultation

Fetal heart rate (FHR) :... Beats/Mint : ....

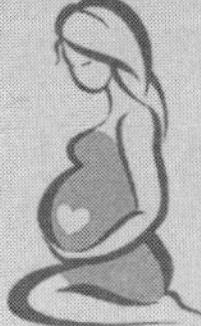

Laboratory Investigations

Date: .... Blood: Hb .... Group .... Sugar .... Urine: Albumin ....
HIV: .... HbsAg :..................... Malaria: VDRL .... Any other specify ....

Treatment

Drugs: .... Dose/Route: ....

Health Education

....

....

....

....

Remark

....

....

....

....

....

....

Signature of Sister in Charge **Signature of Supervisor**

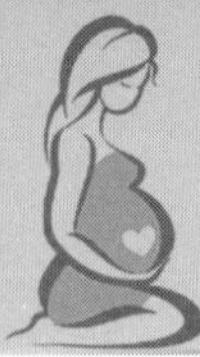

Antenatal Assessment (Case No. 26)

Client's Profile

Name	:	Education	: ....
Age	:	Occupation	: ....
Hospital name	:	Income per month	: ....
Date of booking	:	Marriage duration	: ....
Reg. No.	:	W/o	: ....
Religion	:	LMP	: ....
Parity	:	EDD	: ....

Address : ....

Period of gestation : ....

Menstrual History

Age at menarche	:..............................	year of age	Blood flow :	average/scanty/heavy ....
Cycle of	:..............................	days	Dysmenorrhea :	....
Period duration of	:..............................	days		

History of Present Pregnancy

No. of antenatal visits : .... Immunization Status : ....

Tick mark (√), if present

Nausea/Vomiting/Back ache/Constipation/Frequency of Micturition/Leaking of watery fluid through vagina/Vaginal bleeding/Severe headache/Blurred vision/Difficulty in breathing/Palpitation/Decrease or absent fetal movement/ Acidity/generalized swelling of body or face/Fever

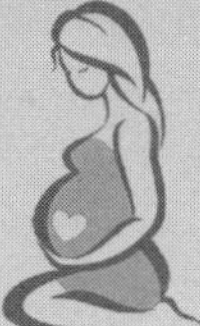

Obstetric History

S. No	Year	Term/ preterm	Abortion/ stillbirth	Nature of delivery	Child		Immunization	Growth and development	Nature of puerperium	Remark
					Alive	Sex/ weight				

Personal History

Allergies to drug : .... Body built : ....
Habit : Smoking/alcohol/betel chewing/any drug addiction : ....
Dietary habits : Vegetarian/nonvegetarian : ....
Hobbies : .... Diet per day - 2/3/4/5/6 : ....

Present and Past Medical History

Hypertension/diabetes/breathlessness on exertion/palpitation/tuberculosis/asthma/renal disease/convulsion/jaundice/malaria/RTI/STI/HIV/AIDS/no any/if any other specify ....

Family History

Family history of systemic illness: Hypertension/Diabetes/Tuberculosis/No any ....
Blood disorder: Thalassemia/Repeated blood transfusion
Delivery of: Twins/Congenital abnormalities

Examinations of Client

General Examinations

Height : ....cm Temperature : ......F Respiration : ....breath/mint
Weight : ....kg Pulse : ....beats/mint BP : ....mm Hg

Physical Examinations

General appearance : Sick/active/anemic/pallor
Body built : Moderate/thin/obsess
Head : Dandruff/pediculosis/flakes/dryness/itching/normal
Eye : Pupil—normal/dilated/constricted, Conjunctiva—pink/white
Ear : Normal/wax impaction/abnormal auricle development
Nose : Normal/nasal septum deviation/polyps/rhinitis
Lips : Normal/cheilosis/dry/pale lips
Tongue : White and smooth/pallor
Nail : Pink/pallor
Breast examination : Breast—normal/lump/tenderness
Nipple : Normal/inverted or flat nipples/crust or sore nipple
Micturition : Scanty/retention/incontinence/painful/frequent/normal
Digestion : Heart burn/constipation/diarrhea/hemorrhoids/normal

Abdominal Examinations

Inspection

Abdomen : Size : .... Shape : ....
Counter : Fundal notching/convex/flattened anterior wall/cylindrical/spherical ....
Umbilicus : Striae gravidarum: ....
Linea nigra : ....

Palpation

Abdominal girth : ....cm
Fundal height of uterus : ....cm ....weeks
Fetal lie and presentation :

- Fundal palpation/grip
  Presentation—hard and globular (head)/soft and irregular (breech)
- Lateral palpation/grip
  Left—continuous hard/irregular small knobs
  Right—continuous hard/irregular small knobs
- Superficial pelvic grip
  Head (hard and globular)/breech (soft and irregular)/empty
- Deep pelvic grip (only in 3rd trimester)
  Head engagement—head engaged/not engaged

Auscultation

Fetal heart rate (FHR) :.. Beats/Mint : ....

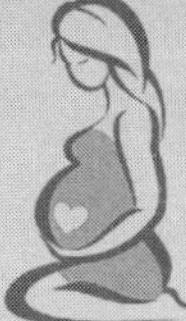

Laboratory Investigations

Date: .... Blood: Hb .... Group .... Sugar .... Urine: Albumin ....
HIV: .... HbsAg :..................... Malaria: VDRL .... Any other specify ....

Treatment

Drugs: .... Dose/Route: ....

Health Education

....

....

....

....

Remark

....

....

....

....

....

....

Signature of Sister in Charge

____

Signature of Supervisor

____

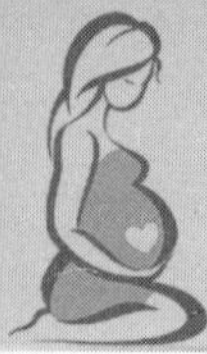

Antenatal Assessment (Case No. 27)

Client's Profile

Name : .... Education : ....

Age : .... Occupation : ....

Hospital name : .... Income per month : ....

Date of booking : .... Marriage duration : ....

Reg. No. : .... W/o : ....

Religion : .... LMP : ....

Parity : .... EDD : ....

Address : ....

Period of gestation : ....

Menstrual History

Age at menarche : .... year of age Blood flow : average/scanty/heavy ....

Cycle of : .... days Dysmenorrhea : ....

Period duration of : .... days

History of Present Pregnancy

No. of antenatal visits : .... Immunization Status : ....

Tick mark (√), if present

Nausea/Vomiting/Back ache/Constipation/Frequency of Micturition/Leaking of watery fluid through vagina/Vaginal bleeding/Severe headache/Blurred vision/Difficulty in breathing/Palpitation/Decrease or absent fetal movement/Acidity/generalized swelling of body or face/Fever

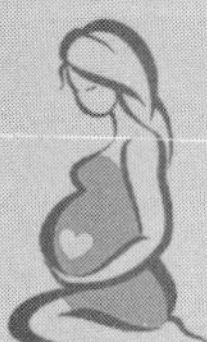

Obstetric History

S. No	Year	Term/ preterm	Abortion/ stillbirth	Nature of delivery	Child		Immunization	Growth and development	Nature of puerperium	Remark
					Alive	Sex/ weight				

Personal History

Allergies to drug : .... Body built : ....

Habit : Smoking/alcohol/betel chewing/any drug addiction : ....

Dietary habits : Vegetarian/nonvegetarian : ....

Hobbies : .... Diet per day - 2/3/4/5/6 : ....

Present and Past Medical History

Hypertension/diabetes/breathlessness on exertion/palpitation/tuberculosis/asthma/renal disease/convulsion/jaundice/malaria/RTI/STI/HIV/AIDS/no any/if any other specify ....

Family History

Family history of systemic illness: Hypertension/Diabetes/Tuberculosis/No any ....
Blood disorder: Thalassemia/Repeated blood transfusion
Delivery of: Twins/Congenital abnormalities

Examinations of Client

General Examinations

Height : ....cm Temperature : ......F Respiration : ....breath/mint

Weight : ....kg Pulse : ....beats/mint BP : ....mm Hg

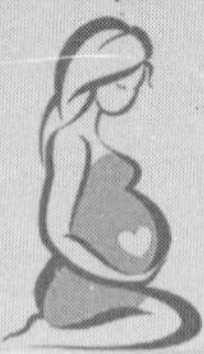

Physical Examinations

General appearance	:	Sick/active/anemic/pallor
Body built	:	Moderate/thin/obsess
Head	:	Dandruff/pediculosis/flakes/dryness/itching/normal
Eye	:	Pupil—normal/dilated/constricted, Conjunctiva—pink/white
Ear	:	Normal/wax impaction/abnormal auricle development
Nose	:	Normal/nasal septum deviation/polyps/rhinitis
Lips	:	Normal/cheilosis/dry/pale lips
Tongue	:	White and smooth/pallor
Nail	:	Pink/pallor
Breast examination	:	Breast—normal/lump/tenderness
Nipple	:	Normal/inverted or flat nipples/crust or sore nipple
Micturition	:	Scanty/retention/incontinence/painful/frequent/normal
Digestion	:	Heart burn/constipation/diarrhea/hemorrhoids/normal

Abdominal Examinations

Inspection

Abdomen : Size : .... Shape : ....

Counter : Fundal notching/convex/flattened anterior wall/cylindrical/spherical ....

Umbilicus : Striae gravidarum: ....

Linea nigra : ....

Palpation

Abdominal girth : ....cm

Fundal height of uterus : ....cm ....weeks

Fetal lie and presentation :

- Fundal palpation/grip
  Presentation—hard and globular (head)/soft and irregular (breech)
- Lateral palpation/grip
  Left—continuous hard/irregular small knobs
  Right—continuous hard/irregular small knobs
- Superficial pelvic grip
  Head (hard and globular)/breech (soft and irregular)/empty
- Deep pelvic grip (only in 3rd trimester)
  Head engagement—head engaged/not engaged

Auscultation

Fetal heart rate (FHR) :.. Beats/Mint : ....

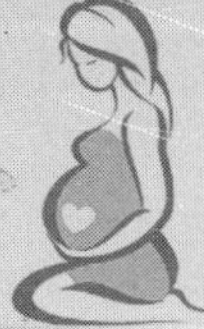

Laboratory Investigations

Date: .... Blood: Hb .... Group .... Sugar .... Urine: Albumin ....
HIV: .... HbsAg :..................... Malaria: VDRL .... Any other specify ....

Treatment

Drugs: .... Dose/Route: ....

Health Education

....

....

....

....

Remark

....

....

....

....

....

....

Signature of Sister in Charge **Signature of Supervisor**

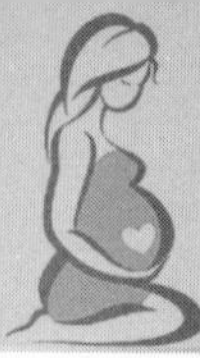

Antenatal Assessment (Case No. 28)

Client's Profile

Name : .... Education : ....

Age : .... Occupation : ....

Hospital name : .... Income per month : ....

Date of booking : .... Marriage duration : ....

Reg. No. : .... W/o : ....

Religion : .... LMP : ....

Parity : .... EDD : ....

Address : ....

Period of gestation : ....

Menstrual History

Age at menarche : .... year of age Blood flow : average/scanty/heavy ....

Cycle of : .... days Dysmenorrhea : ....

Period duration of : .... days

History of Present Pregnancy

No. of antenatal visits : .... Immunization Status : ....

Tick mark (√), if present

Nausea/Vomiting/Back ache/Constipation/Frequency of Micturition/Leaking of watery fluid through vagina/Vaginal bleeding/Severe headache/Blurred vision/Difficulty in breathing/Palpitation/Decrease or absent fetal movement/Acidity/generalized swelling of body or face/Fever

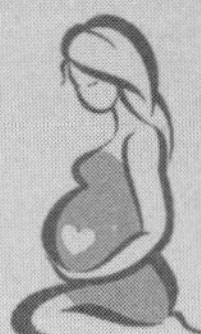

Obstetric History

S. No	Year	Term/ preterm	Abortion/ stillbirth	Nature of delivery	Child		Immunization	Growth and development	Nature of puerperium	Remark
					Alive	Sex/ weight				

Personal History

Allergies to drug : .... Body built : ....
Habit : Smoking/alcohol/betel chewing/any drug addiction : ....
Dietary habits : Vegetarian/nonvegetarian : ....
Hobbies : .... Diet per day - 2/3/4/5/6 : ....

Present and Past Medical History

Hypertension/diabetes/breathlessness on exertion/palpitation/tuberculosis/asthma/renal disease/convulsion/jaundice/malaria/RTI/STI/HIV/AIDS/no any/if any other specify ....

Family History

Family history of systemic illness: Hypertension/Diabetes/Tuberculosis/No any ....
Blood disorder: Thalassemia/Repeated blood transfusion
Delivery of: Twins/Congenital abnormalities

Examinations of Client

General Examinations

Height : ....cm Temperature : ......F Respiration : ....breath/mint
Weight : ....kg Pulse : ....beats/mint BP : ....mm Hg

Physical Examinations

General appearance	:	Sick/active/anemic/pallor
Body built	:	Moderate/thin/obsess
Head	:	Dandruff/pediculosis/flakes/dryness/itching/normal
Eye	:	Pupil—normal/dilated/constricted, Conjunctiva—pink/white
Ear	:	Normal/wax impaction/abnormal auricle development
Nose	:	Normal/nasal septum deviation/polyps/rhinitis
Lips	:	Normal/cheilosis/dry/pale lips
Tongue	:	White and smooth/pallor
Nail	:	Pink/pallor
Breast examination	:	Breast—normal/lump/tenderness
Nipple	:	Normal/inverted or flat nipples/crust or sore nipple
Micturition	:	Scanty/retention/incontinence/painful/frequent/normal
Digestion	:	Heart burn/constipation/diarrhea/hemorrhoids/normal

Abdominal Examinations

Inspection

Abdomen : Size : .... Shape : ....

Counter : Fundal notching/convex/flattened anterior wall/cylindrical/spherical ....

Umbilicus : Striae gravidarum: ....

Linea nigra : ....

Palpation

Abdominal girth : ....cm

Fundal height of uterus : ....cm ....weeks

Fetal lie and presentation :

- Fundal palpation/grip
  Presentation—hard and globular (head)/soft and irregular (breech)
- Lateral palpation/grip
  Left—continuous hard/irregular small knobs
  Right—continuous hard/irregular small knobs
- Superficial pelvic grip
  Head (hard and globular)/breech (soft and irregular)/empty
- Deep pelvic grip (only in 3rd trimester)
  Head engagement—head engaged/not engaged

Auscultation

Fetal heart rate (FHR) :.. Beats/Mint : ....

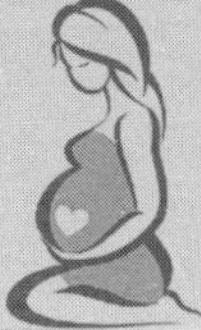

Laboratory Investigations

Date: .... Blood: Hb .... Group .... Sugar .... Urine: Albumin ....

HIV: .... HbsAg :..................... Malaria: VDRL .... Any other specify ....

Treatment

Drugs: .... Dose/Route: ....

Health Education

....

....

....

....

Remark

....

....

....

....

....

....

Signature of Sister in Charge

Signature of Supervisor

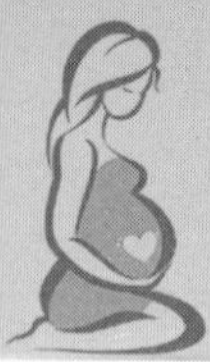

Antenatal Assessment (Case No. 29)

Client's Profile

Name	:	Education	: ....
Age	:	Occupation	: ....
Hospital name	:	Income per month	: ....
Date of booking	:	Marriage duration	: ....
Reg. No.	:	W/o	: ....
Religion	:	LMP	: ....
Parity	:	EDD	: ....

Address : ....

Period of gestation : ....

Menstrual History

Age at menarche	:...............................	year of age	Blood flow :	average/scanty/heavy ....
Cycle of	:...............................	days	Dysmenorrhea :	....
Period duration of	:...............................	days		

History of Present Pregnancy

No. of antenatal visits : .... Immunization Status : ....

Tick mark (√), if present

Nausea/Vomiting/Back ache/Constipation/Frequency of Micturition/Leaking of watery fluid through vagina/Vaginal bleeding/Severe headache/Blurred vision/Difficulty in breathing/Palpitation/Decrease or absent fetal movement/Acidity/generalized swelling of body or face/Fever

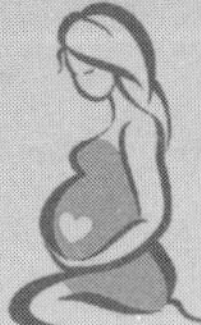

Obstetric History

S. No	Year	Term/ preterm	Abortion/ stillbirth	Nature of delivery	Child		Immunization	Growth and development	Nature of puerperium	Remark
					Alive	Sex/ weight				

Personal History

Allergies to drug : .... Body built : ....

Habit : Smoking/alcohol/betel chewing/any drug addiction : ....

Dietary habits : Vegetarian/nonvegetarian : ....

Hobbies : .... Diet per day - 2/3/4/5/6 : ....

Present and Past Medical History

Hypertension/diabetes/breathlessness on exertion/palpitation/tuberculosis/asthma/renal disease/convulsion/jaundice/malaria/RTI/STI/HIV/AIDS/no any/if any other specify ....

Family History

Family history of systemic illness: Hypertension/Diabetes/Tuberculosis/No any ....

Blood disorder: Thalassemia/Repeated blood transfusion

Delivery of: Twins/Congenital abnormalities

Examinations of Client

General Examinations

Height	:	........cm	Temperature	:	......F	Respiration	: ....breath/mint
Weight	:	........kg	Pulse	:	.......beats/mint	BP	: ....mm Hg

Physical Examinations

General appearance	:	Sick/active/anemic/pallor
Body built	:	Moderate/thin/obsess
Head	:	Dandruff/pediculosis/flakes/dryness/itching/normal
Eye	:	Pupil—normal/dilated/constricted, Conjunctiva—pink/white
Ear	:	Normal/wax impaction/abnormal auricle development
Nose	:	Normal/nasal septum deviation/polyps/rhinitis
Lips	:	Normal/cheilosis/dry/pale lips
Tongue	:	White and smooth/pallor
Nail	:	Pink/pallor
Breast examination	:	Breast—normal/lump/tenderness
Nipple	:	Normal/inverted or flat nipples/crust or sore nipple
Micturition	:	Scanty/retention/incontinence/painful/frequent/normal
Digestion	:	Heart burn/constipation/diarrhea/hemorrhoids/normal

Abdominal Examinations

Inspection

Abdomen : Size : .... Shape : ....

Counter : Fundal notching/convex/flattened anterior wall/cylindrical/spherical ....

Umbilicus : Striae gravidarum: ....

Linea nigra : ....

Palpation

Abdominal girth : ....cm

Fundal height of uterus : ....cm ....weeks

Fetal lie and presentation :

- Fundal palpation/grip
  Presentation—hard and globular (head)/soft and irregular (breech)
- Lateral palpation/grip
  Left—continuous hard/irregular small knobs
  Right—continuous hard/irregular small knobs
- Superficial pelvic grip
  Head (hard and globular)/breech (soft and irregular)/empty
- Deep pelvic grip (only in 3rd trimester)
  Head engagement—head engaged/not engaged

Auscultation

Fetal heart rate (FHR) :.. Beats/Mint : ....

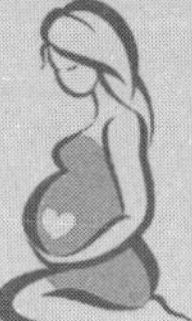

Laboratory Investigations

Date: .... Blood: Hb .... Group .... Sugar .... Urine: Albumin ....
HIV: .... HbsAg :..................... Malaria: VDRL .... Any other specify ....

Treatment

Drugs: .... Dose/Route: ....

Health Education

....

....

....

....

Remark

....

....

....

....

....

....

Signature of Sister in Charge **Signature of Supervisor**

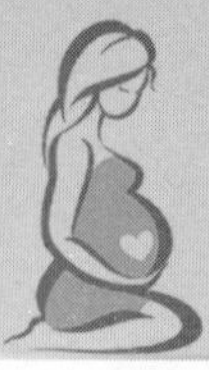

Antenatal Assessment (Case No. 30)

Client's Profile

Name	:	Education	: ....
Age	:	Occupation	: ....
Hospital name	:	Income per month	: ....
Date of booking	:	Marriage duration	: ....
Reg. No.	:	W/o	: ....
Religion	:	LMP	: ....
Parity	:	EDD	: ....

Address : ....

Period of gestation : ....

Menstrual History

Age at menarche	:............................	year of age	Blood flow :	average/scanty/heavy ....
Cycle of	:............................	days	Dysmenorrhea :	....
Period duration of	:............................	days		

History of Present Pregnancy

No. of antenatal visits : .... Immunization Status : ....

Tick mark (√), if present

Nausea/Vomiting/Back ache/Constipation/Frequency of Micturition/Leaking of watery fluid through vagina/Vaginal bleeding/Severe headache/Blurred vision/Difficulty in breathing/Palpitation/Decrease or absent fetal movement/ Acidity/generalized swelling of body or face/Fever

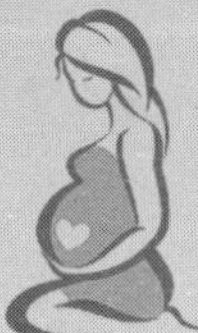

Obstetric History

S. No	Year	Term/ preterm	Abortion/ stillbirth	Nature of delivery	Child		Immunization	Growth and development	Nature of puerperium	Remark
					Alive	Sex/ weight				

Personal History

Allergies to drug : .... Body built : ....

Habit : Smoking/alcohol/betel chewing/any drug addiction : ....

Dietary habits : Vegetarian/nonvegetarian : ....

Hobbies : .... Diet per day - 2/3/4/5/6 : ....

Present and Past Medical History

Hypertension/diabetes/breathlessness on exertion/palpitation/tuberculosis/asthma/renal disease/convulsion/jaundice/malaria/RTI/STI/HIV/AIDS/no any/if any other specify ....

Family History

Family history of systemic illness: Hypertension/Diabetes/Tuberculosis/No any ....

Blood disorder: Thalassemia/Repeated blood transfusion

Delivery of: Twins/Congenital abnormalities

Examinations of Client

General Examinations

Height : ....cm Temperature : ......F Respiration : ....breath/mint

Weight : ....kg Pulse : ....beats/mint BP : ....mm Hg

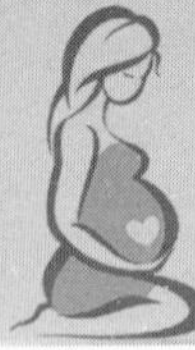

Physical Examinations

General appearance : Sick/active/anemic/pallor
Body built : Moderate/thin/obsess
Head : Dandruff/pediculosis/flakes/dryness/itching/normal
Eye : Pupil—normal/dilated/constricted, Conjunctiva—pink/white
Ear : Normal/wax impaction/abnormal auricle development
Nose : Normal/nasal septum deviation/polyps/rhinitis
Lips : Normal/cheilosis/dry/pale lips
Tongue : White and smooth/pallor
Nail : Pink/pallor
Breast examination : Breast—normal/lump/tenderness
Nipple : Normal/inverted or flat nipples/crust or sore nipple
Micturition : Scanty/retention/incontinence/painful/frequent/normal
Digestion : Heart burn/constipation/diarrhea/hemorrhoids/normal

Abdominal Examinations

Inspection

Abdomen : Size : .... Shape : ....
Counter : Fundal notching/convex/flattened anterior wall/cylindrical/spherical ....
Umbilicus : Striae gravidarum: ....
Linea nigra : ....

Palpation

Abdominal girth : ....cm
Fundal height of uterus : ....cm ....weeks
Fetal lie and presentation :

- Fundal palpation/grip
  Presentation—hard and globular (head)/soft and irregular (breech)
- Lateral palpation/grip
  Left—continuous hard/irregular small knobs
  Right—continuous hard/irregular small knobs
- Superficial pelvic grip
  Head (hard and globular)/breech (soft and irregular)/empty
- Deep pelvic grip (only in 3rd trimester)
  Head engagement—head engaged/not engaged

Auscultation

Fetal heart rate (FHR) :.. Beats/Mint : ....

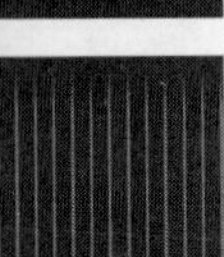

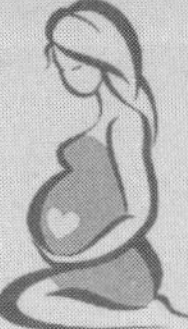

Laboratory Investigations

Date: .... Blood: Hb .... Group .... Sugar .... Urine: Albumin ....
HIV: .... HbsAg :.................... Malaria: VDRL .... Any other specify ....

Treatment

Drugs: .... Dose/Route: ....

Health Education

....

....

....

....

Remark

....

....

....

....

....

....

Signature of Sister in Charge **Signature of Supervisor**

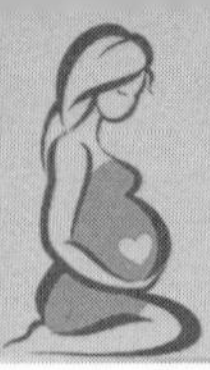

Conducted Normal Delivery (Case No. 1)

Client's Profile

Name : .... Religion : .... W/o : ....

Age : .... Education : .... Parity : ....

Hospital name : .... Occupation : .... LMP : ....

Date of booking : .... Income per month : .... EDD................................

Reg. No : .... Marriage duration : .... Period of gestation ....

Address : ....

....

Date and time of admission : ....

Date and time of discharge or transfer : ....

Admission Note

General Examinations

i. Temperature: ....

iii. Respiration: ....

ii. Pulse: ....

iv. BP: ....

Hydration: ....

Anemia: (Present/absent) ....

Labor pain: (Present/absent)..................................

Edema: (Generalized/ankle edema) ....

Abdominal Examination/Obstetrical Examination by Palpation

Height of uterus: .... cm Lie: .... Superficial grip: ....

Gestational weeks: .... Presentation: .... Deep pelvic grip: ....

Abdominal girth: ....cm Position of fetus: .... FHR: ....

Scar:... Lateral grip: ....

Time/date of onset of contraction : ....

Uterine contraction: Present/absent/well contracted : ....

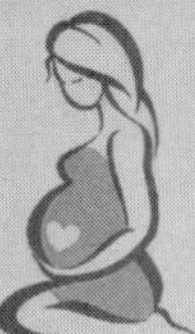

Investigation

Date	Hemoglobin	Blood Group/ Sugar	Urine		Bowel	Bladder	Any Other
			Albumin	Sugar			

Vaginal Examination

S.No	Date and time	Finding	Remark

Previous Obstetrical History

S.No	Year	Term/ preterm	Abortion/ stillbirth	Nature of delivery	Child		Immunization	Growth and development	Nature of puerperium	Remark
					Alive	Sex/ weight				

Admission History

Pregnancy complaints	
Menstrual history	
Medical history	
Surgical history	

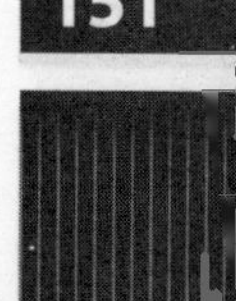

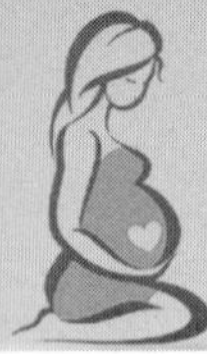

Old Pattern Partograph

Parity: *Reg No:* *Date and Time of Admission:* *Date and Time of ROM:*

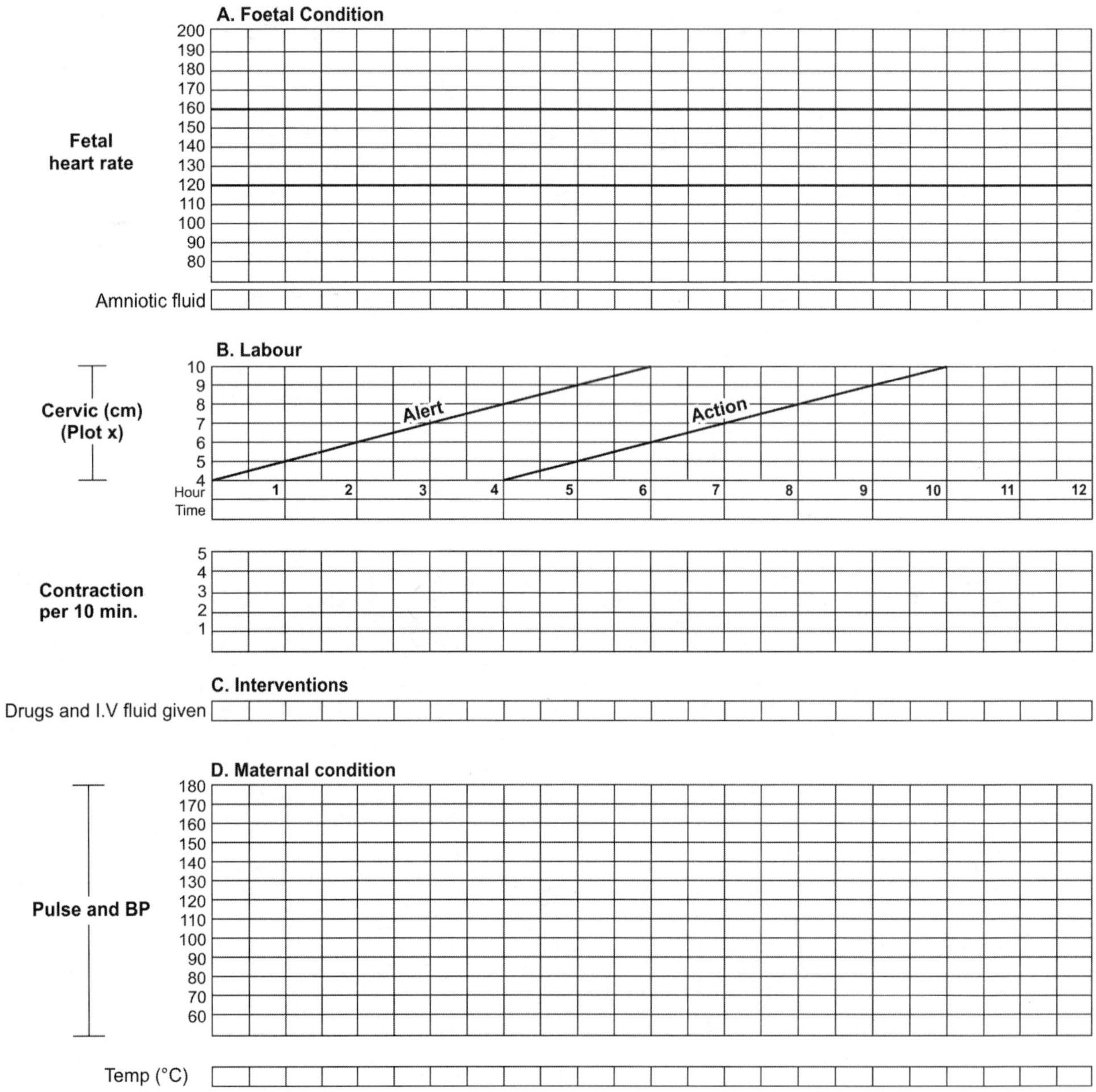

A. Foetal Condition

Fetal heart rate: 200, 190, 180, 170, 160, 150, 140, 130, 120, 110, 100, 90, 80

Amniotic fluid

B. Labour

Cervic (cm) (Plot x): 10, 9, 8, 7, 6, 5, 4

Alert

Action

Hour	1	2	3	4	5	6	7	8	9	10	11	12
Time												

Contraction per 10 min.: 5, 4, 3, 2, 1

C. Interventions

Drugs and I.V fluid given

D. Maternal condition

Pulse and BP: 180, 170, 160, 150, 140, 130, 120, 110, 100, 90, 80, 70, 60

Temp (°C)

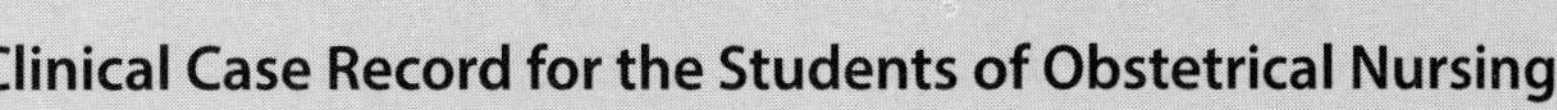

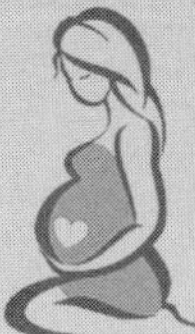

WHO Modified Partograph

Parity: *Reg No:* *Date and Time of Admission:* *Date and Time of ROM:*

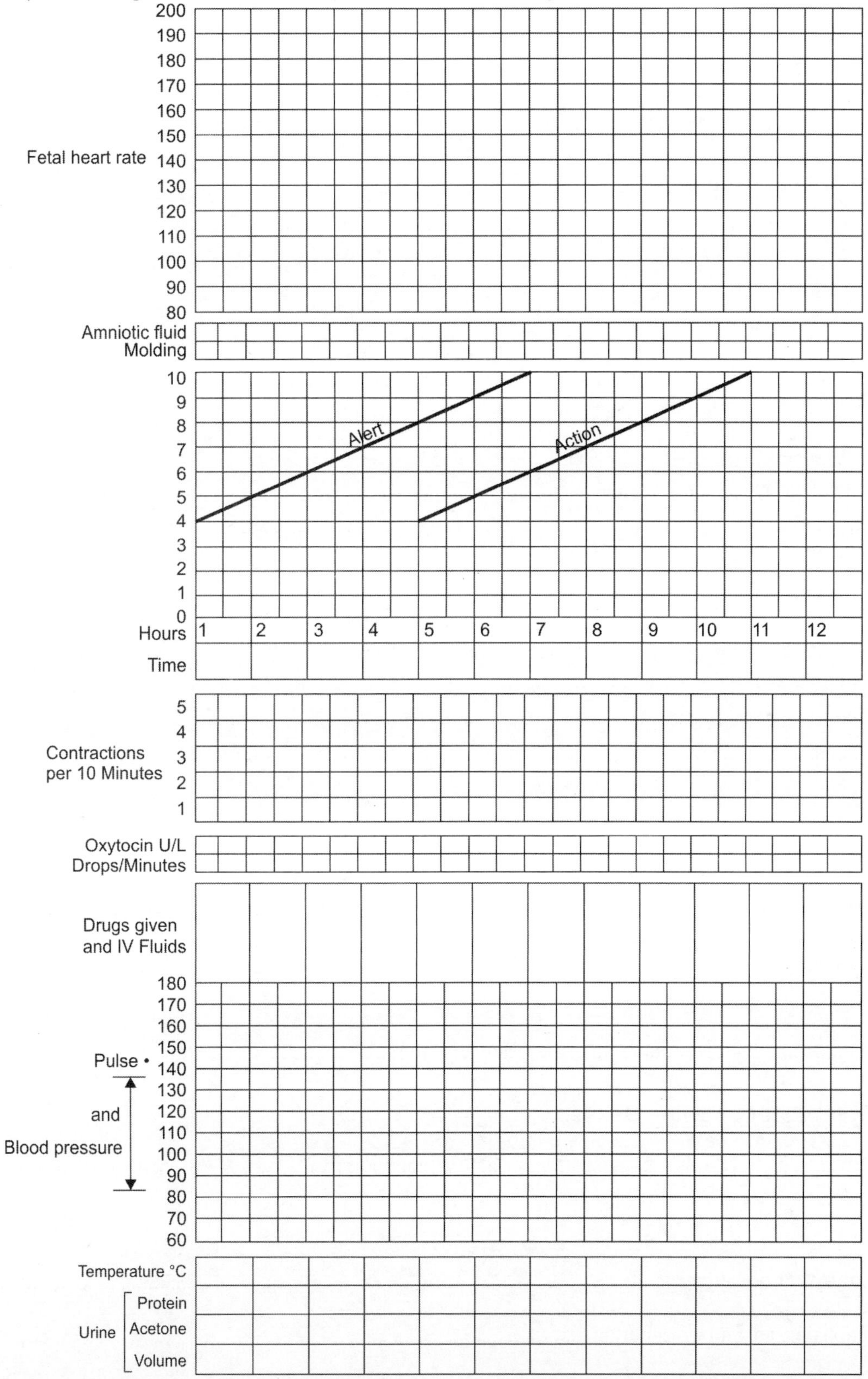

Fetal heart rate: 200, 190, 180, 170, 160, 150, 140, 130, 120, 110, 100, 90, 80

Amniotic fluid

Molding

Cervical dilatation: 10, 9, 8, 7, 6, 5, 4, 3, 2, 1, 0 (Alert, Action)

Hours: 1, 2, 3, 4, 5, 6, 7, 8, 9, 10, 11, 12

Time

Contractions per 10 Minutes: 5, 4, 3, 2, 1

Oxytocin U/L

Drops/Minutes

Drugs given and IV Fluids

Pulse • and Blood pressure: 180, 170, 160, 150, 140, 130, 120, 110, 100, 90, 80, 70, 60

Temperature °C

Urine: Protein, Acetone, Volume

Delivery Note

Labor Progress Note Date and Time of Onset of Pain

Onset of true labor: On .... At: ....
Date and time of full cervix dilatation: .... Effacement: ....
Membrane ruptured (spontaneous/artificial/PROM) on .... At ....
Total duration of: 1st stage .... Hrs .... Min ....
2nd stage .... Hrs .... Min ....
3rd stage .... Hrs .... Min ....
Total hours = ... Hrs .... Min ....

Baby at Birth

Mode of delivery: .... Score at one minute ....
Baby born on:.................... At: .... Sex: ....
Apgar scoring: .... Score at five minute.................... Anus patent: ....
Initiation of breastfeeding: ....
Drug administration: ....

Delivery of Placenta and Membrane

Delivery of placenta on:.................... At:.................... Cord insertion: ....
Spontaneous/helped/manually removed .... Examination of placenta: Complete/Incomplete ....
Weight of placenta:..
Cord length: .... Examination of membrane: ....

Blood Loss

Before delivery of placenta : ....
During delivery of placenta : ....
After delivery of placenta : ....

Perineum

Intact : .... Episiotomy :.............. Laceration :.................... Repair : ....

Condition of Mother Following Delivery

Pulse: .... BP: .... Uterus: .... Vaginal bleeding: .... Breastfeeding initiated at: ....

Condition of Mother on Transfer

Healthy/unhealthy (if unhealthy specify): ....

Condition of baby on transfer or discharge: ....

Nursing Care Plan

S.No.	Assessment	Nursing Diagnosis	Goal/Expected Out Come	Nursing Intervention	Rational	Implementation	Evaluation

Signature of Sister in Charge

Signature of Supervisor

Conducted Normal Delivery (Case No. 2)

Client's Profile

Name : .... Religion : .... W/o : ....

Age : .... Education : .... Parity : ....

Hospital name : .... Occupation : .... LMP : ....

Date of booking : .... Income per month : .... EDD.................................

Reg. No : .... Marriage duration : .... Period of gestation ....

Address : ....

....

Date and time of admission : ....

Date and time of discharge or transfer : ....

Admission Note

General Examinations

i. Temperature: ....

ii. Pulse: ....

iii. Respiration: ....

iv. BP: ....

Hydration: ....

Anemia: (Present/absent) ....

Labor pain: (Present/absent)..................................

Edema: (Generalized/ankle edema) ....

Abdominal Examination/Obstetrical Examination by Palpation

Height of uterus: .... cm Lie: .... Superficial grip: ....

Gestational weeks: .... Presentation: .... Deep pelvic grip: ....

Abdominal girth: ....cm Position of fetus: .... FHR: ....

Scar: .... Lateral grip: ....

Time/date of onset of contraction : ....

Uterine contraction: Present/absent/well contracted : ....

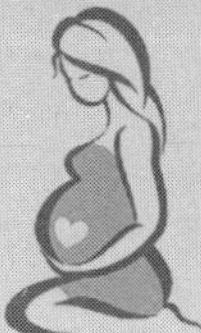

Investigation

Date	Hemoglobin	Blood Group/ Sugar	Urine		Bowel	Bladder	Any Other
			Albumin	Sugar			

Vaginal Examination

S.No	Date and time	Finding	Remark

Previous Obstetrical History

S.No	Year	Term/ preterm	Abortion/ stillbirth	Nature of delivery	Child		Immunization	Growth and development	Nature of puerperium	Remark
					Alive	Sex/ weight				

Admission History

Pregnancy complaints	
Menstrual history	
Medical history	
Surgical history	

Old Pattern Partograph

Parity: *Reg No:* *Date and Time of Admission:* *Date and Time of ROM:*

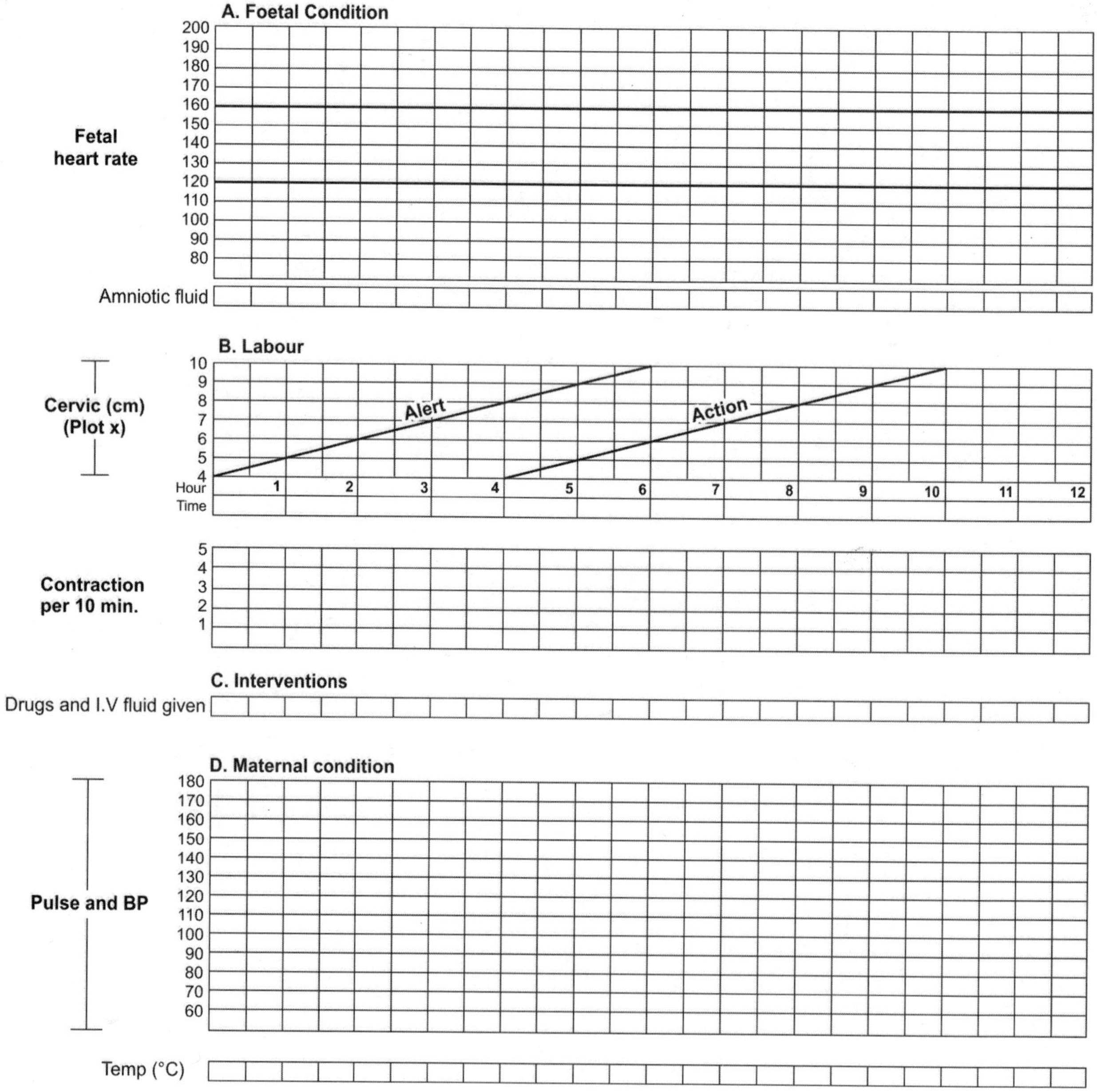

A. Foetal Condition

Fetal heart rate

200
190
180
170
160
150
140
130
120
110
100
90
80

Amniotic fluid

B. Labour

Cervic (cm) (Plot x)

10
9
8
7
6
5
4

Alert

Action

Hour	1	2	3	4	5	6	7	8	9	10	11	12
Time												

Contraction per 10 min.

5
4
3
2
1

C. Interventions

Drugs and I.V fluid given

D. Maternal condition

Pulse and BP

180
170
160
150
140
130
120
110
100
90
80
70
60

Temp (°C)

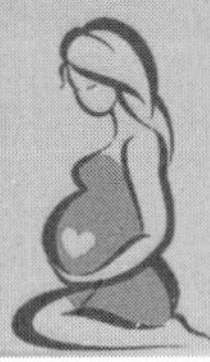

WHO Modified Partograph

Parity: *Reg No:* *Date and Time of Admission:* *Date and Time of ROM:*

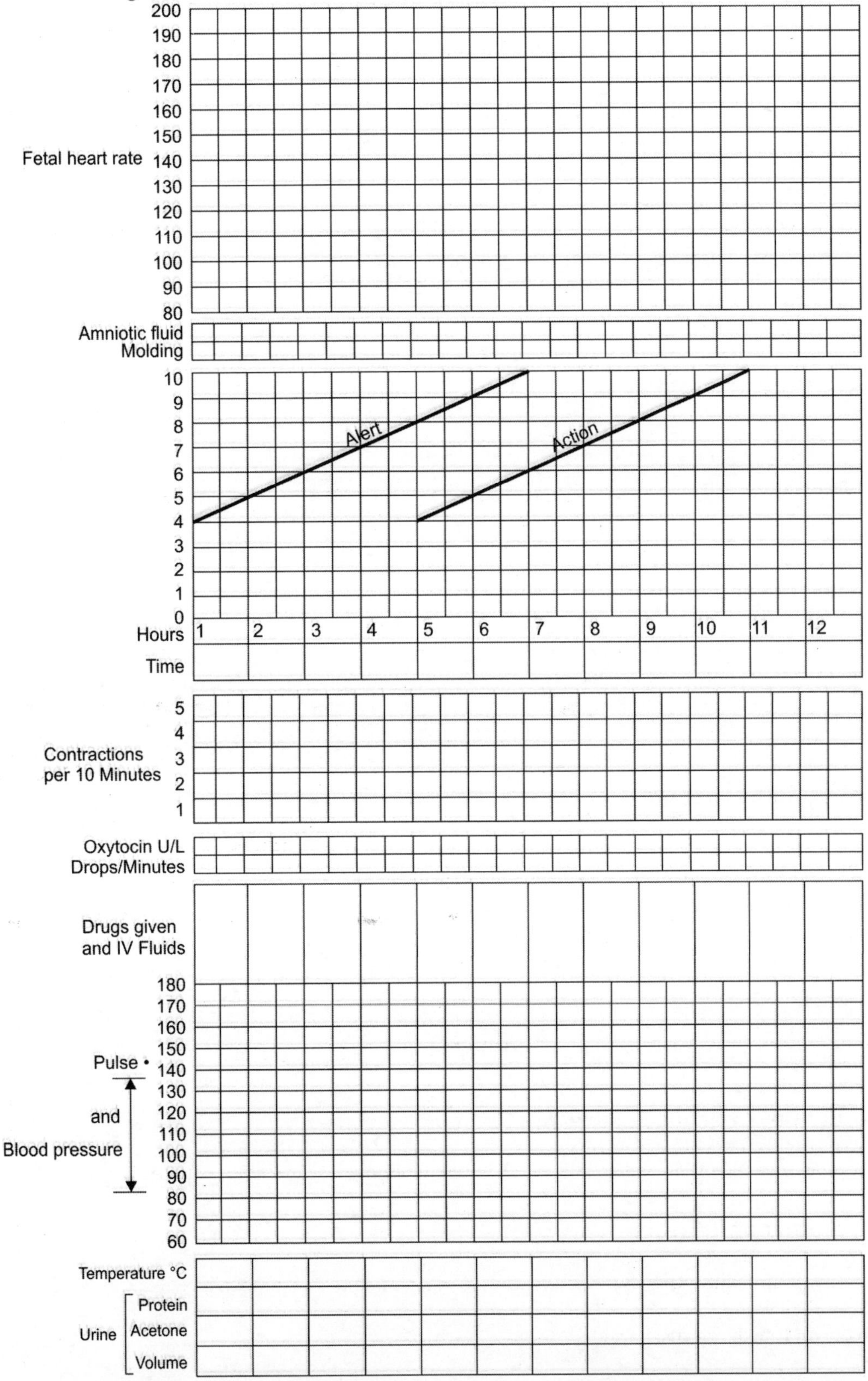

Fetal heart rate: 200, 190, 180, 170, 160, 150, 140, 130, 120, 110, 100, 90, 80

Amniotic fluid

Molding

10, 9, 8, 7, 6, 5, 4, 3, 2, 1, 0

Alert

Action

Hours: 1, 2, 3, 4, 5, 6, 7, 8, 9, 10, 11, 12

Time

Contractions per 10 Minutes: 5, 4, 3, 2, 1

Oxytocin U/L

Drops/Minutes

Drugs given and IV Fluids

Pulse • and Blood pressure: 180, 170, 160, 150, 140, 130, 120, 110, 100, 90, 80, 70, 60

Temperature °C

Urine: Protein, Acetone, Volume

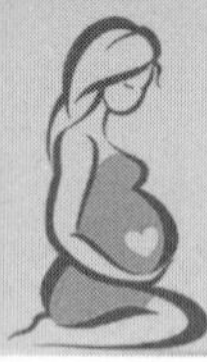

Delivery Note

Labor Progress Note Date and Time of Onset of Pain

Onset of true labor: On .... At: ....
Date and time of full cervix dilatation: .... Effacement: ....
Membrane ruptured (spontaneous/artificial/PROM) on .... At ....

Total duration of:
1st stage .... Hrs .... Min ....
2nd stage .... Hrs .... Min ....
3rd stage .... Hrs .... Min ....
Total hours = ... Hrs .... Min ....

Baby at Birth

Mode of delivery: .... Score at one minute ....
Baby born on:.................................... At: .... Sex: ....
Apgar scoring: .... Score at five minute.................................... Anus patent: ....
Initiation of breastfeeding: ....
Drug administration: ....

Delivery of Placenta and Membrane

Delivery of placenta on:.......................... At:.......................... Cord insertion: ....
Spontaneous/helped/manually removed .... Examination of placenta: Complete/Incomplete ....
Weight of placenta:..
Cord length: .... Examination of membrane: ....

Blood Loss

Before delivery of placenta : ....
During delivery of placenta : ....
After delivery of placenta : ....

Perineum

Intact : .... Episiotomy :............. Laceration :............................... Repair : ....

Condition of Mother Following Delivery

Pulse: .... BP: .... Uterus: .... Vaginal bleeding: .... Breastfeeding initiated at: ....

Condition of Mother on Transfer

Healthy/unhealthy (if unhealthy specify): ....

Condition of baby on transfer or discharge: ....

Nursing Care Plan

S.No.	Assessment	Nursing Diagnosis	Goal/Expected Out Come	Nursing Intervention	Rational	Implementation	Evaluation

Signature of Sister in Charge

Signature of Supervisor

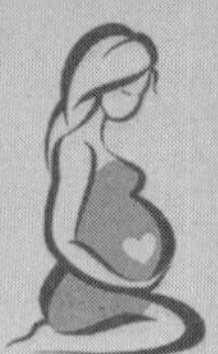

Conducted Normal Delivery (Case No. 3)

Client's Profile

Name : .... Religion : .... W/o : ....

Age : .... Education : .... Parity : ....

Hospital name : .... Occupation : .... LMP : ....

Date of booking : .... Income per month : .... EDD.................................

Reg. No : .... Marriage duration : .... Period of gestation ....

Address : ....

....

Date and time of admission : ....

Date and time of discharge or transfer : ....

Admission Note

General Examinations

i. Temperature: ....

ii. Pulse: ....

iii. Respiration: ....

iv. BP: ....

Hydration: ....

Labor pain: (Present/absent).................................

Anemia: (Present/absent) ....

Edema: (Generalized/ankle edema) ....

Abdominal Examination/Obstetrical Examination by Palpation

Height of uterus: .... cm Lie: .... Superficial grip: ....

Gestational weeks: .... Presentation: .... Deep pelvic grip: ....

Abdominal girth: ....cm Position of fetus: .... FHR: ....

Scar: .... Lateral grip: ....

Time/date of onset of contraction : ....

Uterine contraction: Present/absent/well contracted : ....

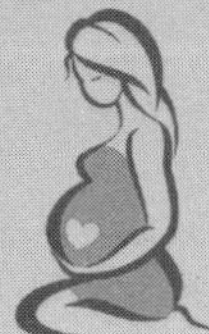

Investigation

Date	Hemoglobin	Blood Group/ Sugar	Urine		Bowel	Bladder	Any Other
			Albumin	Sugar			

Vaginal Examination

S.No	Date and time	Finding	Remark

Previous Obstetrical History

S.No	Year	Term/ preterm	Abortion/ stillbirth	Nature of delivery	Child		Immunization	Growth and development	Nature of puerperium	Remark
					Alive	Sex/ weight				

Admission History

Pregnancy complaints	
Menstrual history	
Medical history	
Surgical history	

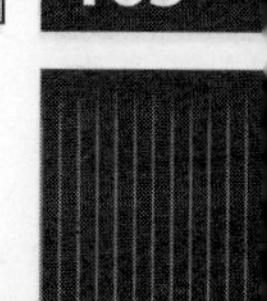

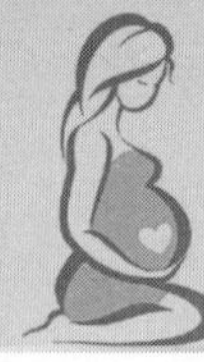

Old Pattern Partograph

Parity: *Reg No:* *Date and Time of Admission:* *Date and Time of ROM:*

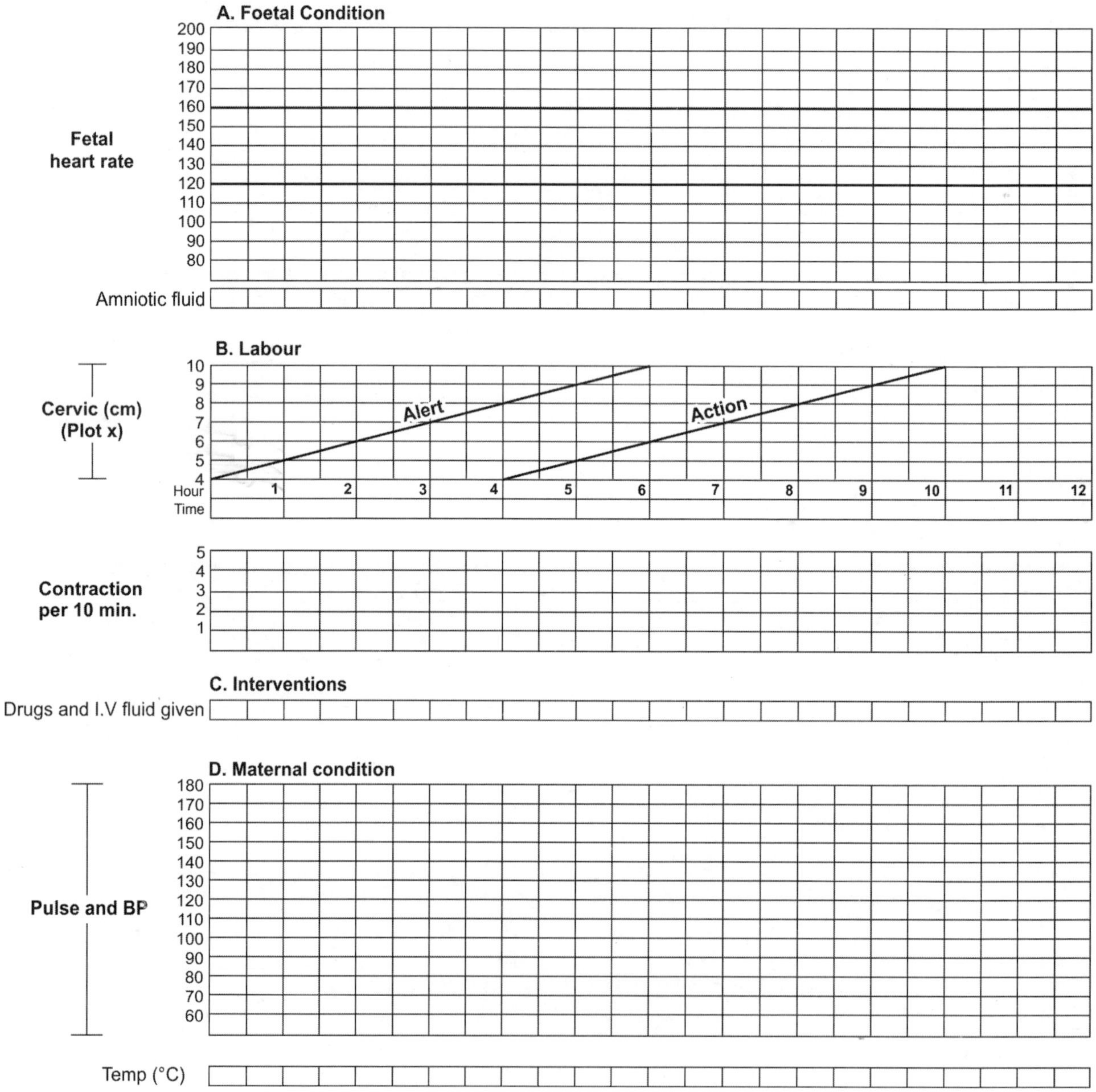

A. Foetal Condition

Fetal heart rate

200
190
180
170
160
150
140
130
120
110
100
90
80

Amniotic fluid

B. Labour

Cervic (cm) (Plot x)

10
9
8
7
6
5
4

Alert

Action

Hour 1 2 3 4 5 6 7 8 9 10 11 12

Time

Contraction per 10 min.

5
4
3
2
1

C. Interventions

Drugs and I.V fluid given

D. Maternal condition

Pulse and BP

180
170
160
150
140
130
120
110
100
90
80
70
60

Temp (°C)

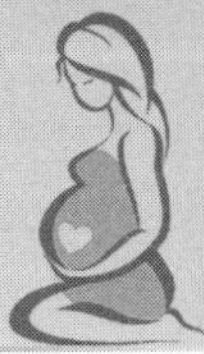

WHO Modified Partograph

Parity: *Reg No:* *Date and Time of Admission:* *Date and Time of ROM:*

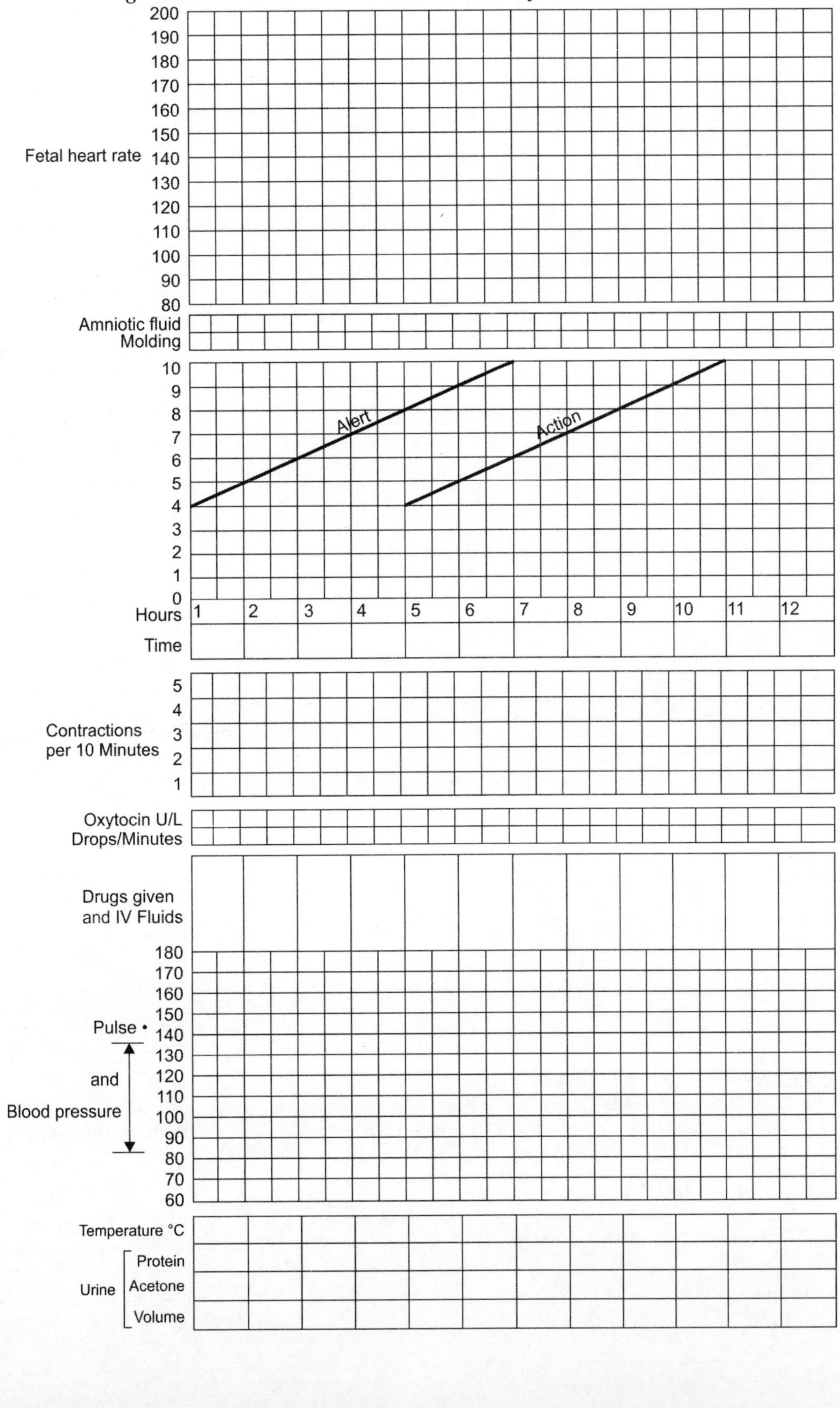

Fetal heart rate
200
190
180
170
160
150
140
130
120
110
100
90
80

Amniotic fluid
Molding

10
9
8
7
6
5
4
3
2
1
0

Hours 1 2 3 4 5 6 7 8 9 10 11 12

Time

Contractions per 10 Minutes
5
4
3
2
1

Oxytocin U/L
Drops/Minutes

Drugs given and IV Fluids

Pulse •
and
Blood pressure
180
170
160
150
140
130
120
110
100
90
80
70
60

Temperature °C

Urine
Protein
Acetone
Volume

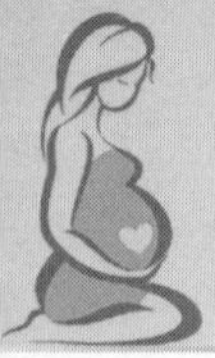

Delivery Note

Labor Progress Note Date and Time of Onset of Pain

Onset of true labor: On .... At: ....

Date and time of full cervix dilatation: .... Effacement: ....

Membrane ruptured (spontaneous/artificial/PROM) on .... At ....

Total duration of: 1st stage .... Hrs .... Min ....

2nd stage .... Hrs .... Min ....

3rd stage .... Hrs .... Min ....

Total hours = ... Hrs .... Min ....

Baby at Birth

Mode of delivery: .... Score at one minute ....

Baby born on:.. At: .... Sex: ....

Apgar scoring: .... Score at five minute.. Anus patent: ....

Initiation of breastfeeding: ....

Drug administration: ....

Delivery of Placenta and Membrane

Delivery of placenta on: .... At:.......................... Cord insertion: ....

Spontaneous/helped/manually removed .... Examination of placenta: Complete/Incomplete ....

Weight of placenta:..

Cord length: .... Examination of membrane: ....

Blood Loss

Before delivery of placenta : ....

During delivery of placenta : ....

After delivery of placenta : ....

Perineum

Intact : .... Episiotomy : .... Laceration : .... Repair : ....

Condition of Mother Following Delivery

Pulse: .... BP: .... Uterus: .... Vaginal bleeding: .... Breastfeeding initiated at: ....

Condition of Mother on Transfer

Healthy/unhealthy (if unhealthy specify): ....

Condition of baby on transfer or discharge: ....

Nursing Care Plan

S.No.	Assessment	Nursing Diagnosis	Goal/Expected Out Come	Nursing Intervention	Rational	Implementation	Evaluation

Signature of Sister in Charge

Signature of Supervisor

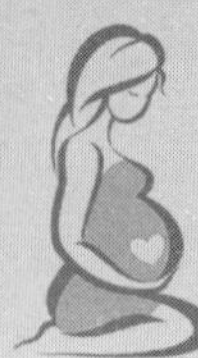

Conducted Normal Delivery (Case No. 4)

Client's Profile

Name : .... Religion : .... W/o : ....

Age : .... Education : .... Parity : ....

Hospital name : .... Occupation : .... LMP : ....

Date of booking : .... Income per month : .... EDD................................

Reg. No : .... Marriage duration : .... Period of gestation ....

Address : ....

....

Date and time of admission : ....

Date and time of discharge or transfer : ....

Admission Note

General Examinations

i. Temperature: .... iii. Respiration: ....

ii. Pulse: .... iv. BP: ....

Hydration: .... Anemia: (Present/absent) ....

Labor pain: (Present/absent).................................. Edema: (Generalized/ankle edema) ....

Abdominal Examination/Obstetrical Examination by Palpation

Height of uterus: .... cm Lie: .... Superficial grip: ....

Gestational weeks: .... Presentation: .... Deep pelvic grip: ....

Abdominal girth: ....cm Position of fetus: .... FHR: ....

Scar:.. Lateral grip: ....

Time/date of onset of contraction : ....

Uterine contraction: Present/absent/well contracted : ....

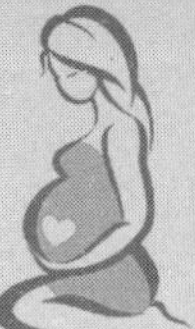

Investigation

Date	Hemoglobin	Blood Group/ Sugar	Urine		Bowel	Bladder	Any Other
			Albumin	Sugar			

Vaginal Examination

S.No	Date and time	Finding	Remark

Previous Obstetrical History

S.No	Year	Term/ preterm	Abortion/ stillbirth	Nature of delivery	Child		Immunization	Growth and development	Nature of puerperium	Remark
					Alive	Sex/ weight				

Admission History

Pregnancy complaints	
Menstrual history	
Medical history	
Surgical history	

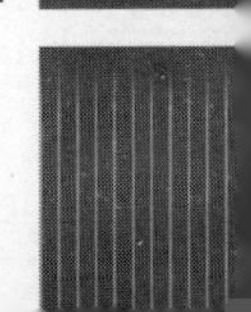

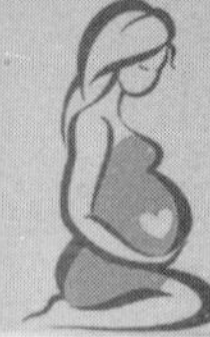

Old Pattern Partograph

Parity: *Reg No:* *Date and Time of Admission:* *Date and Time of ROM:*

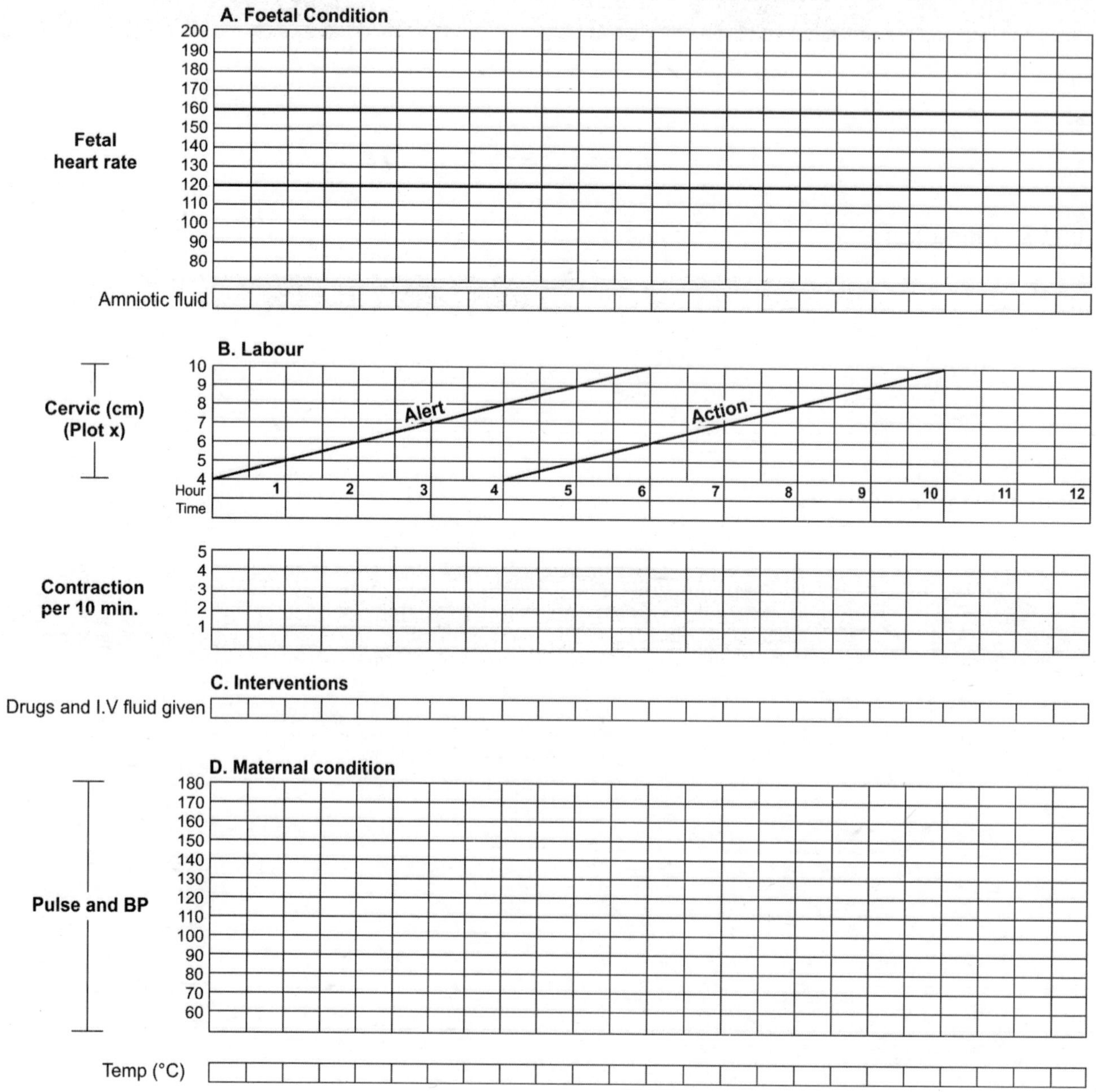

A. Foetal Condition

Fetal heart rate

200 190 180 170 160 150 140 130 120 110 100 90 80

Amniotic fluid

B. Labour

Cervic (cm) (Plot x)

10 9 8 7 6 5 4

Alert

Action

Hour 1 2 3 4 5 6 7 8 9 10 11 12

Time

Contraction per 10 min.

5 4 3 2 1

C. Interventions

Drugs and I.V fluid given

D. Maternal condition

Pulse and BP

180 170 160 150 140 130 120 110 100 90 80 70 60

Temp (°C)

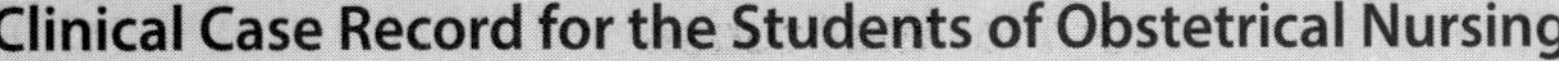

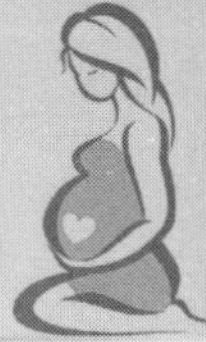

WHO Modified Partograph

Parity: *Reg No:* *Date and Time of Admission:* *Date and Time of ROM:*

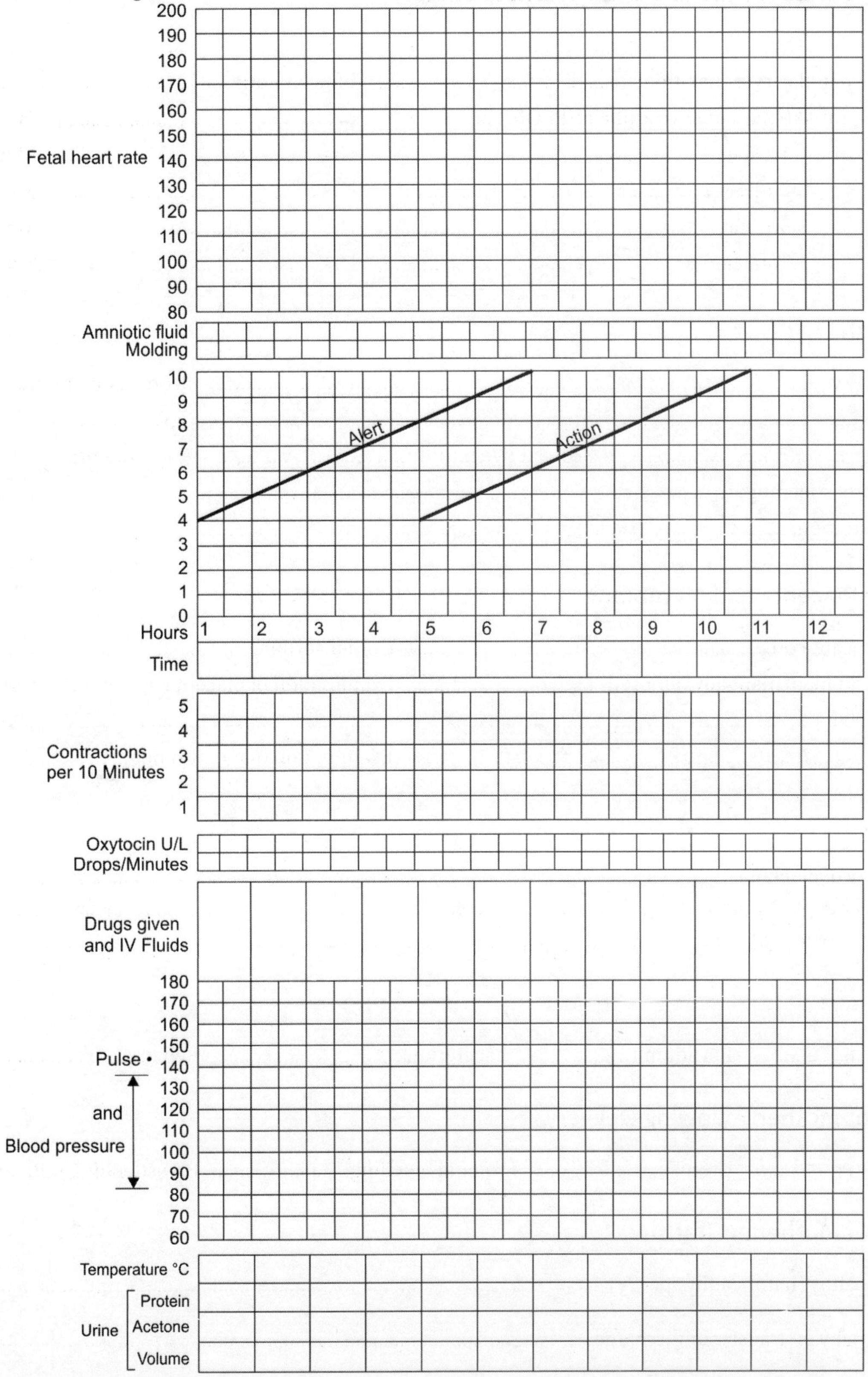

Fetal heart rate: 200, 190, 180, 170, 160, 150, 140, 130, 120, 110, 100, 90, 80

Amniotic fluid

Molding

10
9
8
7
6
5
4
3
2
1
0

Alert

Action

Hours: 1, 2, 3, 4, 5, 6, 7, 8, 9, 10, 11, 12

Time

Contractions per 10 Minutes: 5, 4, 3, 2, 1

Oxytocin U/L

Drops/Minutes

Drugs given and IV Fluids

Pulse • and Blood pressure: 180, 170, 160, 150, 140, 130, 120, 110, 100, 90, 80, 70, 60

Temperature °C

Urine: Protein, Acetone, Volume

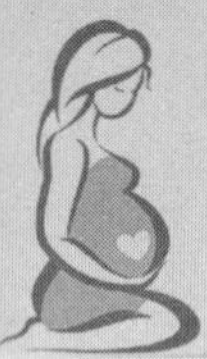

Delivery Note

Labor Progress Note Date and Time of Onset of Pain

Onset of true labor: On .... At: ....

Date and time of full cervix dilatation: .... Effacement: ....

Membrane ruptured (spontaneous/artificial/PROM) on .... At ....

Total duration of: 1st stage .... Hrs .... Min ....

2nd stage .... Hrs .... Min ....

3rd stage .... Hrs .... Min ....

Total hours = ... Hrs .... Min ....

Baby at Birth

Mode of delivery: .... Score at one minute ....

Baby born on:.................................... At: .... Sex: ....

Apgar scoring: .... Score at five minute.................................... Anus patent: ....

Initiation of breastfeeding: ....

Drug administration: ....

Delivery of Placenta and Membrane

Delivery of placenta on: .... At:.......................... Cord insertion: ....

Spontaneous/helped/manually removed .... Examination of placenta: Complete/Incomplete ....

Weight of placenta:..

Cord length: .... Examination of membrane: ....

Blood Loss

Before delivery of placenta : ....

During delivery of placenta : ....

After delivery of placenta : ....

Perineum

Intact : .... Episiotomy :............. Laceration :.............................. Repair : ....

Condition of Mother Following Delivery

Pulse: .... BP: .... Uterus: .... Vaginal bleeding: .... Breastfeeding initiated at: ....

Condition of Mother on Transfer

Healthy/unhealthy (if unhealthy specify): ....

Condition of baby on transfer or discharge: ....

Nursing Care Plan

S.No.	Assessment	Nursing Diagnosis	Goal/Expected Out Come	Nursing Intervention	Rational	Implementation	Evaluation

Signature of Sister in Charge

Signature of Supervisor

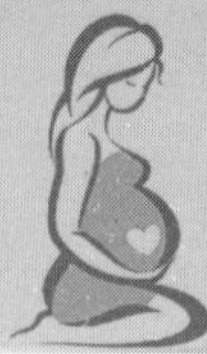

Conducted Normal Delivery (Case No. 5)

Client's Profile

Name	:	Religion	:	W/o	: ....
Age	:	Education	:	Parity	: ....
Hospital name	:	Occupation	:	LMP	: ....
Date of booking	:	Income per month	:	EDD	....
Reg. No	:	Marriage duration	:	Period of gestation	....

Address : ....

....

Date and time of admission : ....

Date and time of discharge or transfer : ....

Admission Note

General Examinations

i. Temperature: .... iii. Respiration: ....

ii. Pulse: .... iv. BP: ....

Hydration: .... Anemia: (Present/absent) ....

Labor pain: (Present/absent) .... Edema: (Generalized/ankle edema) ....

Abdominal Examination/Obstetrical Examination by Palpation

Height of uterus: .... cm Lie: .... Superficial grip: ....

Gestational weeks: .... Presentation: .... Deep pelvic grip: ....

Abdominal girth: ....cm Position of fetus: .... FHR: ....

Scar: .... Lateral grip: ....

Time/date of onset of contraction : ....

Uterine contraction: Present/absent/well contracted : ....

Investigation

Date	Hemoglobin	Blood Group/ Sugar	Urine		Bowel	Bladder	Any Other
			Albumin	Sugar			

Vaginal Examination

S.No	Date and time	Finding	Remark

Previous Obstetrical History

S.No	Year	Term/ preterm	Abortion/ stillbirth	Nature of delivery	Child		Immunization	Growth and development	Nature of puerperium	Remark
					Alive	Sex/ weight				

Admission History

Pregnancy complaints	
Menstrual history	
Medical history	
Surgical history	

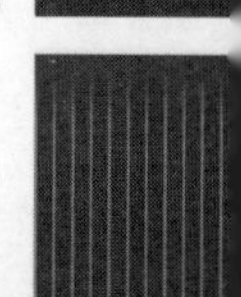

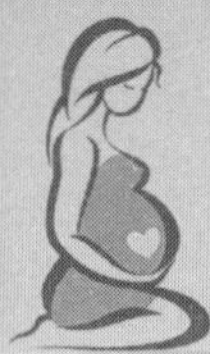

Old Pattern Partograph

Parity: *Reg No:* *Date and Time of Admission:* *Date and Time of ROM:*

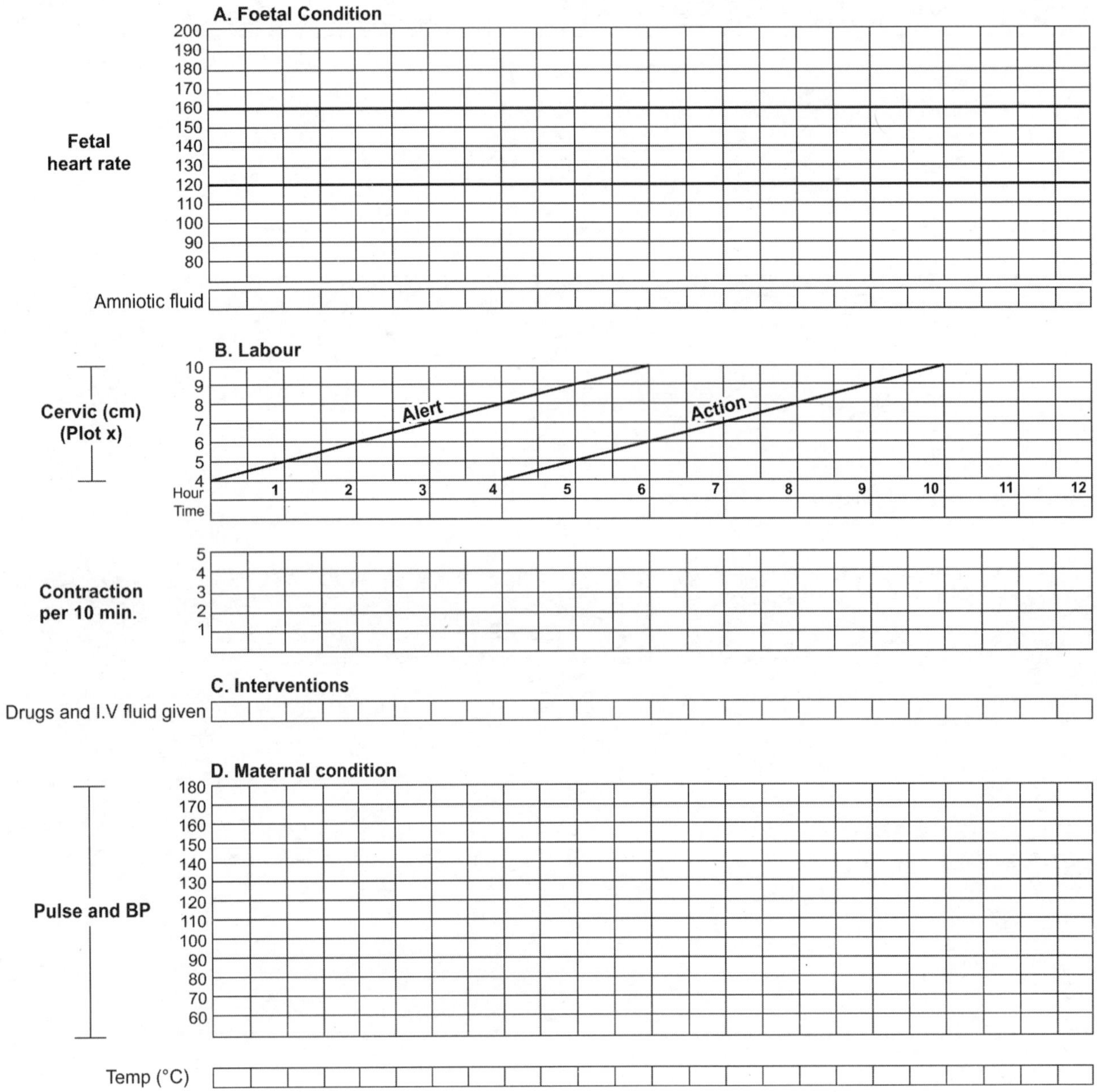

A. Foetal Condition

Fetal heart rate

200
190
180
170
160
150
140
130
120
110
100
90
80

Amniotic fluid

B. Labour

Cervic (cm) (Plot x)

10
9
8
7
6
5
4

Alert

Action

Hour	1	2	3	4	5	6	7	8	9	10	11	12
Time												

Contraction per 10 min.

5
4
3
2
1

C. Interventions

Drugs and I.V fluid given

D. Maternal condition

Pulse and BP

180
170
160
150
140
130
120
110
100
90
80
70
60

Temp (°C)

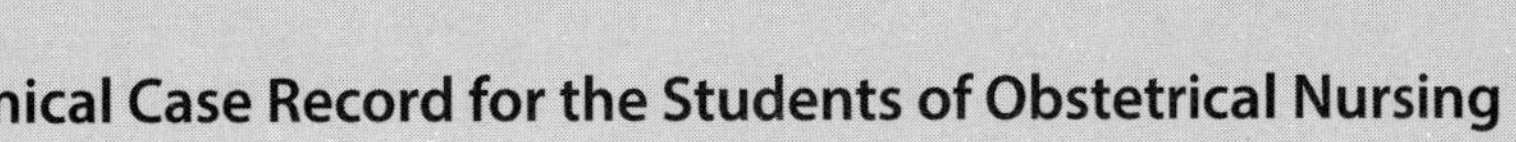

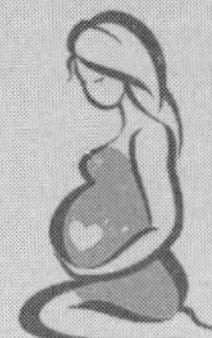

WHO Modified Partograph

Parity: *Reg No:* *Date and Time of Admission:* *Date and Time of ROM:*

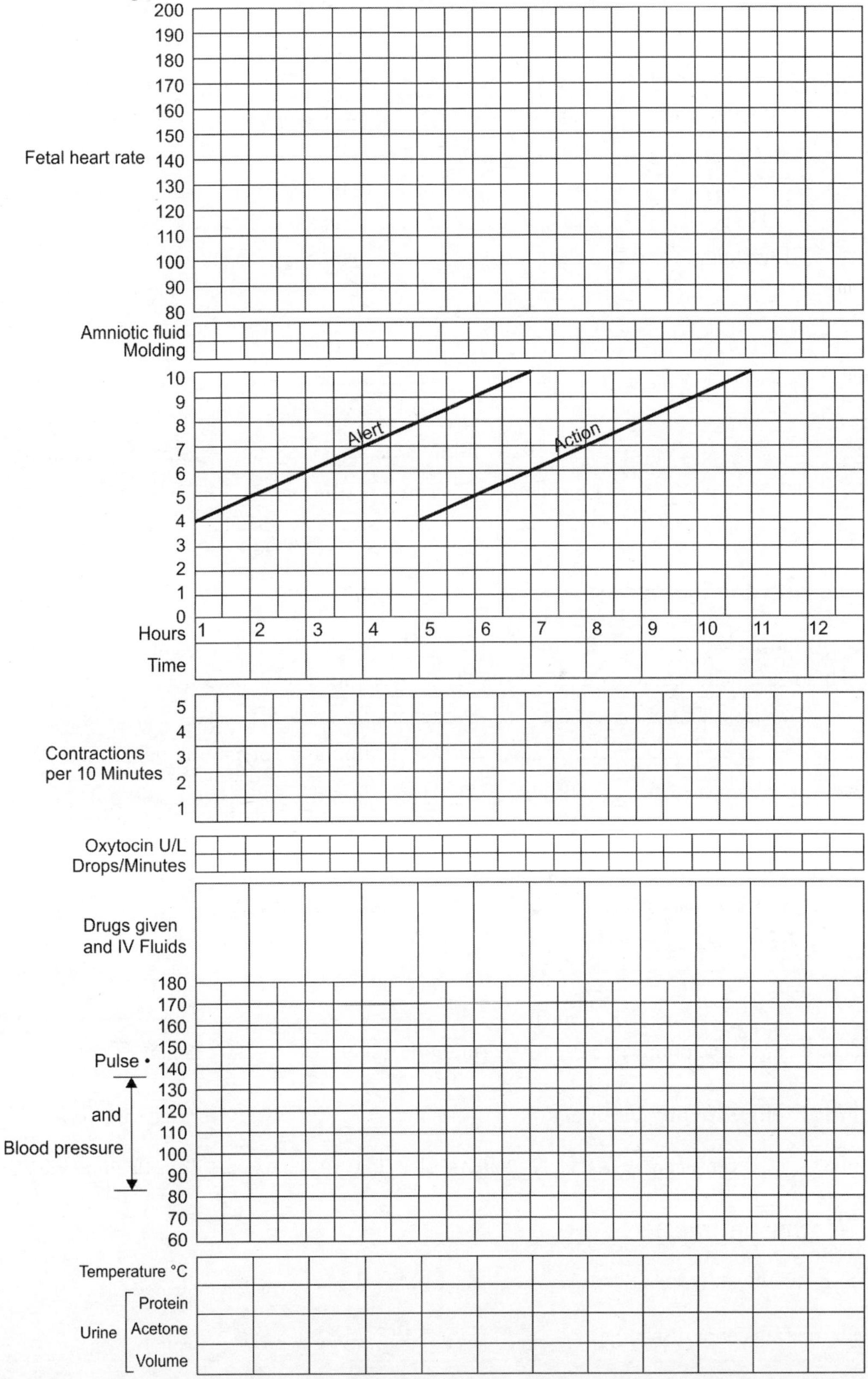

Fetal heart rate

200
190
180
170
160
150
140
130
120
110
100
90
80

Amniotic fluid
Molding

10
9
8
7
6
5
4
3
2
1
0

Alert

Action

Hours	1	2	3	4	5	6	7	8	9	10	11	12
Time												

Contractions per 10 Minutes

5
4
3
2
1

Oxytocin U/L
Drops/Minutes

Drugs given and IV Fluids

Pulse •

and

Blood pressure

180
170
160
150
140
130
120
110
100
90
80
70
60

Temperature °C

Urine
- Protein
- Acetone
- Volume

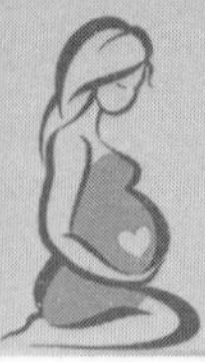

Delivery Note

Labor Progress Note Date and Time of Onset of Pain

Onset of true labor: On .... At: ....

Date and time of full cervix dilatation: .... Effacement: ....

Membrane ruptured (spontaneous/artificial/PROM) on .... At ....

Total duration of: 1st stage .... Hrs .... Min ....

2nd stage .... Hrs .... Min ....

3rd stage .... Hrs .... Min ....

Total hours = ... Hrs .... Min ....

Baby at Birth

Mode of delivery: .... Score at one minute ....

Baby born on:.................................... At: .... Sex: ....

Apgar scoring: .... Score at five minute.................................... Anus patent: ....

Initiation of breastfeeding: ....

Drug administration: ....

Delivery of Placenta and Membrane

Delivery of placenta on: .... At:.......................... Cord insertion: ....

Spontaneous/helped/manually removed .... Examination of placenta: Complete/Incomplete ....

Weight of placenta:...

Cord length: .... Examination of membrane: ....

Blood Loss

Before delivery of placenta : ....

During delivery of placenta : ....

After delivery of placenta : ....

Perineum

Intact : .... Episiotomy : .... Laceration : .... Repair : ....

Condition of Mother Following Delivery

Pulse: .... BP: .... Uterus: .... Vaginal bleeding: .... Breastfeeding initiated at: ....

Condition of Mother on Transfer

Healthy/unhealthy (if unhealthy specify): ....

Condition of baby on transfer or discharge: ....

Nursing Care Plan

S.No.	Assessment	Nursing Diagnosis	Goal/Expected Out Come	Nursing Intervention	Rational	Implementation	Evaluation

Signature of Sister in Charge

Signature of Supervisor

Conducted Normal Delivery (Case No. 6)

Client's Profile

Name : .... Religion : .... W/o : ....

Age : .... Education : .... Parity : ....

Hospital name : .... Occupation : .... LMP : ....

Date of booking : .... Income per month : .... EDD ....

Reg. No : .... Marriage duration : .... Period of gestation ....

Address : ....

....

Date and time of admission : ....

Date and time of discharge or transfer : ....

Admission Note

General Examinations

i. Temperature: .... iii. Respiration: ....

ii. Pulse: .... iv. BP: ....

Hydration: .... Anemia: (Present/absent) ....

Labor pain: (Present/absent).................................. Edema: (Generalized/ankle edema) ....

Abdominal Examination/Obstetrical Examination by Palpation

Height of uterus: .... cm Lie: .... Superficial grip: ....

Gestational weeks: .... Presentation: .... Deep pelvic grip: ....

Abdominal girth: ....cm Position of fetus: .... FHR: ....

Scar: .... Lateral grip: ....

Time/date of onset of contraction : ....

Uterine contraction: Present/absent/well contracted : ....

Investigation

Date	Hemoglobin	Blood Group/ Sugar	Urine		Bowel	Bladder	Any Other
			Albumin	Sugar			

Vaginal Examination

S.No	Date and time	Finding	Remark

Previous Obstetrical History

S.No	Year	Term/ preterm	Abortion/ stillbirth	Nature of delivery	Child		Immunization	Growth and development	Nature of puerperium	Remark
					Alive	Sex/ weight				

Admission History

Pregnancy complaints	
Menstrual history	
Medical history	
Surgical history	

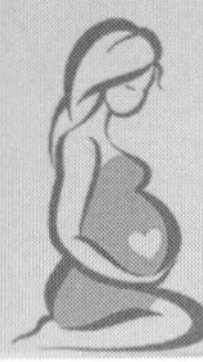

Old Pattern Partograph

Parity: *Reg No:* *Date and Time of Admission:* *Date and Time of ROM:*

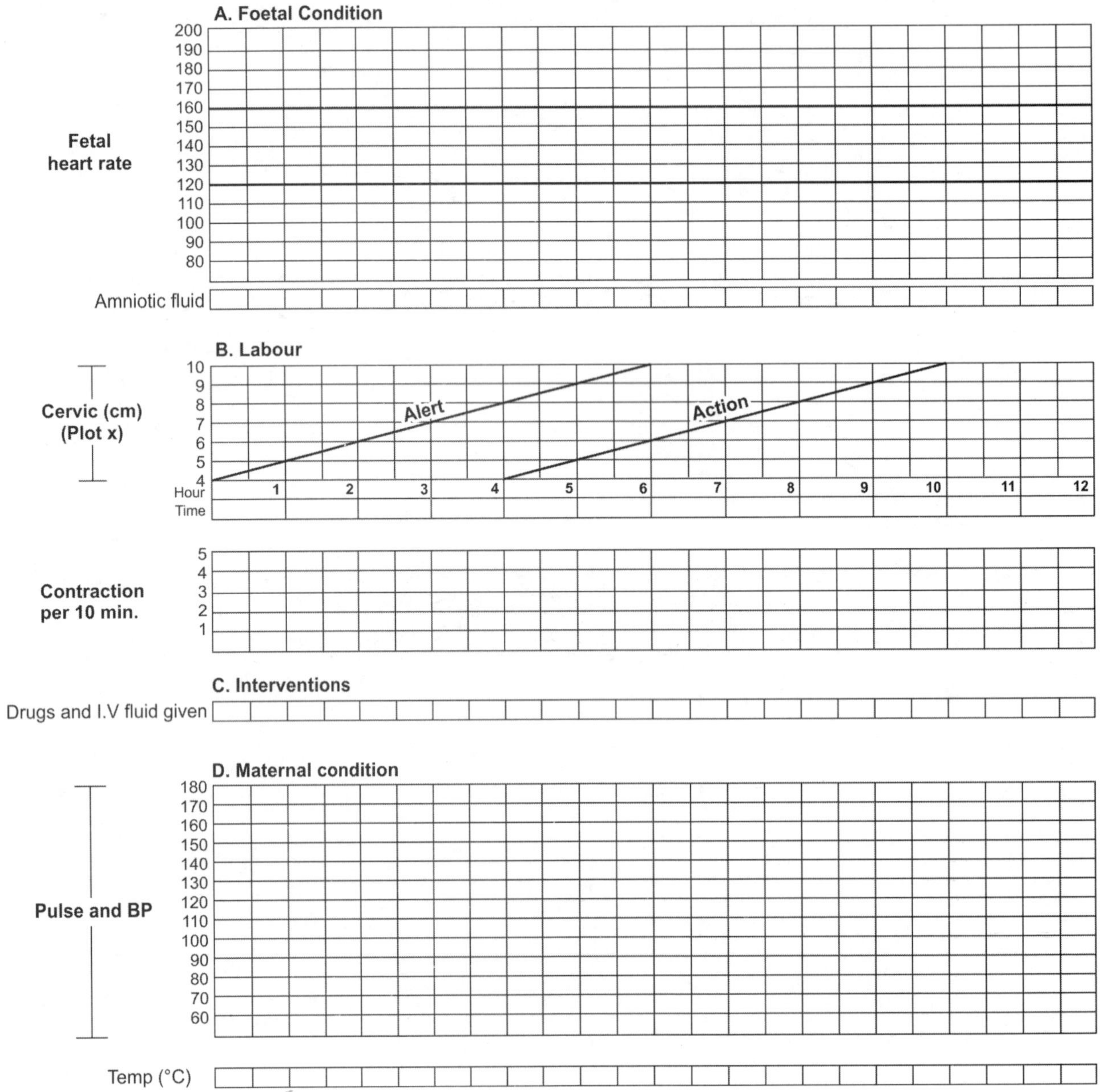

A. Foetal Condition

Fetal heart rate 200 190 180 170 160 150 140 130 120 110 100 90 80

Amniotic fluid

B. Labour

Cervic (cm) (Plot x) 10 9 8 7 6 5 4

Alert

Action

Hour 1 2 3 4 5 6 7 8 9 10 11 12

Time

Contraction per 10 min. 5 4 3 2 1

C. Interventions

Drugs and I.V fluid given

D. Maternal condition

Pulse and BP 180 170 160 150 140 130 120 110 100 90 80 70 60

Temp (°C)

WHO Modified Partograph

Parity: *Reg No:* *Date and Time of Admission:* *Date and Time of ROM:*

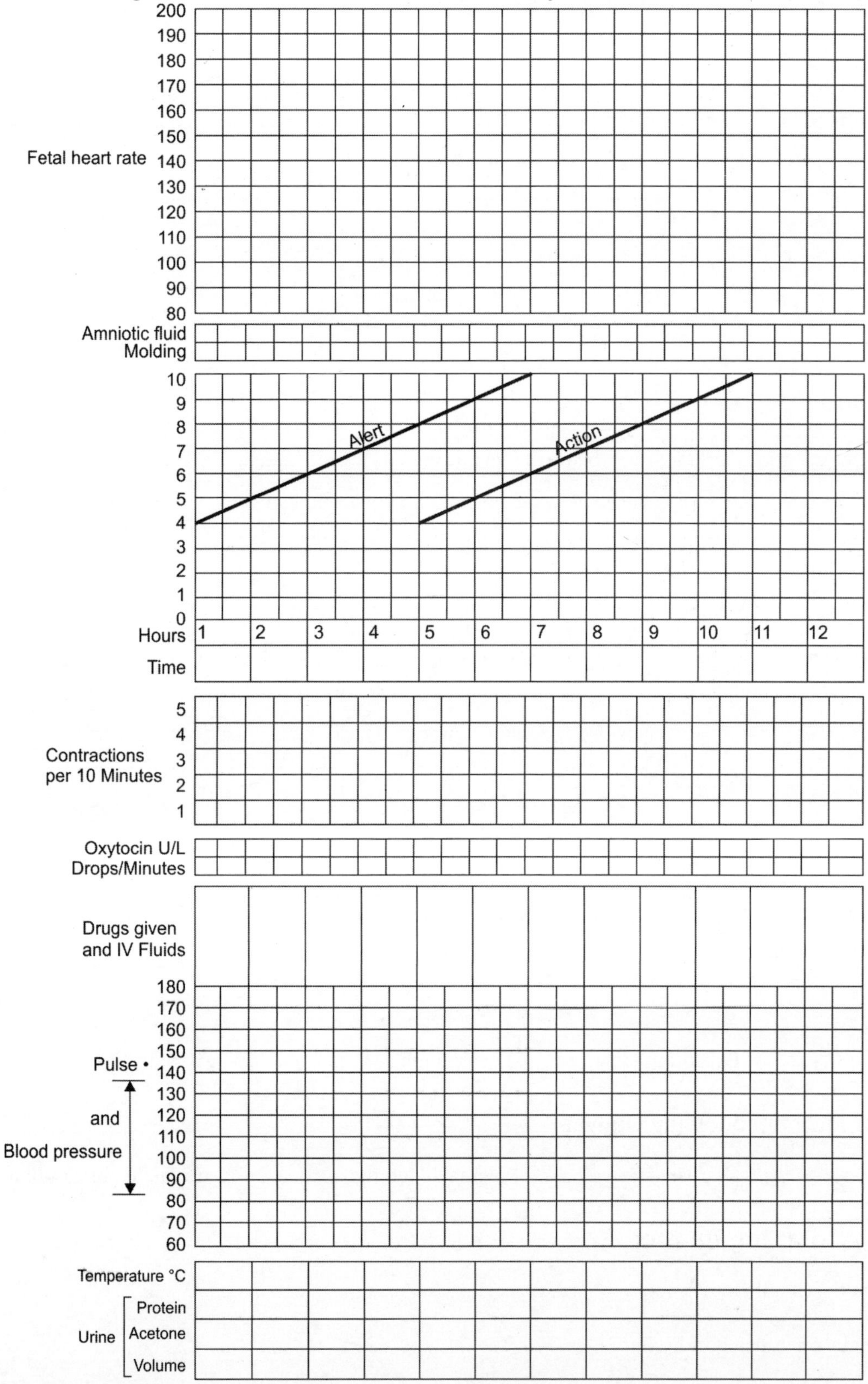

Fetal heart rate: 200, 190, 180, 170, 160, 150, 140, 130, 120, 110, 100, 90, 80

Amniotic fluid

Molding

10, 9, 8, 7, 6, 5, 4, 3, 2, 1, 0

Alert

Action

Hours	1	2	3	4	5	6	7	8	9	10	11	12
Time												

Contractions per 10 Minutes: 5, 4, 3, 2, 1

Oxytocin U/L

Drops/Minutes

Drugs given and IV Fluids

Pulse • and Blood pressure: 180, 170, 160, 150, 140, 130, 120, 110, 100, 90, 80, 70, 60

Temperature °C

Urine: Protein, Acetone, Volume

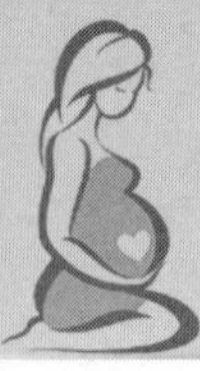

Delivery Note

Labor Progress Note Date and Time of Onset of Pain

Onset of true labor: On .... At: ....

Date and time of full cervix dilatation: .... Effacement: ....

Membrane ruptured (spontaneous/artificial/PROM) on .... At ....

Total duration of: 1st stage .... Hrs .... Min ....

2nd stage .... Hrs .... Min ....

3rd stage .... Hrs .... Min ....

Total hours = ... Hrs .... Min ....

Baby at Birth

Mode of delivery: .... Score at one minute ....

Baby born on:.. At: .... Sex: ....

Apgar scoring: .... Score at five minute.. Anus patent: ....

Initiation of breastfeeding: ....

Drug administration: ....

Delivery of Placenta and Membrane

Delivery of placenta on: .... At:.......................... Cord insertion: ....

Spontaneous/helped/manually removed .... Examination of placenta: Complete/Incomplete ....

Weight of placenta:..

Cord length: .... Examination of membrane: ....

Blood Loss

Before delivery of placenta : ....

During delivery of placenta : ....

After delivery of placenta : ....

Perineum

Intact : .... Episiotomy : .... Laceration :.......................... Repair : ....

Condition of Mother Following Delivery

Pulse: .... BP: .... Uterus: .... Vaginal bleeding: .... Breastfeeding initiated at: ....

Condition of Mother on Transfer

Healthy/unhealthy (if unhealthy specify): ....

Condition of baby on transfer or discharge: ....

Nursing Care Plan

S.No.	Assessment	Nursing Diagnosis	Goal/Expected Out Come	Nursing Intervention	Rational	Implementation	Evaluation

Signature of Sister in Charge

Signature of Supervisor

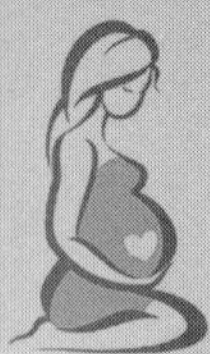

Conducted Normal Delivery (Case No. 7)

Client's Profile

Name : .... Religion : .... W/o : ....

Age : .... Education : .... Parity : ....

Hospital name : .... Occupation : .... LMP : ....

Date of booking : .... Income per month : .... EDD ....

Reg. No : .... Marriage duration : .... Period of gestation ....

Address : ....

....

Date and time of admission : ....

Date and time of discharge or transfer : ....

Admission Note

General Examinations

i. Temperature: ....

iii. Respiration: ....

ii. Pulse: ....

iv. BP: ....

Hydration: ....

Anemia: (Present/absent) ....

Labor pain: (Present/absent).................................

Edema: (Generalized/ankle edema) ....

Abdominal Examination/Obstetrical Examination by Palpation

Height of uterus: .... cm Lie: .... Superficial grip: ....

Gestational weeks: .... Presentation: .... Deep pelvic grip: ....

Abdominal girth: ....cm Position of fetus: .... FHR: ....

Scar: .... Lateral grip: ....

Time/date of onset of contraction : ....

Uterine contraction: Present/absent/well contracted : ....

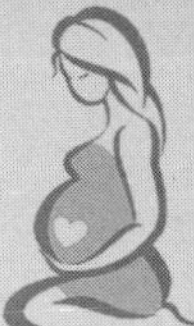

Investigation

Date	Hemoglobin	Blood Group/ Sugar	Urine		Bowel	Bladder	Any Other
			Albumin	Sugar			

Vaginal Examination

S.No	Date and time	Finding	Remark

Previous Obstetrical History

S.No	Year	Term/ preterm	Abortion/ stillbirth	Nature of delivery	Child		Immunization	Growth and development	Nature of puerperium	Remark
					Alive	Sex/ weight				

Admission History

Pregnancy complaints	
Menstrual history	
Medical history	
Surgical history	

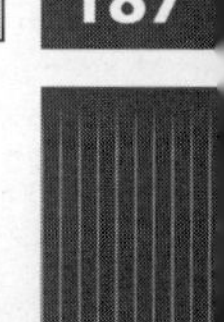

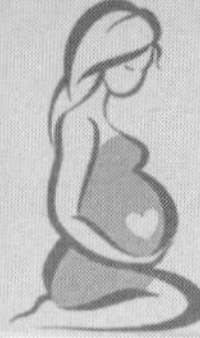

Old Pattern Partograph

Parity: *Reg No:* *Date and Time of Admission:* *Date and Time of ROM:*

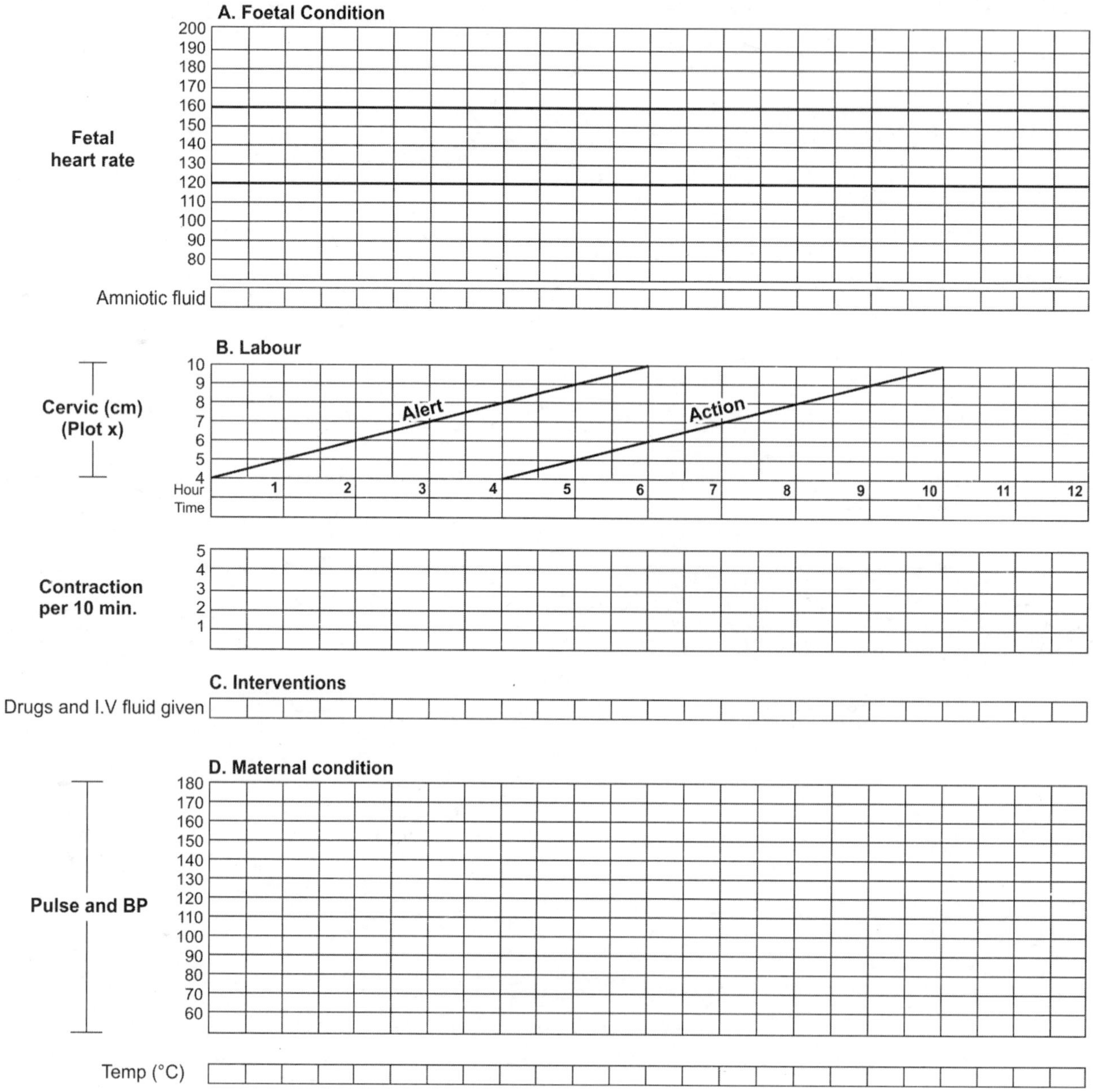

A. Foetal Condition

Fetal heart rate

200
190
180
170
160
150
140
130
120
110
100
90
80

Amniotic fluid

B. Labour

Cervic (cm) (Plot x)

10
9
8
7
6
5
4

Alert

Action

Hour	1	2	3	4	5	6	7	8	9	10	11	12
Time												

Contraction per 10 min.

5
4
3
2
1

C. Interventions

Drugs and I.V fluid given

D. Maternal condition

Pulse and BP

180
170
160
150
140
130
120
110
100
90
80
70
60

Temp (°C)

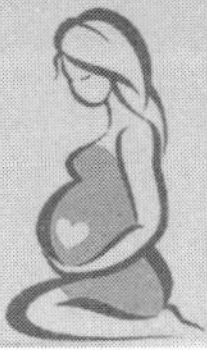

WHO Modified Partograph

Parity: *Reg No:* *Date and Time of Admission:* *Date and Time of ROM:*

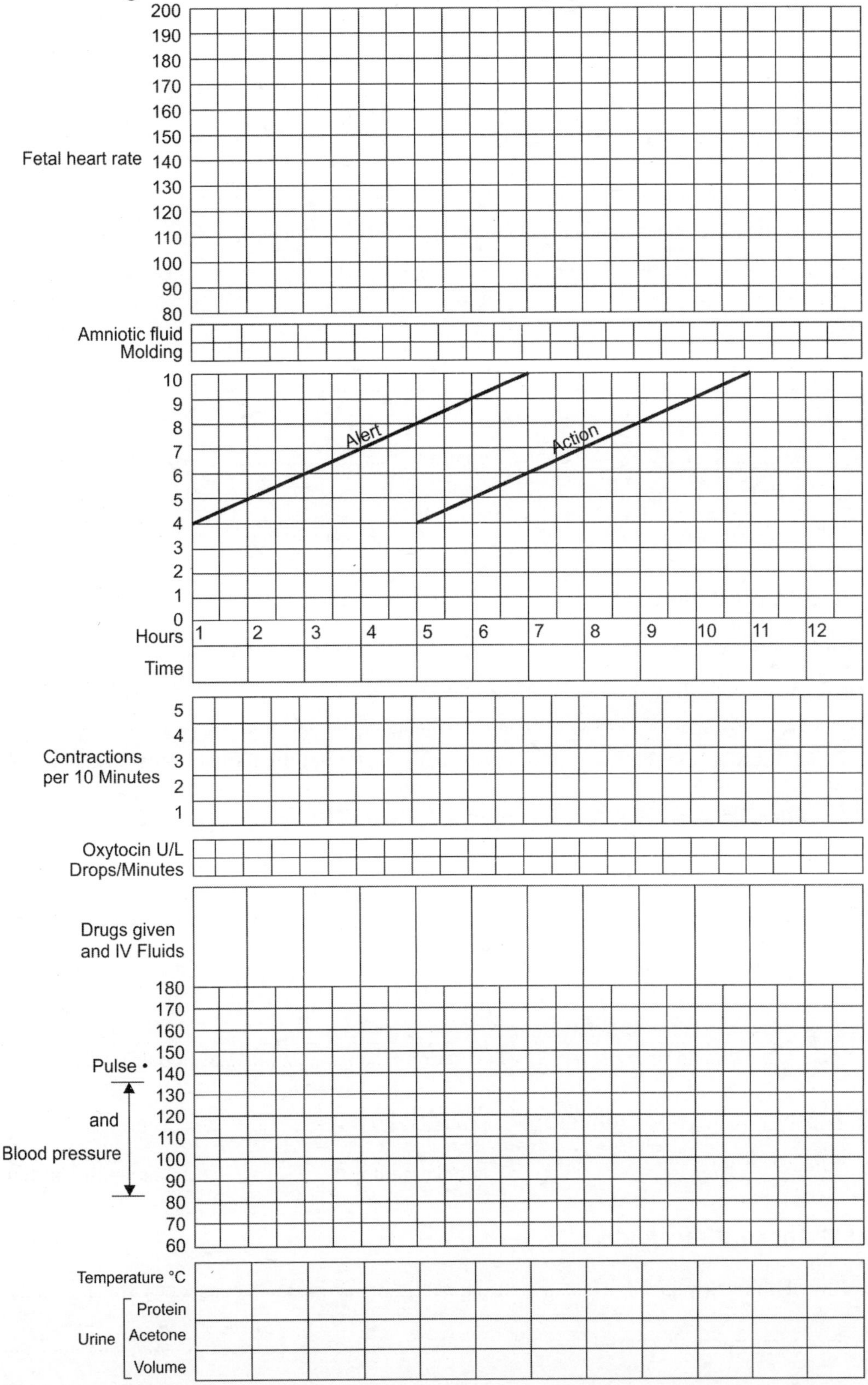

Fetal heart rate: 200, 190, 180, 170, 160, 150, 140, 130, 120, 110, 100, 90, 80

Amniotic fluid

Molding

10, 9, 8, 7, 6, 5, 4, 3, 2, 1, 0

Alert

Action

Hours	1	2	3	4	5	6	7	8	9	10	11	12
Time												

Contractions per 10 Minutes: 5, 4, 3, 2, 1

Oxytocin U/L

Drops/Minutes

Drugs given and IV Fluids

Pulse • and Blood pressure ↕: 180, 170, 160, 150, 140, 130, 120, 110, 100, 90, 80, 70, 60

Temperature °C

Urine: Protein, Acetone, Volume

Delivery Note

Labor Progress Note Date and Time of Onset of Pain

Onset of true labor: On .... At: ....

Date and time of full cervix dilatation: .... Effacement: ....

Membrane ruptured (spontaneous/artificial/PROM) on .... At ....

Total duration of: 1st stage .... Hrs .... Min ....

2nd stage .... Hrs .... Min ....

3rd stage .... Hrs .... Min ....

Total hours = ... Hrs .... Min ....

Baby at Birth

Mode of delivery: .... Score at one minute ....

Baby born on:.................................... At: .... Sex: ....

Apgar scoring: .... Score at five minute.............................. Anus patent: ....

Initiation of breastfeeding: ....

Drug administration: ....

Delivery of Placenta and Membrane

Delivery of placenta on: .... At:......................... Cord insertion: ....

Spontaneous/helped/manually removed .... Examination of placenta: Complete/Incomplete ....

Weight of placenta:...

Cord length: .... Examination of membrane: ....

Blood Loss

Before delivery of placenta : ....

During delivery of placenta : ....

After delivery of placenta : ....

Perineum

Intact : .... Episiotomy : .... Laceration : .... Repair : ....

Condition of Mother Following Delivery

Pulse: .... BP: .... Uterus: .... Vaginal bleeding: .... Breastfeeding initiated at: ....

Condition of Mother on Transfer

Healthy/unhealthy (if unhealthy specify): ....

Condition of baby on transfer or discharge: ....

Nursing Care Plan

S.No.	Assessment	Nursing Diagnosis	Goal/Expected Out Come	Nursing Intervention	Rational	Implementation	Evaluation

Signature of Sister in Charge

Signature of Supervisor

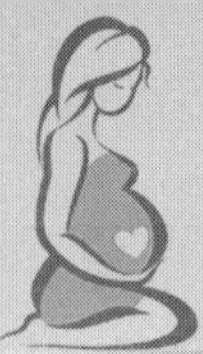

Conducted Normal Delivery (Case No. 8)

Client's Profile

Name : .... Religion : .... W/o : ....

Age : .... Education : .... Parity : ....

Hospital name : .... Occupation : .... LMP : ....

Date of booking : .... Income per month : .... EDD................................

Reg. No : .... Marriage duration : .... Period of gestation ....

Address : ....

....

Date and time of admission : ....

Date and time of discharge or transfer : ....

Admission Note

General Examinations

i. Temperature: .... iii. Respiration: ....

ii. Pulse: .... iv. BP: ....

Hydration: .... Anemia: (Present/absent) ....

Labor pain: (Present/absent).................................. Edema: (Generalized/ankle edema) ....

Abdominal Examination/Obstetrical Examination by Palpation

Height of uterus: .... cm Lie: .... Superficial grip: ....

Gestational weeks: .... Presentation: .... Deep pelvic grip: ....

Abdominal girth: ....cm Position of fetus: .... FHR: ....

Scar: .... Lateral grip: ....

Time/date of onset of contraction : ....

Uterine contraction: Present/absent/well contracted : ....

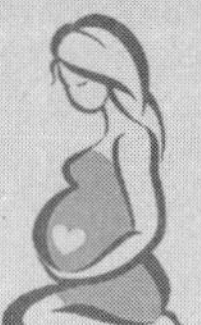

Investigation

Date	Hemoglobin	Blood Group/ Sugar	Urine		Bowel	Bladder	Any Other
			Albumin	Sugar			

Vaginal Examination

S.No	Date and time	Finding	Remark

Previous Obstetrical History

S.No	Year	Term/ preterm	Abortion/ stillbirth	Nature of delivery	Child		Immunization	Growth and development	Nature of puerperium	Remark
					Alive	Sex/ weight				

Admission History

Pregnancy complaints	
Menstrual history	
Medical history	
Surgical history	

Old Pattern Partograph

Parity: *Reg No:* *Date and Time of Admission:* *Date and Time of ROM:*

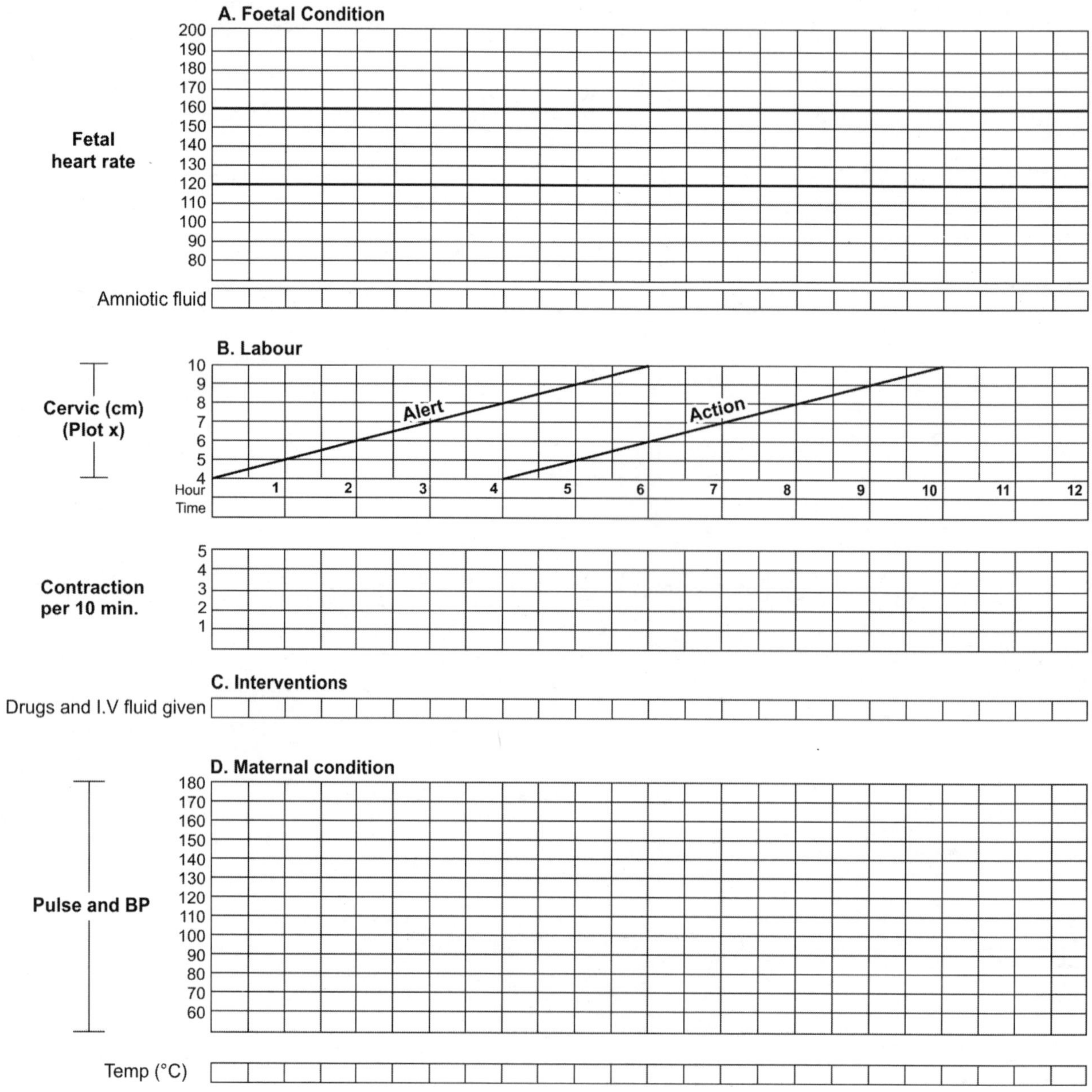

A. Foetal Condition

Fetal heart rate

200
190
180
170
160
150
140
130
120
110
100
90
80

Amniotic fluid

B. Labour

Cervic (cm) (Plot x)

10
9
8
7
6
5
4

Alert

Action

Hour 1 2 3 4 5 6 7 8 9 10 11 12

Time

Contraction per 10 min.

5
4
3
2
1

C. Interventions

Drugs and I.V fluid given

D. Maternal condition

Pulse and BP

180
170
160
150
140
130
120
110
100
90
80
70
60

Temp (°C)

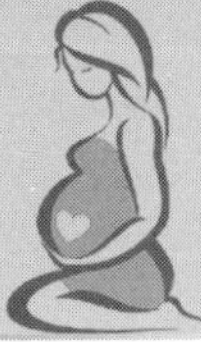

WHO Modified Partograph

Parity: *Reg No:* *Date and Time of Admission:* *Date and Time of ROM:*

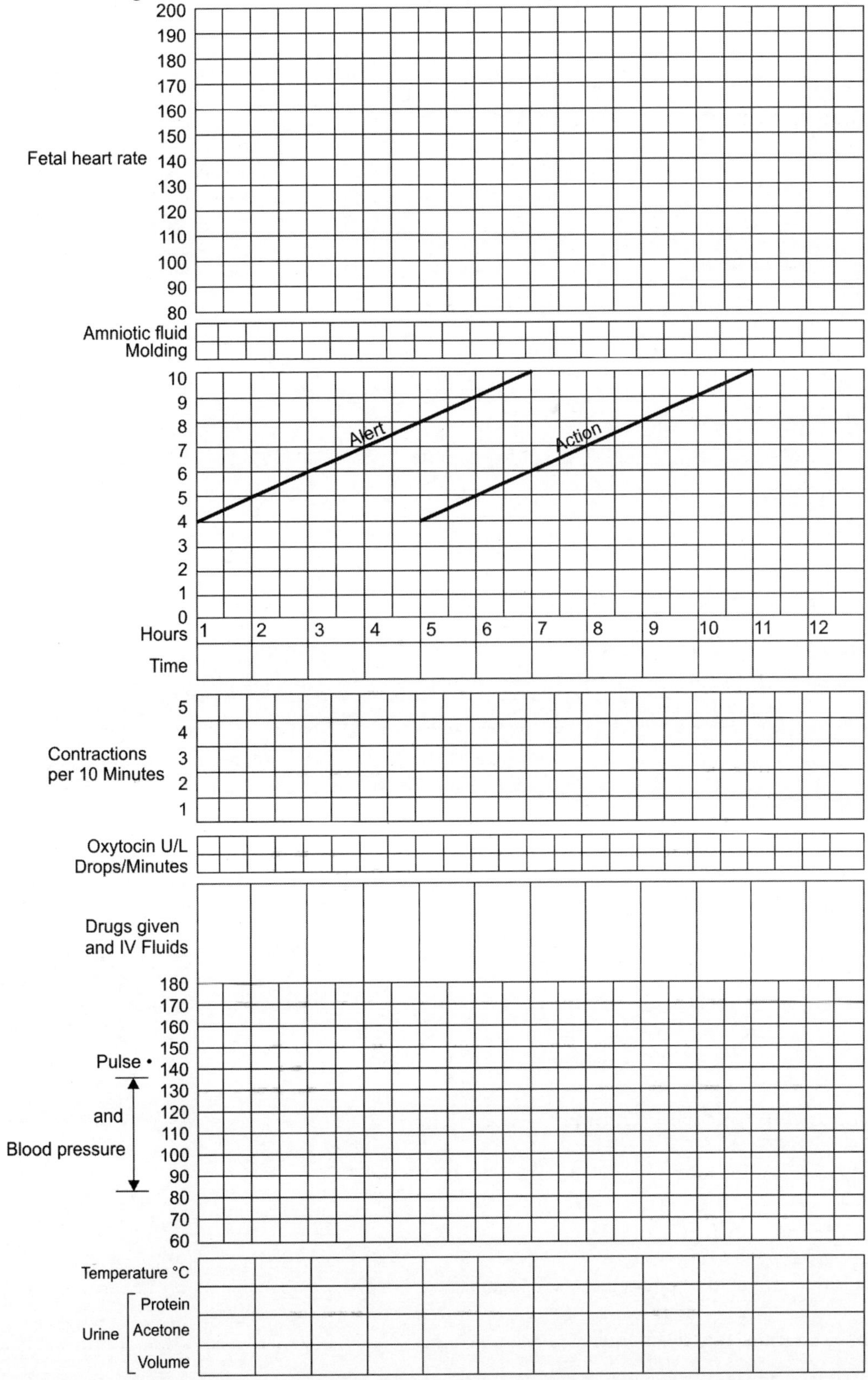

Fetal heart rate: 200, 190, 180, 170, 160, 150, 140, 130, 120, 110, 100, 90, 80

Amniotic fluid

Molding

10, 9, 8, 7, 6, 5, 4, 3, 2, 1, 0

Alert

Action

Hours	1	2	3	4	5	6	7	8	9	10	11	12
Time												

Contractions per 10 Minutes: 5, 4, 3, 2, 1

Oxytocin U/L

Drops/Minutes

Drugs given and IV Fluids

Pulse • and Blood pressure: 180, 170, 160, 150, 140, 130, 120, 110, 100, 90, 80, 70, 60

Temperature °C

Urine: Protein, Acetone, Volume

Delivery Note

Labor Progress Note Date and Time of Onset of Pain

Onset of true labor: On .... At: ....

Date and time of full cervix dilatation: .... Effacement: ....

Membrane ruptured (spontaneous/artificial/PROM) on .... At ....

Total duration of: 1st stage .... Hrs .... Min ....

2nd stage .... Hrs .... Min ....

3rd stage .... Hrs .... Min ....

Total hours = ... Hrs .... Min ....

Baby at Birth

Mode of delivery: .... Score at one minute ....

Baby born on:.. At: .... Sex: ....

Apgar scoring: .... Score at five minute................................ Anus patent: ....

Initiation of breastfeeding: ....

Drug administration: ....

Delivery of Placenta and Membrane

Delivery of placenta on: .... At:.......................... Cord insertion: ....

Spontaneous/helped/manually removed .... Examination of placenta: Complete/Incomplete ....

Weight of placenta:...

Cord length: .... Examination of membrane: ....

Blood Loss

Before delivery of placenta : ....

During delivery of placenta : ....

After delivery of placenta : ....

Perineum

Intact : .... Episiotomy :............. Laceration :.............................. Repair : ....

Condition of Mother Following Delivery

Pulse: .... BP: .... Uterus: .... Vaginal bleeding: .... Breastfeeding initiated at: ....

Condition of Mother on Transfer

Healthy/unhealthy (if unhealthy specify): ....

Condition of baby on transfer or discharge: ....

Nursing Care Plan

S.No.	Assessment	Nursing Diagnosis	Goal/Expected Out Come	Nursing Intervention	Rational	Implementation	Evaluation

Signature of Sister in Charge

Signature of Supervisor

Conducted Normal Delivery (Case No. 9)

Client's Profile

Name	:	Religion	:	W/o	: ....
Age	:	Education	:	Parity	: ....
Hospital name	:	Occupation	:	LMP	: ....
Date of booking	:	Income per month	:	EDD	....
Reg. No	:	Marriage duration	:	Period of gestation	....

Address : ....

....

Date and time of admission : ....

Date and time of discharge or transfer : ....

Admission Note

General Examinations

i. Temperature: ....

ii. Pulse: ....

iii. Respiration: ....

iv. BP: ....

Hydration: ....

Anemia: (Present/absent) ....

Labor pain: (Present/absent)......................................

Edema: (Generalized/ankle edema) ....

Abdominal Examination/Obstetrical Examination by Palpation

Height of uterus: .... cm	Lie:	Superficial grip: ....
Gestational weeks:	Presentation:	Deep pelvic grip: ....
Abdominal girth: ....cm	Position of fetus:	FHR: ....
Scar:	Lateral grip:	

Time/date of onset of contraction : ....

Uterine contraction: Present/absent/well contracted : ....

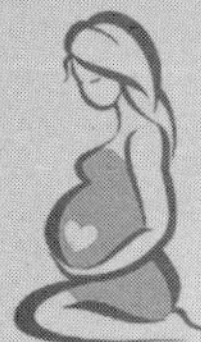

Investigation

Date	Hemoglobin	Blood Group/ Sugar	Urine		Bowel	Bladder	Any Other
			Albumin	Sugar			

Vaginal Examination

S.No	Date and time	Finding	Remark

Previous Obstetrical History

S.No	Year	Term/ preterm	Abortion/ stillbirth	Nature of delivery	Child		Immunization	Growth and development	Nature of puerperium	Remark
					Alive	Sex/ weight				

Admission History

Pregnancy complaints	
Menstrual history	
Medical history	
Surgical history	

Old Pattern Partograph

Parity: *Reg No:* *Date and Time of Admission:* *Date and Time of ROM:*

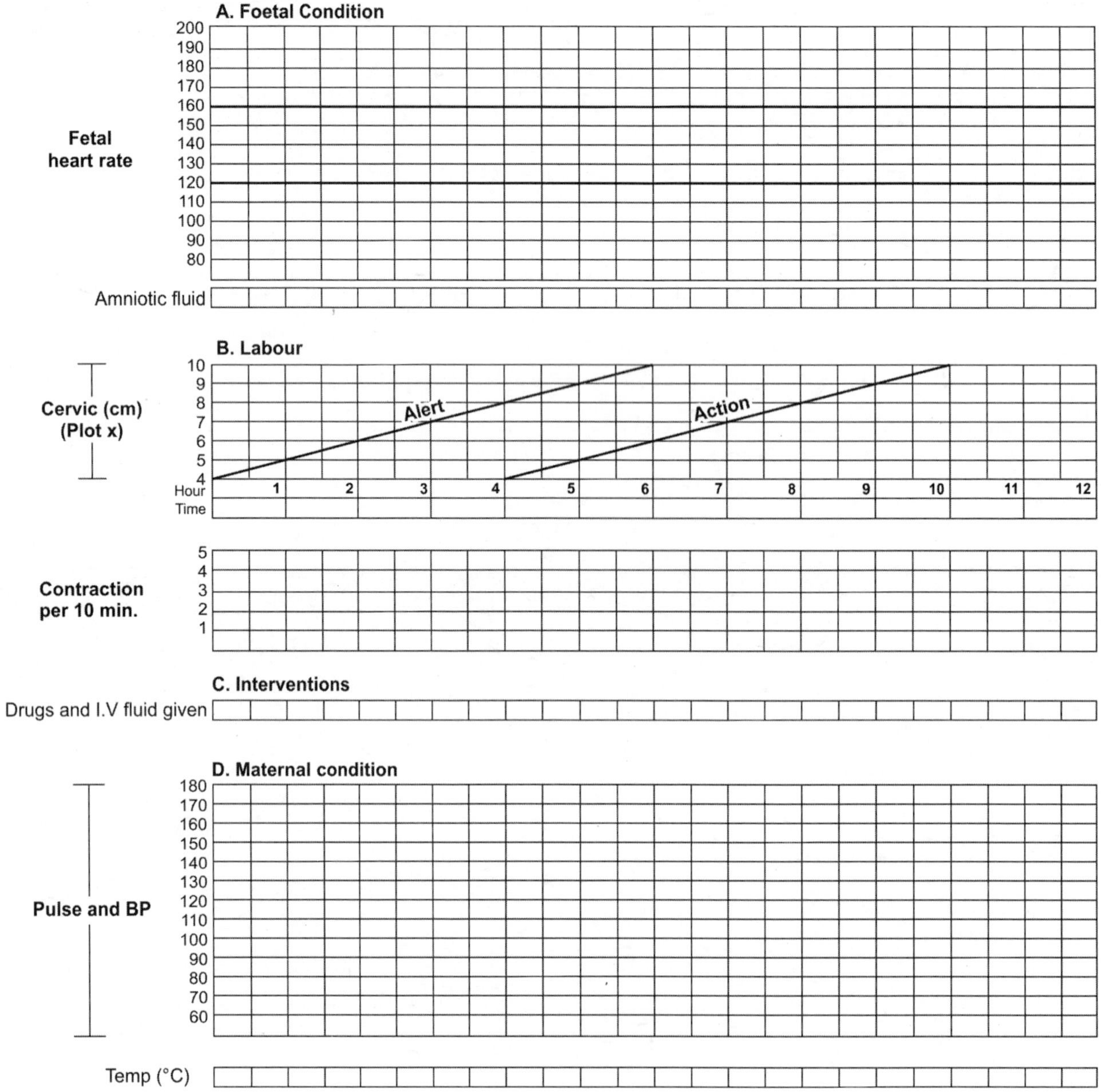

A. Foetal Condition

Fetal heart rate

200
190
180
170
160
150
140
130
120
110
100
90
80

Amniotic fluid

B. Labour

Cervic (cm) (Plot x)

10
9
8
7
6
5
4

Alert

Action

Hour 1 2 3 4 5 6 7 8 9 10 11 12

Time

Contraction per 10 min.

5
4
3
2
1

C. Interventions

Drugs and I.V fluid given

D. Maternal condition

Pulse and BP

180
170
160
150
140
130
120
110
100
90
80
70
60

Temp (°C)

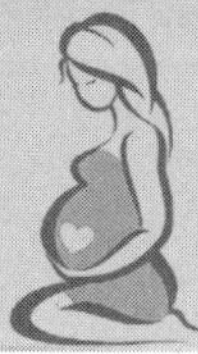

WHO Modified Partograph

Parity: *Reg No:* *Date and Time of Admission:* *Date and Time of ROM:*

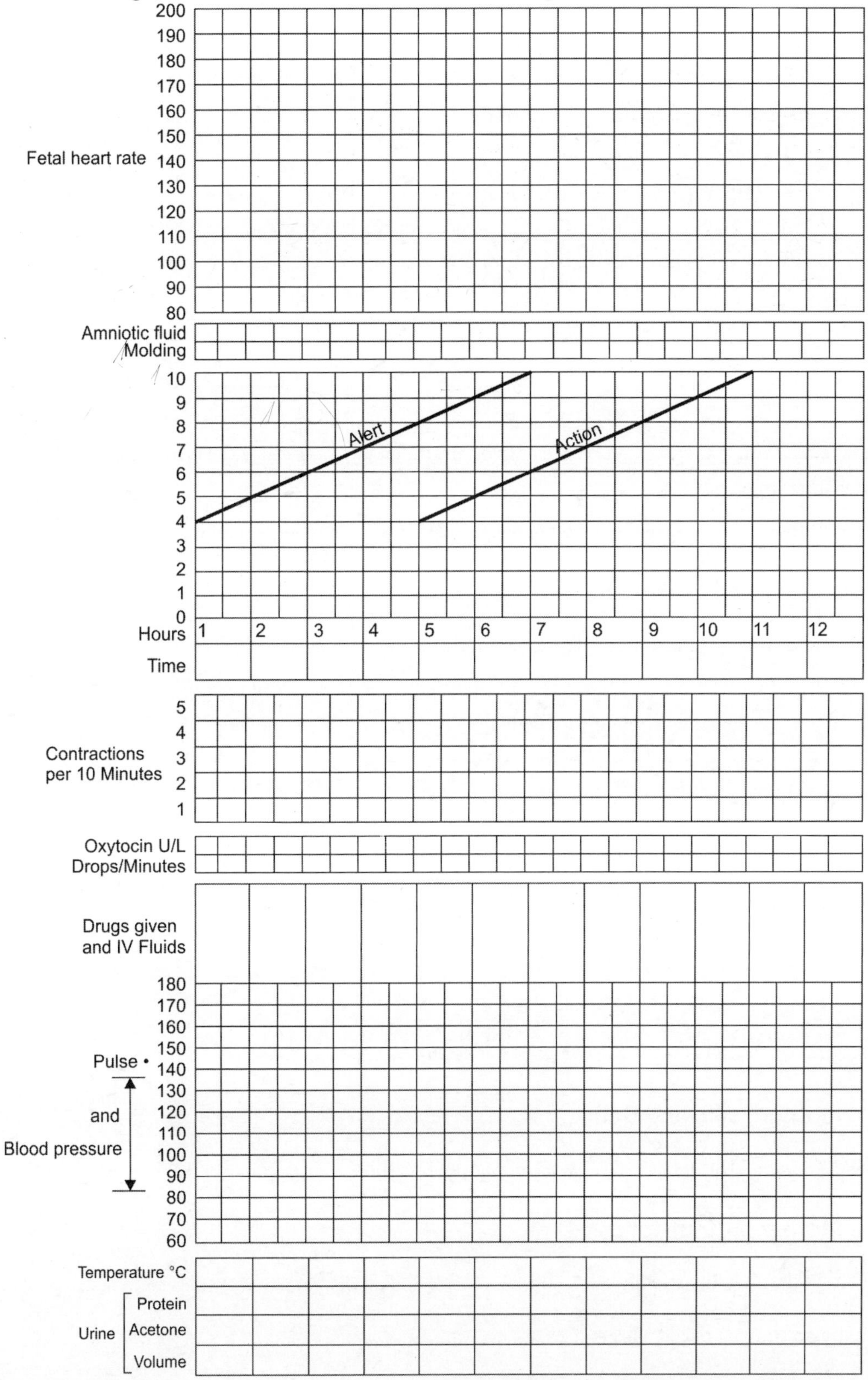

Fetal heart rate: 200, 190, 180, 170, 160, 150, 140, 130, 120, 110, 100, 90, 80

Amniotic fluid

Molding

10, 9, 8, 7, 6, 5, 4, 3, 2, 1, 0

Alert

Action

Hours: 1, 2, 3, 4, 5, 6, 7, 8, 9, 10, 11, 12

Time

Contractions per 10 Minutes: 5, 4, 3, 2, 1

Oxytocin U/L

Drops/Minutes

Drugs given and IV Fluids

Pulse • and Blood pressure: 180, 170, 160, 150, 140, 130, 120, 110, 100, 90, 80, 70, 60

Temperature °C

Urine: Protein, Acetone, Volume

Delivery Note

Labor Progress Note Date and Time of Onset of Pain

Onset of true labor: On .... At: ....

Date and time of full cervix dilatation: .... Effacement: ....

Membrane ruptured (spontaneous/artificial/PROM) on .... At ....

Total duration of: 1st stage .... Hrs .... Min ....

2nd stage .... Hrs .... Min ....

3rd stage .... Hrs .... Min ....

Total hours = ... Hrs .... Min ....

Baby at Birth

Mode of delivery: .... Score at one minute ....

Baby born on:... At: .... Sex: ....

Apgar scoring: .... Score at five minute................................ Anus patent: ....

Initiation of breastfeeding: ....

Drug administration: ....

Delivery of Placenta and Membrane

Delivery of placenta on: .... At:.......................... Cord insertion: ....

Spontaneous/helped/manually removed .... Examination of placenta: Complete/Incomplete ....

Weight of placenta:...

Cord length: .... Examination of membrane: ....

Blood Loss

Before delivery of placenta : ....

During delivery of placenta : ....

After delivery of placenta : ....

Perineum

Intact : .... Episiotomy :............. Laceration :.............................. Repair : ....

Condition of Mother Following Delivery

Pulse: .... BP: .... Uterus: .... Vaginal bleeding: .... Breastfeeding initiated at: ....

Condition of Mother on Transfer

Healthy/unhealthy (if unhealthy specify): ....

Condition of baby on transfer or discharge: ....

Nursing Care Plan

S.No.	Assessment	Nursing Diagnosis	Goal/Expected Out Come	Nursing Intervention	Rational	Implementation	Evaluation

Signature of Sister in Charge

Signature of Supervisor

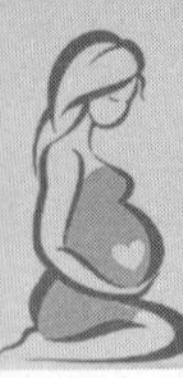

Conducted Normal Delivery (Case No. 10)

Client's Profile

Name : .... Religion : .... W/o : ....

Age : .... Education : .... Parity : ....

Hospital name : .... Occupation : .... LMP : ....

Date of booking : .... Income per month : .... EDD.................................

Reg. No : .... Marriage duration : .... Period of gestation ....

Address : ....

....

Date and time of admission : ....

Date and time of discharge or transfer : ....

Admission Note

General Examinations

i. Temperature: ....

ii. Pulse: ....

iii. Respiration: ....

iv. BP: ....

Hydration: ....

Anemia: (Present/absent) ....

Labor pain: (Present/absent)...................................

Edema: (Generalized/ankle edema) ....

Abdominal Examination/Obstetrical Examination by Palpation

Height of uterus: .... cm Lie: .... Superficial grip: ....

Gestational weeks: .... Presentation: .... Deep pelvic grip: ....

Abdominal girth: ....cm Position of fetus:.. FHR: ....

Scar:... Lateral grip: ....

Time/date of onset of contraction : ....

Uterine contraction: Present/absent/well contracted : ....

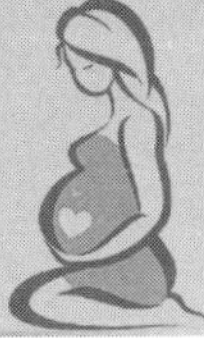

Investigation

Date	Hemoglobin	Blood Group/ Sugar	Urine		Bowel	Bladder	Any Other
			Albumin	Sugar			

Vaginal Examination

S.No	Date and time	Finding	Remark

Previous Obstetrical History

S.No	Year	Term/ preterm	Abortion/ stillbirth	Nature of delivery	Child		Immunization	Growth and development	Nature of puerperium	Remark
					Alive	Sex/ weight				

Admission History

Pregnancy complaints	
Menstrual history	
Medical history	
Surgical history	

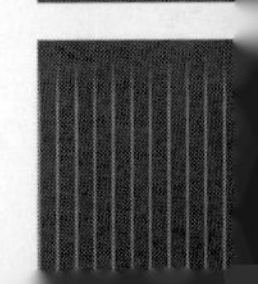

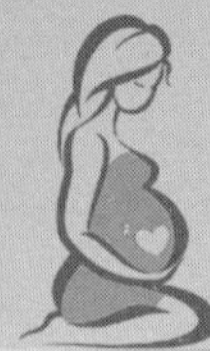

Old Pattern Partograph

Parity: *Reg No:* *Date and Time of Admission:* *Date and Time of ROM:*

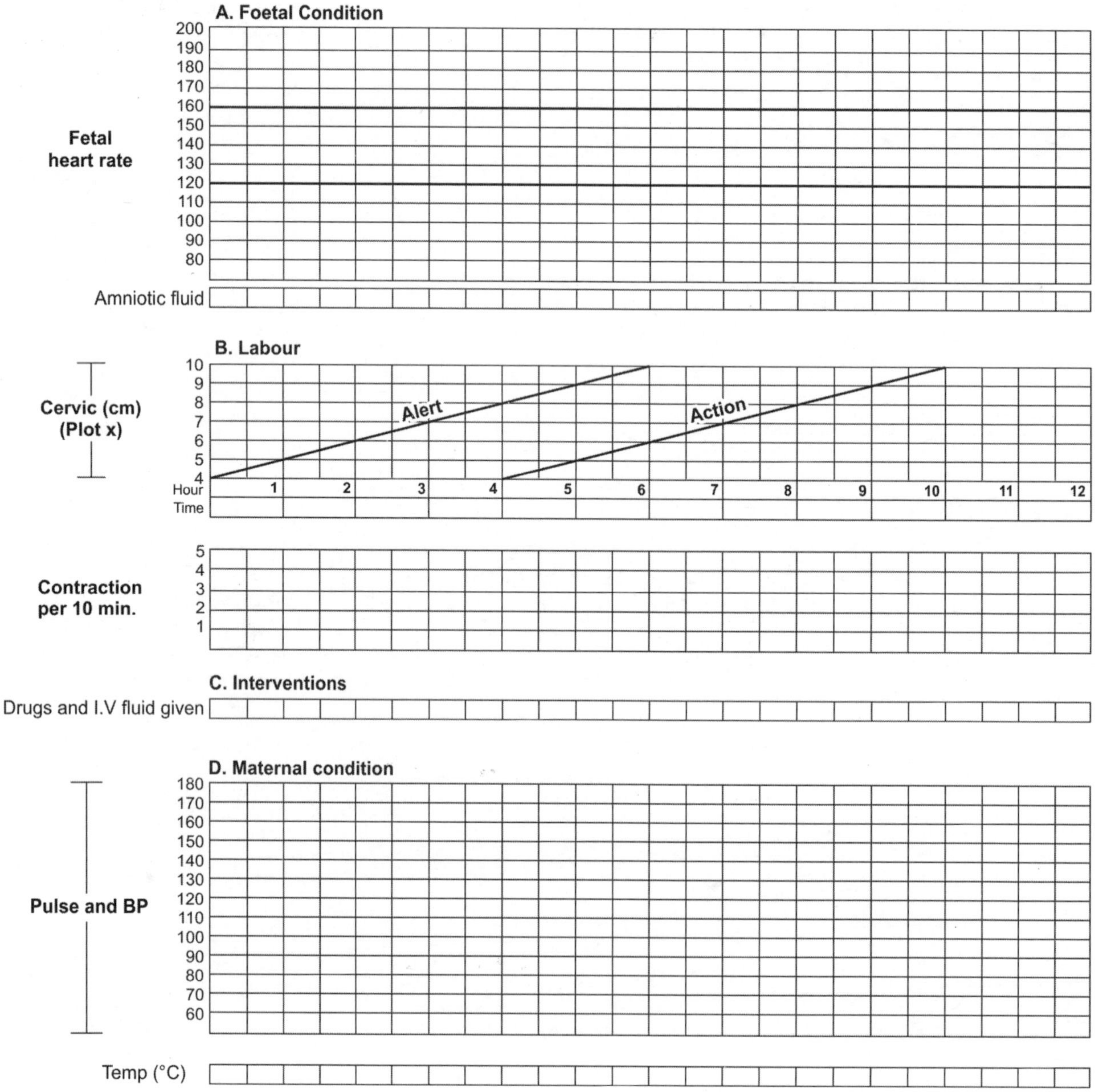

A. Foetal Condition

Fetal heart rate

200
190
180
170
160
150
140
130
120
110
100
90
80

Amniotic fluid

B. Labour

Cervic (cm) (Plot x)

10
9
8
7
6
5
4

Alert

Action

Hour	1	2	3	4	5	6	7	8	9	10	11	12
Time												

Contraction per 10 min.

5
4
3
2
1

C. Interventions

Drugs and I.V fluid given

D. Maternal condition

Pulse and BP

180
170
160
150
140
130
120
110
100
90
80
70
60

Temp (°C)

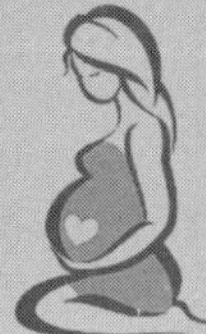

WHO Modified Partograph

Parity: *Reg No:* *Date and Time of Admission:* *Date and Time of ROM:*

Fetal heart rate	1	2	3	4	5	6	7	8	9	10	11	12
200												
190												
180												
170												
160												
150												
140												
130												
120												
110												
100												
90												
80												
Amniotic fluid												
Molding												

Cervix (cm): 10, 9, 8, 7, 6, 5, 4, 3, 2, 1, 0 — Alert — Action

Hours	1	2	3	4	5	6	7	8	9	10	11	12
Time												

Contractions per 10 Minutes												
5												
4												
3												
2												
1												
Oxytocin U/L												
Drops/Minutes												
Drugs given and IV Fluids												

Pulse • and Blood pressure ↕												
180												
170												
160												
150												
140												
130												
120												
110												
100												
90												
80												
70												
60												
Temperature °C												
Urine: Protein												
Urine: Acetone												
Urine: Volume												

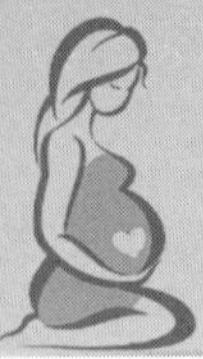

Delivery Note

Labor Progress Note Date and Time of Onset of Pain

Onset of true labor: On .... At: ....

Date and time of full cervix dilatation: .... Effacement: ....

Membrane ruptured (spontaneous/artificial/PROM) on .... At ....

Total duration of: 1st stage .... Hrs .... Min ....

2nd stage .... Hrs .... Min ....

3rd stage .... Hrs .... Min ....

Total hours = ... Hrs .... Min ....

Baby at Birth

Mode of delivery: .... Score at one minute ....

Baby born on:.. At: .... Sex: ....

Apgar scoring: .... Score at five minute .... Anus patent: ....

Initiation of breastfeeding: ....

Drug administration: ....

Delivery of Placenta and Membrane

Delivery of placenta on: .... At:......................... Cord insertion: ....

Spontaneous/helped/manually removed .... Examination of placenta: Complete/Incomplete ....

Weight of placenta:...

Cord length: .... Examination of membrane: ....

Blood Loss

Before delivery of placenta : ....

During delivery of placenta : ....

After delivery of placenta : ....

Perineum

Intact : .... Episiotomy : .... Laceration : .... Repair : ....

Condition of Mother Following Delivery

Pulse: .... BP: .... Uterus: .... Vaginal bleeding: .... Breastfeeding initiated at: ....

Condition of Mother on Transfer

Healthy/unhealthy (if unhealthy specify): ....

Condition of baby on transfer or discharge: ....

Nursing Care Plan

S.No.	Assessment	Nursing Diagnosis	Goal/Expected Out Come	Nursing Intervention	Rational	Implementation	Evaluation

Signature of Sister in Charge

Signature of Supervisor

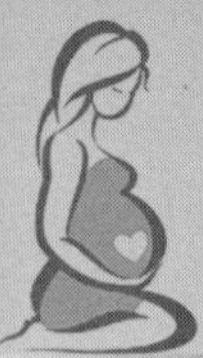

Conducted Normal Delivery (Case No. 11)

Client's Profile

Name : .... Religion : .... W/o : ....

Age : .... Education : .... Parity : ....

Hospital name : .... Occupation : .... LMP : ....

Date of booking : .... Income per month : .... EDD ....

Reg. No : .... Marriage duration : .... Period of gestation ....

Address : ....

....

Date and time of admission : ....

Date and time of discharge or transfer : ....

Admission Note

General Examinations

i. Temperature: .... iii. Respiration: ....

ii. Pulse: .... iv. BP: ....

Hydration: .... Anemia: (Present/absent) ....

Labor pain: (Present/absent)................................... Edema: (Generalized/ankle edema) ....

Abdominal Examination/Obstetrical Examination by Palpation

Height of uterus: .... cm Lie: .... Superficial grip: ....

Gestational weeks: .... Presentation: .... Deep pelvic grip: ....

Abdominal girth: ....cm Position of fetus: .... FHR: ....

Scar: .... Lateral grip: ....

Time/date of onset of contraction : ....

Uterine contraction: Present/absent/well contracted : ....

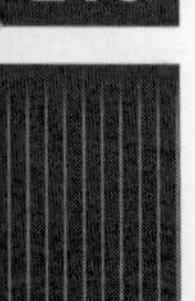

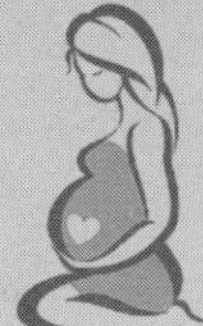

Investigation

Date	Hemoglobin	Blood Group/ Sugar	Urine		Bowel	Bladder	Any Other
			Albumin	Sugar			

Vaginal Examination

S.No	Date and time	Finding	Remark

Previous Obstetrical History

S.No	Year	Term/ preterm	Abortion/ stillbirth	Nature of delivery	Child		Immunization	Growth and development	Nature of puerperium	Remark
					Alive	Sex/ weight				

Admission History

Pregnancy complaints	
Menstrual history	
Medical history	
Surgical history	

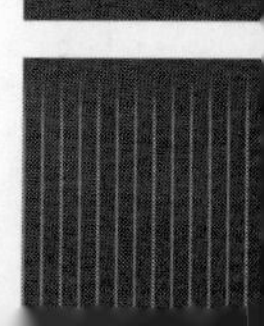

Old Pattern Partograph

Parity: *Reg No:* *Date and Time of Admission:* *Date and Time of ROM:*

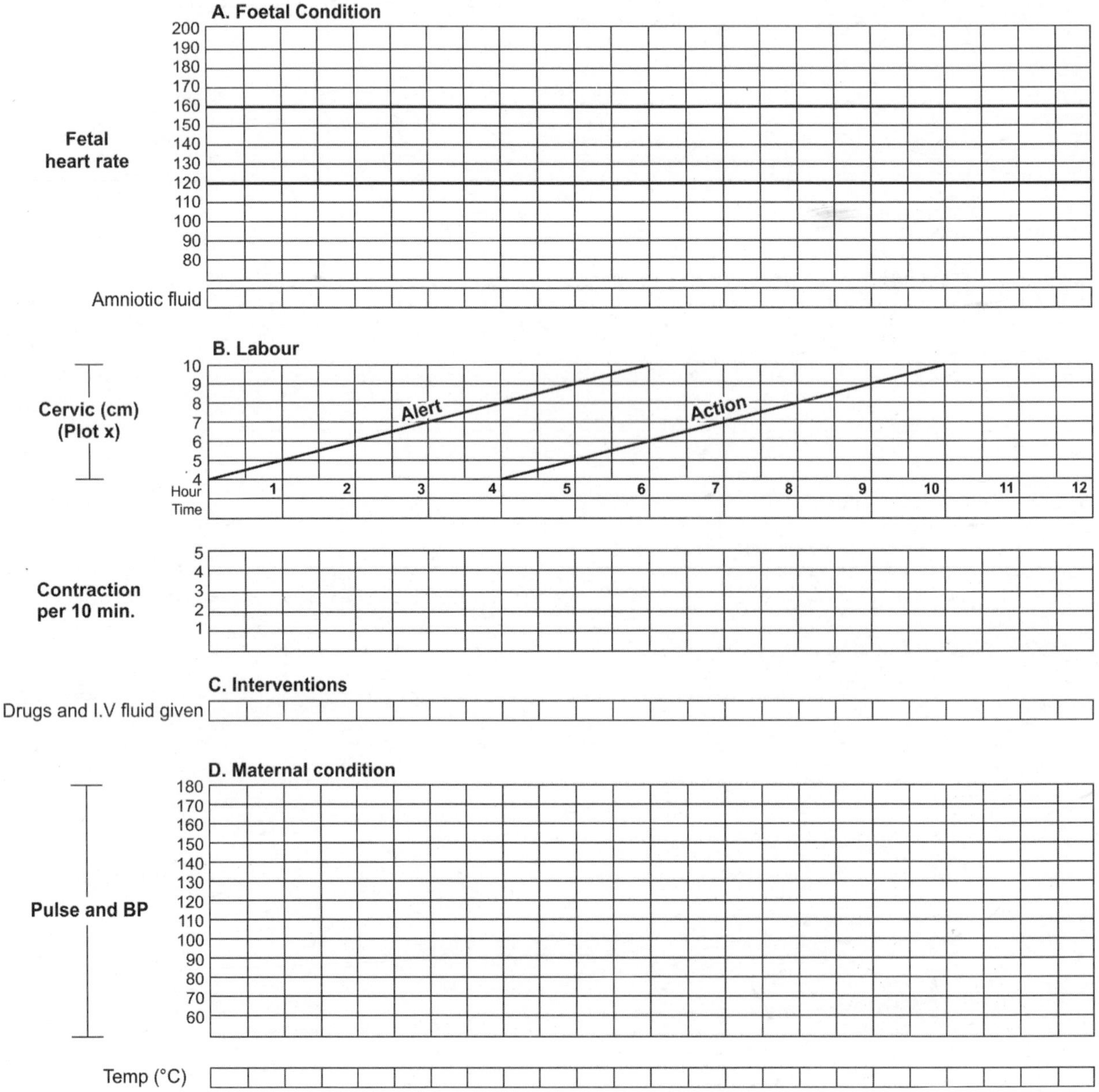

A. Foetal Condition

Fetal heart rate: 200, 190, 180, 170, 160, 150, 140, 130, 120, 110, 100, 90, 80

Amniotic fluid

B. Labour

Cervic (cm) (Plot x): 10, 9, 8, 7, 6, 5, 4

Alert

Action

Hour	1	2	3	4	5	6	7	8	9	10	11	12
Time												

Contraction per 10 min.: 5, 4, 3, 2, 1

C. Interventions

Drugs and I.V fluid given

D. Maternal condition

Pulse and BP: 180, 170, 160, 150, 140, 130, 120, 110, 100, 90, 80, 70, 60

Temp (°C)

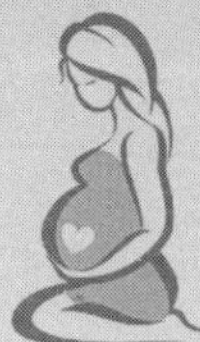

WHO Modified Partograph

Parity: *Reg No:* *Date and Time of Admission:* *Date and Time of ROM:*

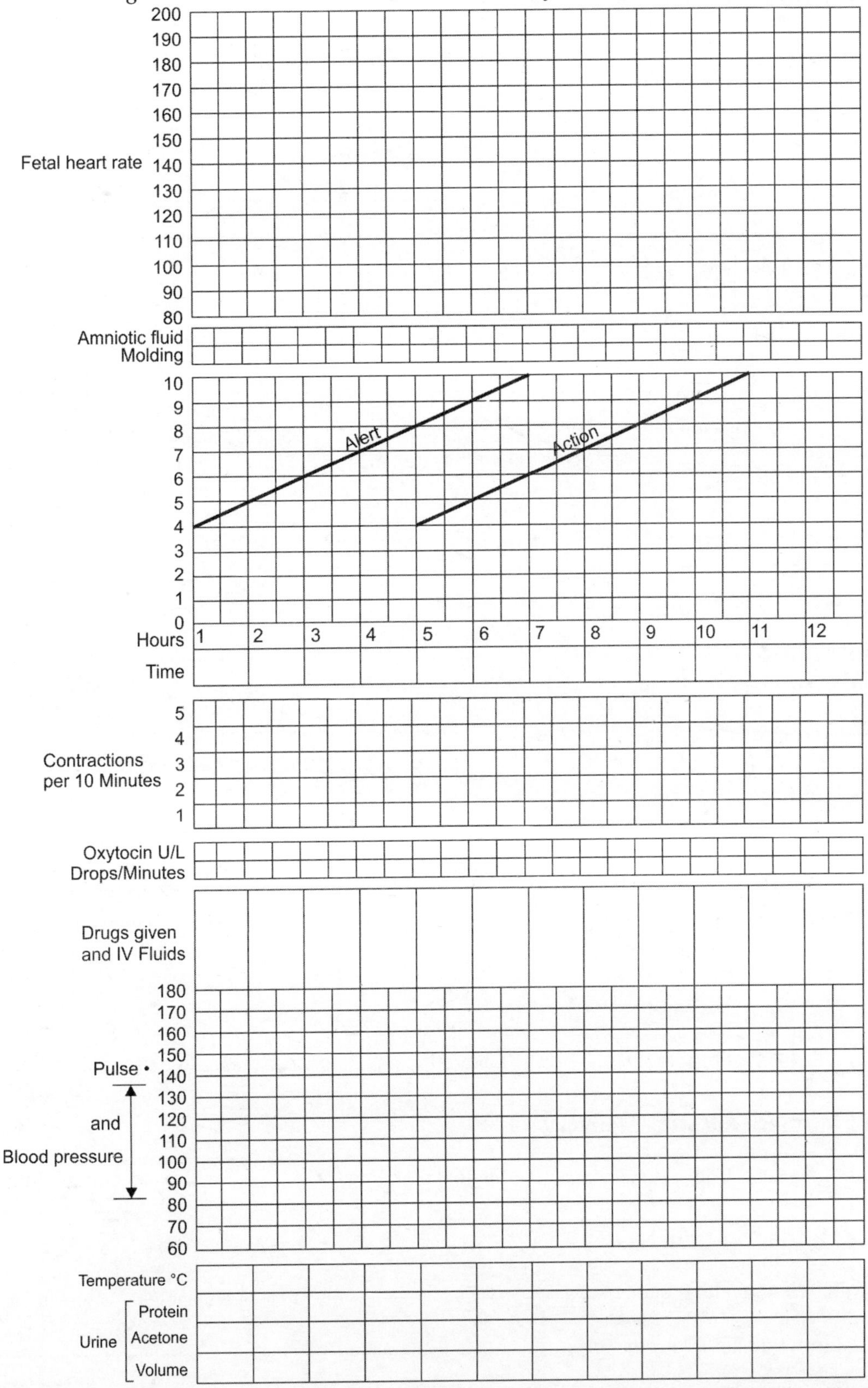

Fetal heart rate: 200, 190, 180, 170, 160, 150, 140, 130, 120, 110, 100, 90, 80

Amniotic fluid
Molding

10, 9, 8, 7, 6, 5, 4, 3, 2, 1, 0

Alert

Action

Hours: 1, 2, 3, 4, 5, 6, 7, 8, 9, 10, 11, 12

Time

Contractions per 10 Minutes: 5, 4, 3, 2, 1

Oxytocin U/L
Drops/Minutes

Drugs given and IV Fluids

Pulse • and Blood pressure: 180, 170, 160, 150, 140, 130, 120, 110, 100, 90, 80, 70, 60

Temperature °C

Urine: Protein, Acetone, Volume

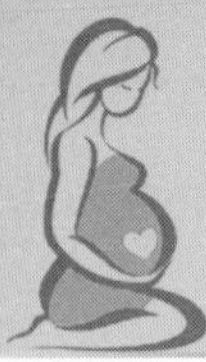

Delivery Note

Labor Progress Note Date and Time of Onset of Pain

Onset of true labor: On .... At: ....
Date and time of full cervix dilatation: .... Effacement: ....
Membrane ruptured (spontaneous/artificial/PROM) on .... At ....
Total duration of: 1st stage .... Hrs .... Min ....
2nd stage .... Hrs .... Min ....
3rd stage .... Hrs .... Min ....
Total hours = ... Hrs .... Min ....

Baby at Birth

Mode of delivery: .... Score at one minute ....
Baby born on:........................ At: .... Sex: ....
Apgar scoring: .... Score at five minute........................ Anus patent: ....
Initiation of breastfeeding: ....
Drug administration: ....

Delivery of Placenta and Membrane

Delivery of placenta on: .... At:........................ Cord insertion: ....
Spontaneous/helped/manually removed .... Examination of placenta: Complete/Incomplete ....
Weight of placenta:..
Cord length: .... Examination of membrane: ....

Blood Loss

Before delivery of placenta : ....
During delivery of placenta : ....
After delivery of placenta : ....

Perineum

Intact : .... Episiotomy : .... Laceration : .... Repair : ....

Condition of Mother Following Delivery

Pulse: .... BP: .... Uterus: .... Vaginal bleeding: .... Breastfeeding initiated at: ....

Condition of Mother on Transfer

Healthy/unhealthy (if unhealthy specify): ....

Condition of baby on transfer or discharge: ....

Nursing Care Plan

S.No.	Assessment	Nursing Diagnosis	Goal/Expected Out Come	Nursing Intervention	Rational	Implementation	Evaluation

Signature of Sister in Charge

Signature of Supervisor

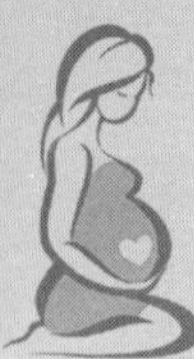

Conducted Normal Delivery (Case No. 12)

Client's Profile

Name : .... Religion : .... W/o : ....

Age : .... Education : .... Parity : ....

Hospital name : .... Occupation : .... LMP : ....

Date of booking : .... Income per month : .... EDD ....

Reg. No : .... Marriage duration : .... Period of gestation ....

Address : ....

....

Date and time of admission : ....

Date and time of discharge or transfer : ....

Admission Note

General Examinations

i. Temperature: .... iii. Respiration: ....

ii. Pulse: .... iv. BP: ....

Hydration: .... Anemia: (Present/absent) ....

Labor pain: (Present/absent).................................. Edema: (Generalized/ankle edema) ....

Abdominal Examination/Obstetrical Examination by Palpation

Height of uterus: .... cm Lie: .... Superficial grip: ....

Gestational weeks: .... Presentation: .... Deep pelvic grip: ....

Abdominal girth: ....cm Position of fetus: .... FHR: ....

Scar: .... Lateral grip: ....

Time/date of onset of contraction : ....

Uterine contraction: Present/absent/well contracted : ....

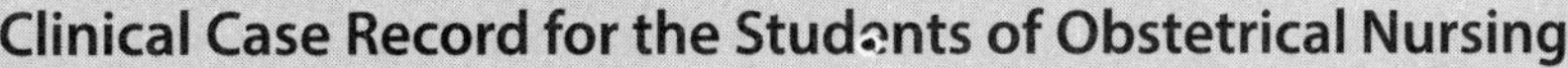
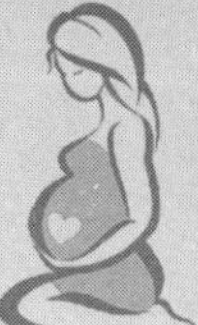

Investigation

Date	Hemoglobin	Blood Group/ Sugar	Urine		Bowel	Bladder	Any Other
			Albumin	Sugar			

Vaginal Examination

S.No	Date and time	Finding	Remark

Previous Obstetrical History

S.No	Year	Term/ preterm	Abortion/ stillbirth	Nature of delivery	Child		Immunization	Growth and development	Nature of puerperium	Remark
					Alive	Sex/ weight				

Admission History

Pregnancy complaints	
Menstrual history	
Medical history	
Surgical history	

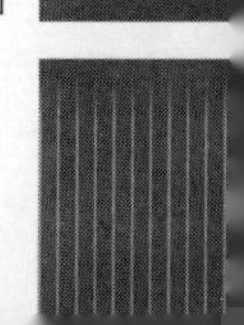

Old Pattern Partograph

Parity: *Reg No:* *Date and Time of Admission:* *Date and Time of ROM:*

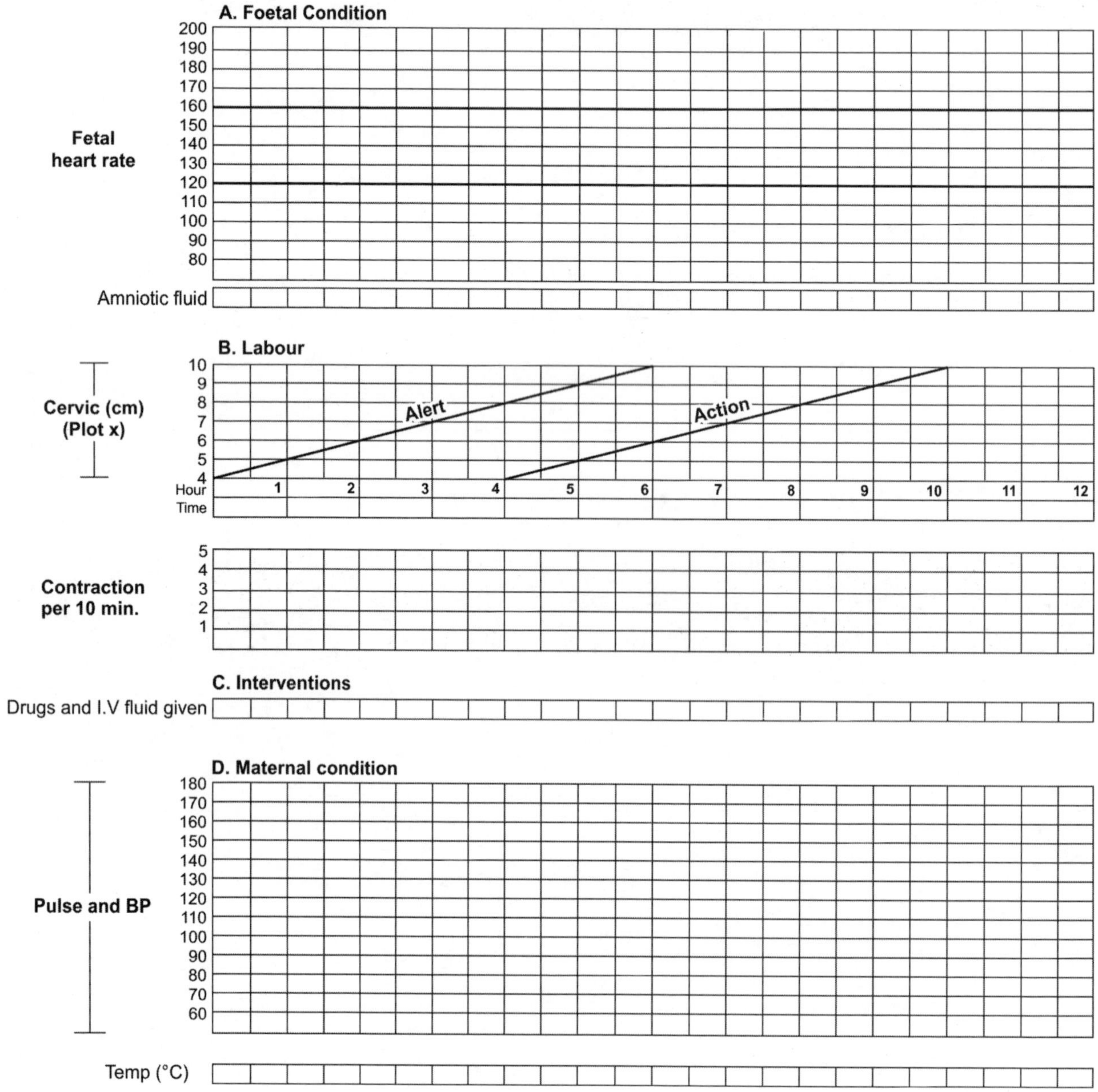

A. Foetal Condition

Fetal heart rate

200
190
180
170
160
150
140
130
120
110
100
90
80

Amniotic fluid

B. Labour

Cervic (cm) (Plot x)

10
9
8
7
6
5
4

Alert

Action

Hour	1	2	3	4	5	6	7	8	9	10	11	12
Time												

Contraction per 10 min.

5
4
3
2
1

C. Interventions

Drugs and I.V fluid given

D. Maternal condition

Pulse and BP

180
170
160
150
140
130
120
110
100
90
80
70
60

Temp (°C)

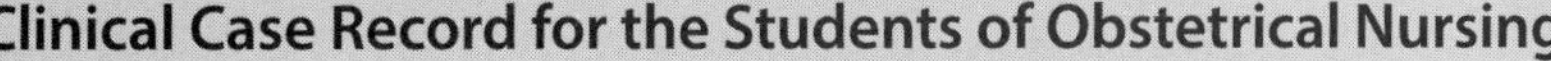

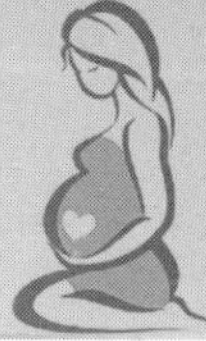

WHO Modified Partograph

Parity: *Reg No:* *Date and Time of Admission:* *Date and Time of ROM:*

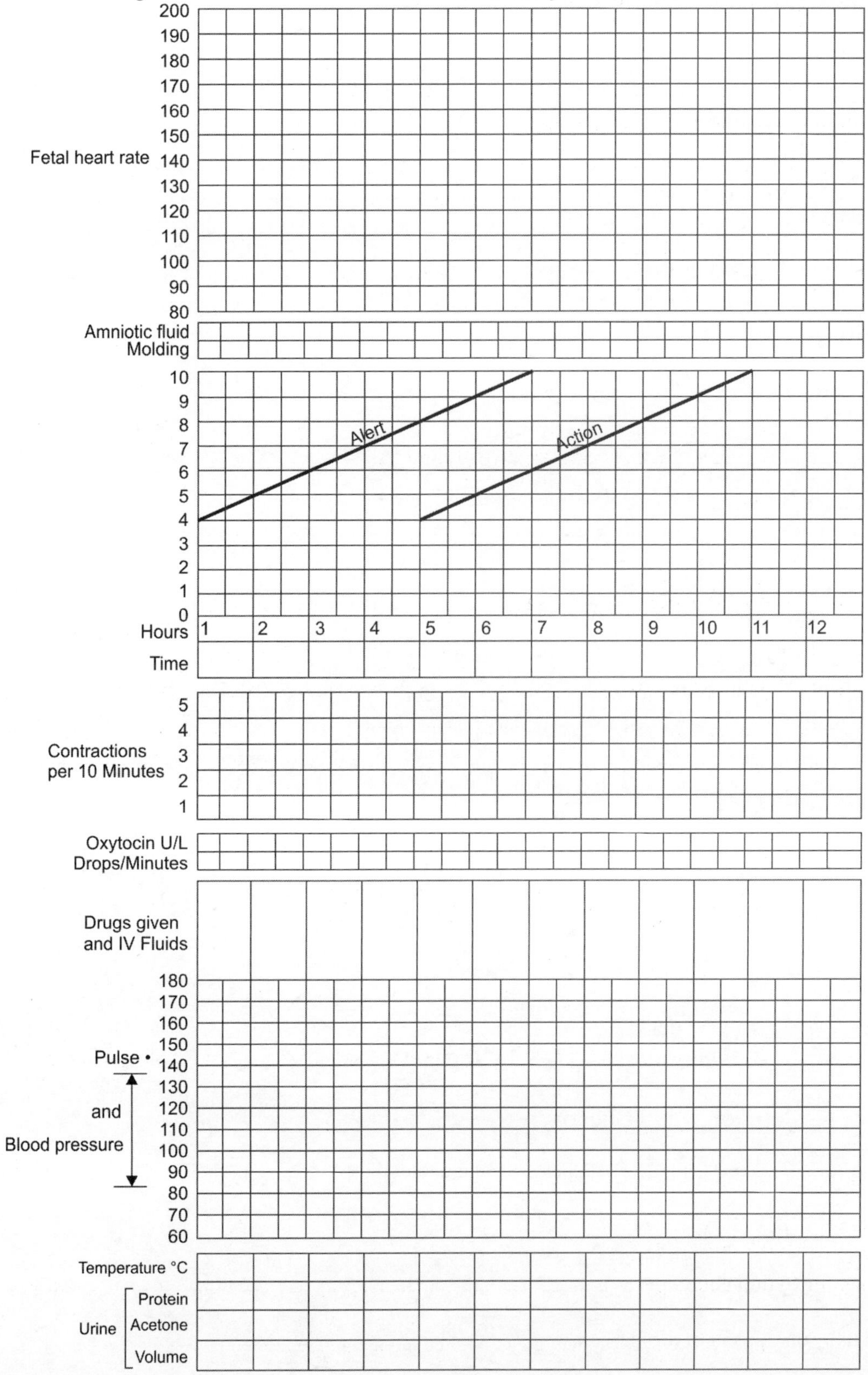

Fetal heart rate: 200, 190, 180, 170, 160, 150, 140, 130, 120, 110, 100, 90, 80

Amniotic fluid

Molding

Cervical dilatation: 10, 9, 8, 7, 6, 5, 4, 3, 2, 1, 0 (Alert line; Action line)

Hours: 1, 2, 3, 4, 5, 6, 7, 8, 9, 10, 11, 12

Time

Contractions per 10 Minutes: 5, 4, 3, 2, 1

Oxytocin U/L

Drops/Minutes

Drugs given and IV Fluids

Pulse • and Blood pressure ↕: 180, 170, 160, 150, 140, 130, 120, 110, 100, 90, 80, 70, 60

Temperature °C

Urine: Protein, Acetone, Volume

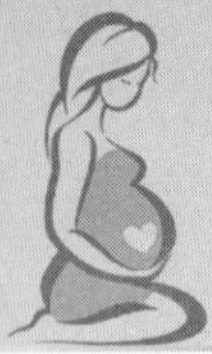

Delivery Note

Labor Progress Note Date and Time of Onset of Pain

Onset of true labor: On .... At: ....

Date and time of full cervix dilatation: .... Effacement: ....

Membrane ruptured (spontaneous/artificial/PROM) on .... At ....

Total duration of: 1st stage .... Hrs .... Min ....

2nd stage .... Hrs .... Min ....

3rd stage .... Hrs .... Min ....

Total hours = ... Hrs .... Min ....

Baby at Birth

Mode of delivery: .... Score at one minute ....

Baby born on:.. At: .... Sex: ....

Apgar scoring: .... Score at five minute.............................. Anus patent: ....

Initiation of breastfeeding: ....

Drug administration: ....

Delivery of Placenta and Membrane

Delivery of placenta on: .... At:.......................... Cord insertion: ....

Spontaneous/helped/manually removed .... Examination of placenta: Complete/Incomplete ....

Weight of placenta:..

Cord length: .... Examination of membrane: ....

Blood Loss

Before delivery of placenta : ....

During delivery of placenta : ....

After delivery of placenta : ....

Perineum

Intact : .... Episiotomy : .... Laceration : .... Repair : ....

Condition of Mother Following Delivery

Pulse: .... BP: .... Uterus: .... Vaginal bleeding: .... Breastfeeding initiated at: ....

Condition of Mother on Transfer

Healthy/unhealthy (if unhealthy specify): ....

Condition of baby on transfer or discharge: ....

Nursing Care Plan

S.No.	Assessment	Nursing Diagnosis	Goal/Expected Out Come	Nursing Intervention	Rational	Implementation	Evaluation

Signature of Sister in Charge

Signature of Supervisor

Conducted Normal Delivery (Case No. 13)

Client's Profile

Name : .... Religion : .... W/o : ....

Age : .... Education : .... Parity : ....

Hospital name : .... Occupation : .... LMP : ....

Date of booking : .... Income per month : .... EDD.................................

Reg. No : .... Marriage duration : .... Period of gestation ....

Address : ....

....

Date and time of admission : ....

Date and time of discharge or transfer : ....

Admission Note

General Examinations

i. Temperature: ....

ii. Pulse: ....

iii. Respiration: ....

iv. BP: ....

Hydration: ....

Anemia: (Present/absent) ....

Labor pain: (Present/absent).....................................

Edema: (Generalized/ankle edema) ....

Abdominal Examination/Obstetrical Examination by Palpation

Height of uterus: .... cm Lie: .... Superficial grip: ....

Gestational weeks: .... Presentation: .... Deep pelvic grip: ....

Abdominal girth: ....cm Position of fetus:... FHR: ....

Scar:.. Lateral grip: ....

Time/date of onset of contraction : ....

Uterine contraction: Present/absent/well contracted : ....

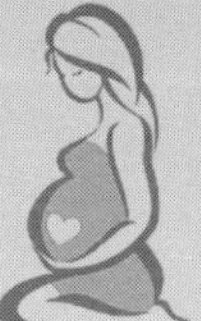

Investigation

Date	Hemoglobin	Blood Group/ Sugar	Urine		Bowel	Bladder	Any Other
			Albumin	Sugar			

Vaginal Examination

S.No	Date and time	Finding	Remark

Previous Obstetrical History

S.No	Year	Term/ preterm	Abortion/ stillbirth	Nature of delivery	Child		Immunization	Growth and development	Nature of puerperium	Remark
					Alive	Sex/ weight				

Admission History

Pregnancy complaints	
Menstrual history	
Medical history	
Surgical history	

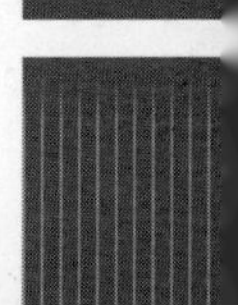

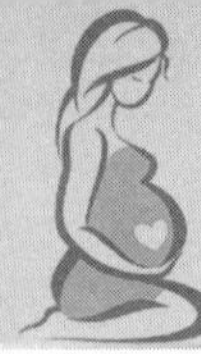

Old Pattern Partograph

Parity: *Reg No:* *Date and Time of Admission:* *Date and Time of ROM:*

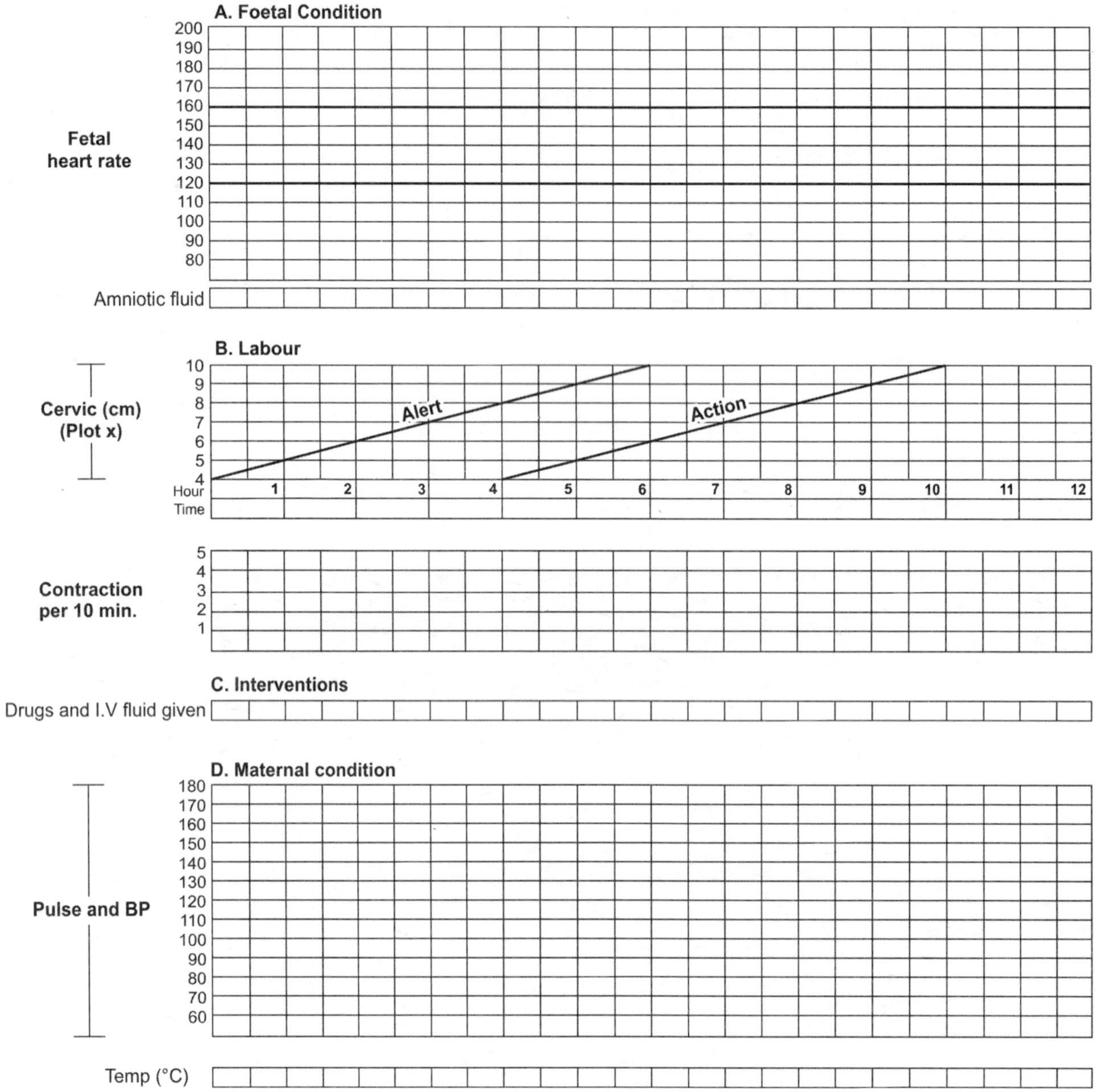

A. Foetal Condition

Fetal heart rate

200
190
180
170
160
150
140
130
120
110
100
90
80

Amniotic fluid

B. Labour

Cervic (cm) (Plot x)

10
9
8
7
6
5
4

Alert

Action

Hour 1 2 3 4 5 6 7 8 9 10 11 12

Time

Contraction per 10 min.

5
4
3
2
1

C. Interventions

Drugs and I.V fluid given

D. Maternal condition

Pulse and BP

180
170
160
150
140
130
120
110
100
90
80
70
60

Temp (°C)

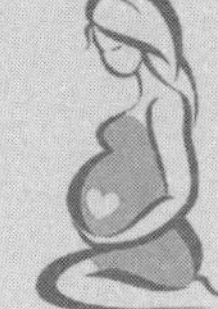

WHO Modified Partograph

Parity: *Reg No:* *Date and Time of Admission:* *Date and Time of ROM:*

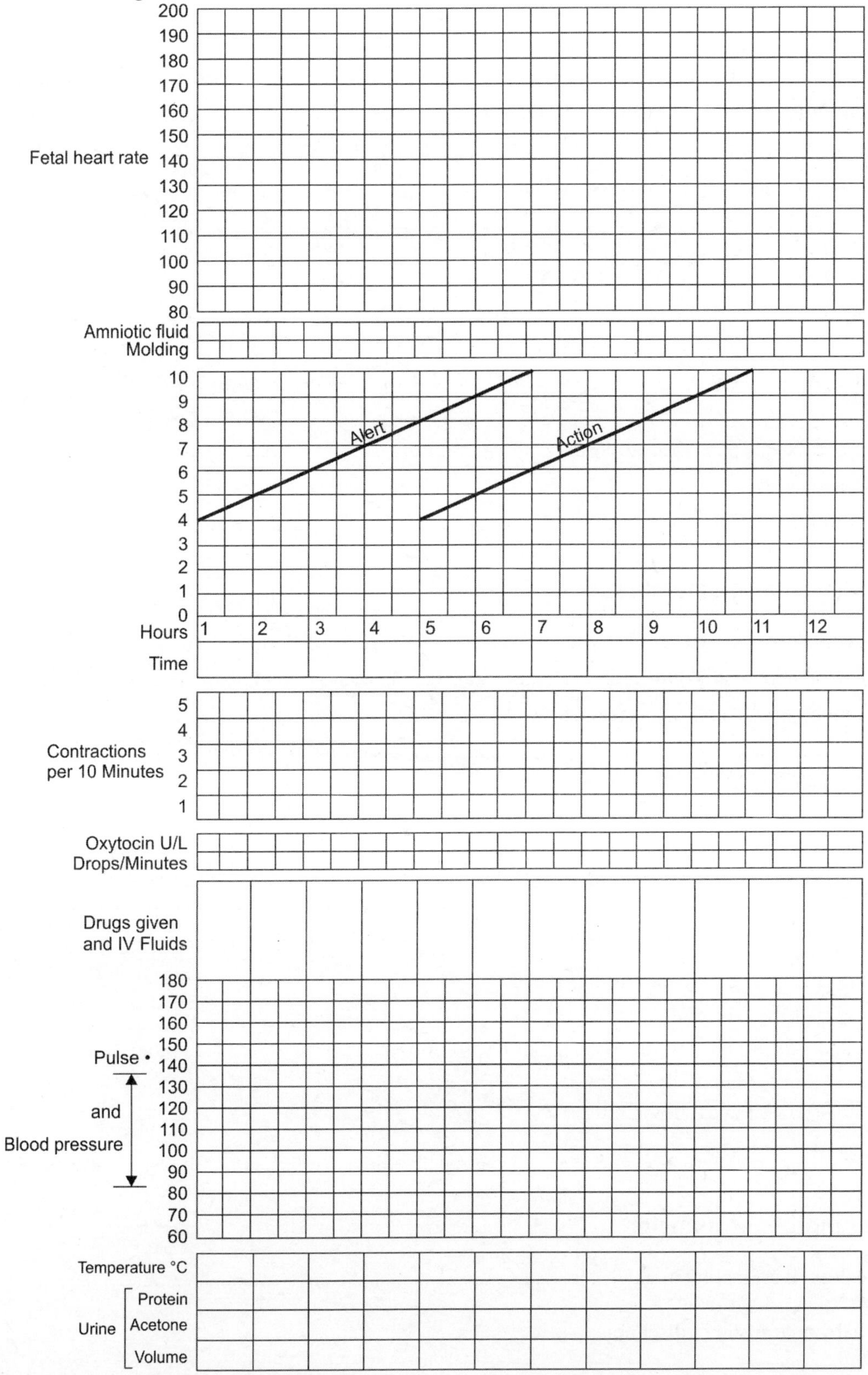

Fetal heart rate: 200, 190, 180, 170, 160, 150, 140, 130, 120, 110, 100, 90, 80

Amniotic fluid

Molding

10, 9, 8, 7, 6, 5, 4, 3, 2, 1, 0

Alert

Action

Hours	1	2	3	4	5	6	7	8	9	10	11	12
Time												

Contractions per 10 Minutes: 5, 4, 3, 2, 1

Oxytocin U/L

Drops/Minutes

Drugs given and IV Fluids

Pulse • and Blood pressure: 180, 170, 160, 150, 140, 130, 120, 110, 100, 90, 80, 70, 60

Temperature °C

Urine: Protein, Acetone, Volume

Delivery Note

Labor Progress Note Date and Time of Onset of Pain

Onset of true labor: On .... At: ....

Date and time of full cervix dilatation: .... Effacement: ....

Membrane ruptured (spontaneous/artificial/PROM) on .... At ....

Total duration of: 1st stage .... Hrs .... Min ....

2nd stage .... Hrs .... Min ....

3rd stage .... Hrs .... Min ....

Total hours = ... Hrs .... Min ....

Baby at Birth

Mode of delivery: .... Score at one minute ....

Baby born on:.................................... At: .... Sex: ....

Apgar scoring: .... Score at five minute................................ Anus patent: ....

Initiation of breastfeeding: ....

Drug administration: ....

Delivery of Placenta and Membrane

Delivery of placenta on: .... At:........................ Cord insertion: ....

Spontaneous/helped/manually removed .... Examination of placenta: Complete/Incomplete ....

Weight of placenta:..

Cord length: .... Examination of membrane: ....

Blood Loss

Before delivery of placenta : ....

During delivery of placenta : ....

After delivery of placenta : ....

Perineum

Intact : .... Episiotomy :............ Laceration :............................ Repair : ....

Condition of Mother Following Delivery

Pulse: .... BP: .... Uterus: .... Vaginal bleeding: .... Breastfeeding initiated at: ....

Condition of Mother on Transfer

Healthy/unhealthy (if unhealthy specify): ....

Condition of baby on transfer or discharge: ....

Nursing Care Plan

S.No.	Assessment	Nursing Diagnosis	Goal/Expected Out Come	Nursing Intervention	Rational	Implementation	Evaluation

Signature of Sister in Charge

Signature of Supervisor

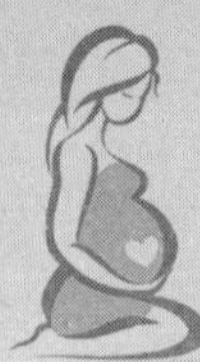

Conducted Normal Delivery (Case No. 14)

Client's Profile

Name : .... Religion : .... W/o : ....

Age : .... Education : .... Parity : ....

Hospital name : .... Occupation : .... LMP : ....

Date of booking : .... Income per month : .... EDD ....

Reg. No : .... Marriage duration : .... Period of gestation ....

Address : ....

....

Date and time of admission : ....

Date and time of discharge or transfer : ....

Admission Note

General Examinations

i. Temperature: ....

ii. Pulse: ....

iii. Respiration: ....

iv. BP: ....

Hydration: ....

Anemia: (Present/absent) ....

Labor pain: (Present/absent)....................................

Edema: (Generalized/ankle edema) ....

Abdominal Examination/Obstetrical Examination by Palpation

Height of uterus: .... cm Lie: .... Superficial grip: ....

Gestational weeks: .... Presentation: .... Deep pelvic grip: ....

Abdominal girth: ....cm Position of fetus: .... FHR: ....

Scar: .... Lateral grip: ....

Time/date of onset of contraction : ....

Uterine contraction: Present/absent/well contracted : ....

Investigation

Date	Hemoglobin	Blood Group/ Sugar	Urine		Bowel	Bladder	Any Other
			Albumin	Sugar			

Vaginal Examination

S.No	Date and time	Finding	Remark

Previous Obstetrical History

S.No	Year	Term/ preterm	Abortion/ stillbirth	Nature of delivery	Child		Immunization	Growth and development	Nature of puerperium	Remark
					Alive	Sex/ weight				

Admission History

Pregnancy complaints	
Menstrual history	
Medical history	
Surgical history	

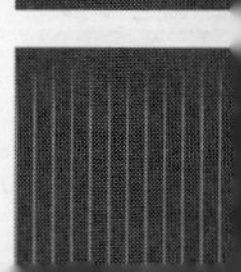

Old Pattern Partograph

Parity: *Reg No:* *Date and Time of Admission:* *Date and Time of ROM:*

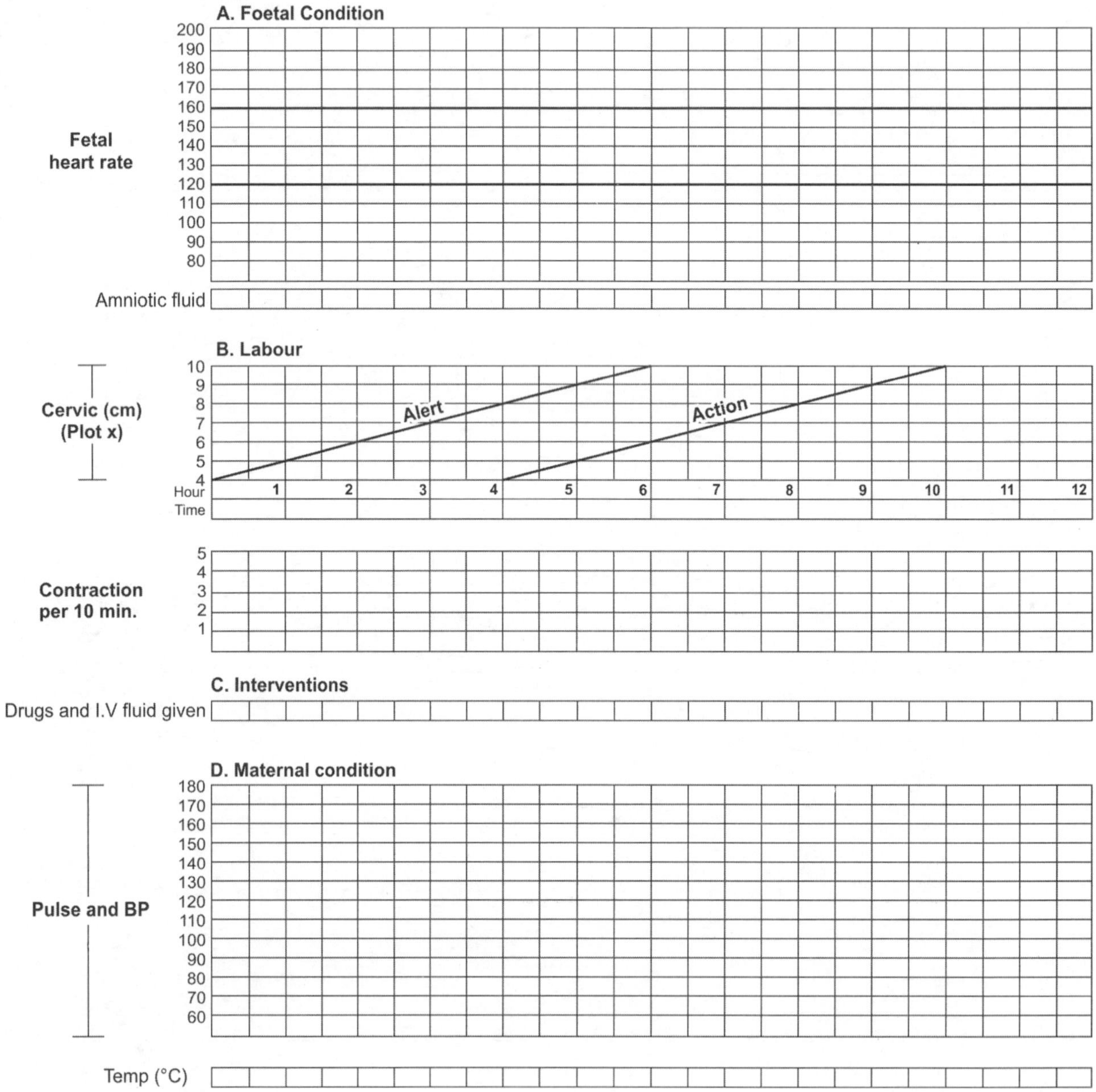

A. Foetal Condition

Fetal heart rate

200
190
180
170
160
150
140
130
120
110
100
90
80

Amniotic fluid

B. Labour

Cervic (cm) (Plot x)

10
9
8
7
6
5
4

Alert

Action

Hour	1	2	3	4	5	6	7	8	9	10	11	12
Time												

Contraction per 10 min.

5
4
3
2
1

C. Interventions

Drugs and I.V fluid given

D. Maternal condition

Pulse and BP

180
170
160
150
140
130
120
110
100
90
80
70
60

Temp (°C)

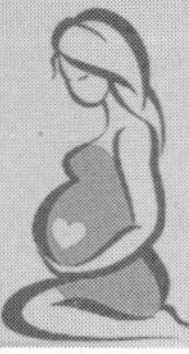

WHO Modified Partograph

Parity: *Reg No:* *Date and Time of Admission:* *Date and Time of ROM:*

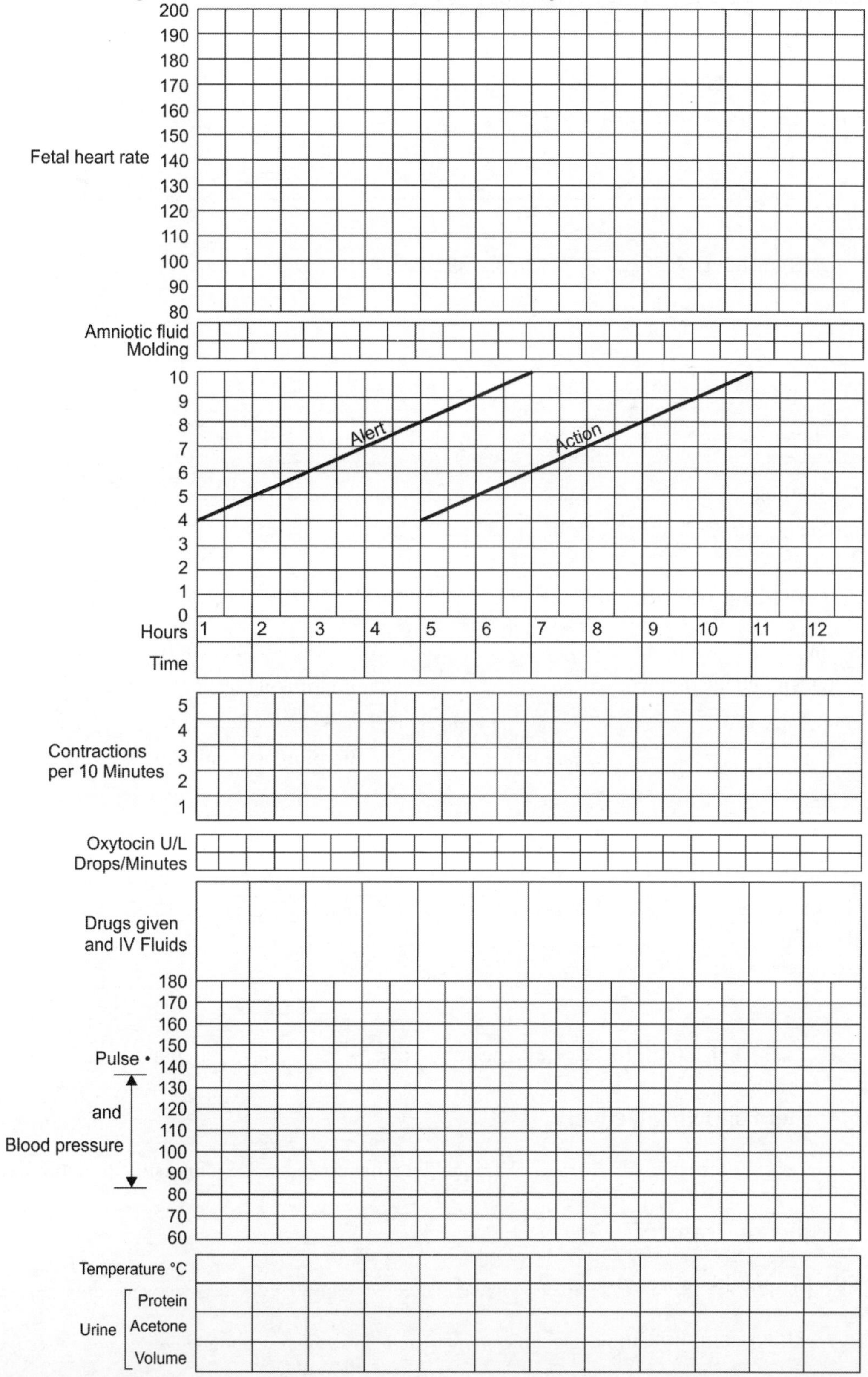

Fetal heart rate	
	200
	190
	180
	170
	160
	150
Fetal heart rate	140
	130
	120
	110
	100
	90
	80

Amniotic fluid
Molding

Cervical dilatation	
	10
	9
	8
	7
	6
	5
	4
	3
	2
	1
	0

Hours	1	2	3	4	5	6	7	8	9	10	11	12
Time												

Contractions per 10 Minutes	
	5
	4
	3
	2
	1

Oxytocin U/L
Drops/Minutes

Drugs given and IV Fluids

Pulse • and Blood pressure ↕	
	180
	170
	160
	150
	140
	130
	120
	110
	100
	90
	80
	70
	60

Temperature °C

Urine: Protein, Acetone, Volume

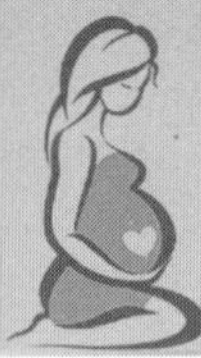

Delivery Note

Labor Progress Note Date and Time of Onset of Pain

Onset of true labor: On .... At: ....

Date and time of full cervix dilatation: .... Effacement: ....

Membrane ruptured (spontaneous/artificial/PROM) on .... At ....

Total duration of: 1st stage .... Hrs .... Min ....

2nd stage .... Hrs .... Min ....

3rd stage .... Hrs .... Min ....

Total hours = ... Hrs .... Min ....

Baby at Birth

Mode of delivery: .... Score at one minute ....

Baby born on:... At: .... Sex: ....

Apgar scoring: .... Score at five minute............................... Anus patent: ....

Initiation of breastfeeding: ....

Drug administration: ....

Delivery of Placenta and Membrane

Delivery of placenta on:.......................... At:.......................... Cord insertion: ....

Spontaneous/helped/manually removed .... Examination of placenta: Complete/Incomplete ....

Weight of placenta:...

Cord length:... Examination of membrane: ....

Blood Loss

Before delivery of placenta : ....

During delivery of placenta : ....

After delivery of placenta : ....

Perineum

Intact : .... Episiotomy :............ Laceration :.............................. Repair : ....

Condition of Mother Following Delivery

Pulse: .... BP: .... Uterus: .... Vaginal bleeding: .... Breastfeeding initiated at: ....

Condition of Mother on Transfer

Healthy/unhealthy (if unhealthy specify): ....

Condition of baby on transfer or discharge: ....

Nursing Care Plan

S.No.	Assessment	Nursing Diagnosis	Goal/Expected Out Come	Nursing Intervention	Rational	Implementation	Evaluation

Signature of Sister in Charge

Signature of Supervisor

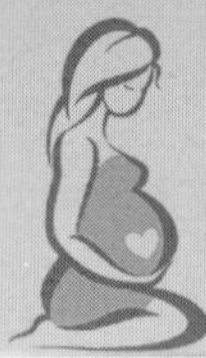

Conducted Normal Delivery (Case No. 15)

Client's Profile

Name : .... Religion : .... W/o : ....

Age : .... Education : .... Parity : ....

Hospital name : .... Occupation : .... LMP : ....

Date of booking : .... Income per month : .... EDD ....

Reg. No : .... Marriage duration : .... Period of gestation ....

Address : ....

....

Date and time of admission : ....

Date and time of discharge or transfer : ....

Admission Note

General Examinations

i. Temperature: .... iii. Respiration: ....

ii. Pulse: .... iv. BP: ....

Hydration: .... Anemia: (Present/absent) ....

Labor pain: (Present/absent)................................... Edema: (Generalized/ankle edema) ....

Abdominal Examination/Obstetrical Examination by Palpation

Height of uterus: .... cm Lie: .... Superficial grip: ....

Gestational weeks: .... Presentation: .... Deep pelvic grip: ....

Abdominal girth: ....cm Position of fetus: .... FHR: ....

Scar: .... Lateral grip: ....

Time/date of onset of contraction : ....

Uterine contraction: Present/absent/well contracted : ....

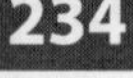

Investigation

Date	Hemoglobin	Blood Group/ Sugar	Urine		Bowel	Bladder	Any Other
			Albumin	Sugar			

Vaginal Examination

S.No	Date and time	Finding	Remark

Previous Obstetrical History

S.No	Year	Term/ preterm	Abortion/ stillbirth	Nature of delivery	Child		Immunization	Growth and development	Nature of puerperium	Remark
					Alive	Sex/ weight				

Admission History

Pregnancy complaints	
Menstrual history	
Medical history	
Surgical history	

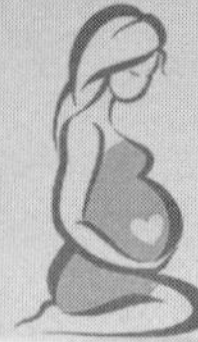

Old Pattern Partograph

Parity: *Reg No:* *Date and Time of Admission:* *Date and Time of ROM:*

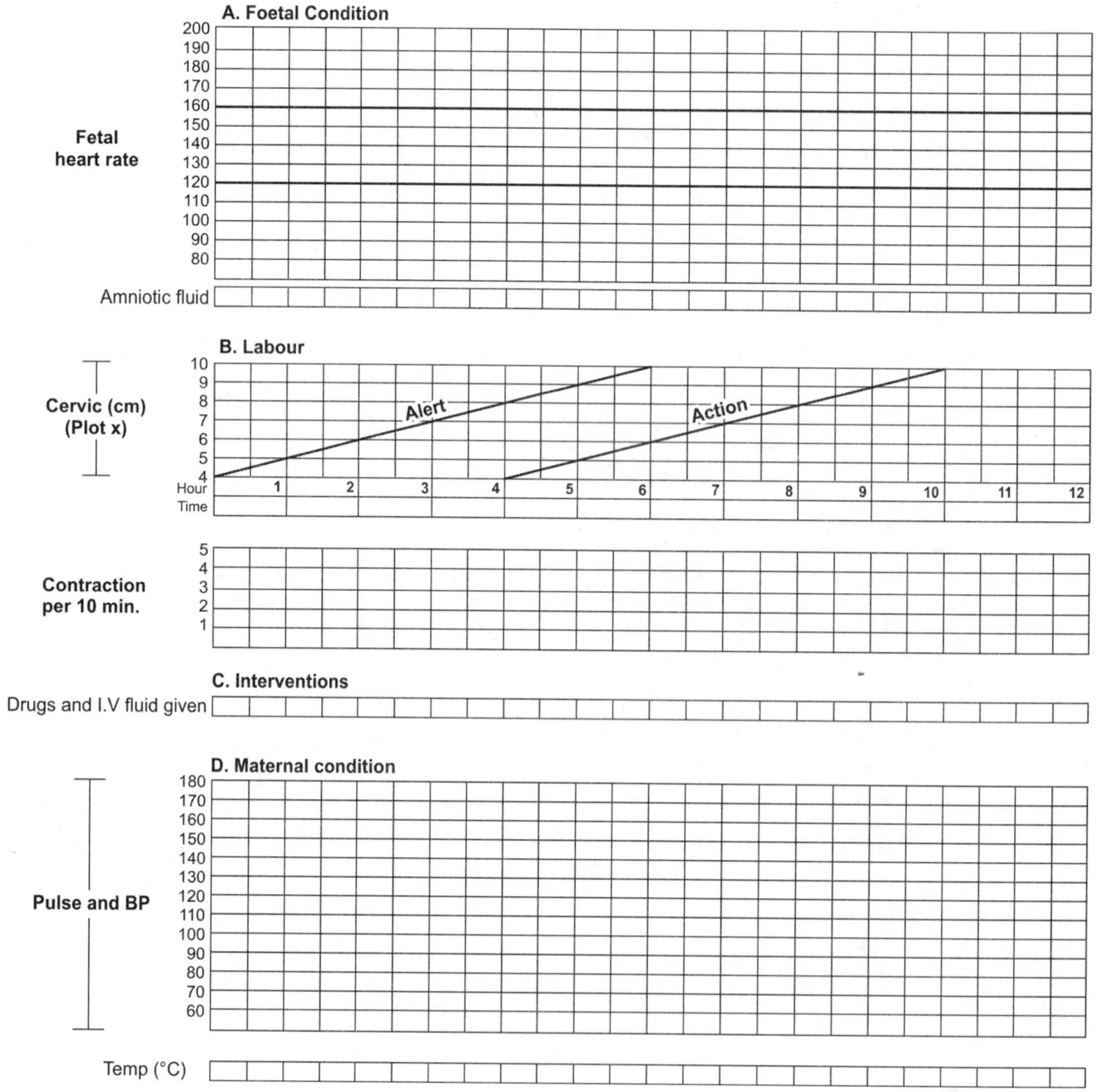

A. Foetal Condition

Fetal heart rate

200
190
180
170
160
150
140
130
120
110
100
90
80

Amniotic fluid

B. Labour

Cervic (cm) (Plot x)

10
9
8
7
6
5
4

Alert

Action

Hour: 1 2 3 4 5 6 7 8 9 10 11 12

Time

Contraction per 10 min.

5
4
3
2
1

C. Interventions

Drugs and I.V fluid given

D. Maternal condition

Pulse and BP

180
170
160
150
140
130
120
110
100
90
80
70
60

Temp (°C)

WHO Modified Partograph

Parity: *Reg No:* *Date and Time of Admission:* *Date and Time of ROM:*

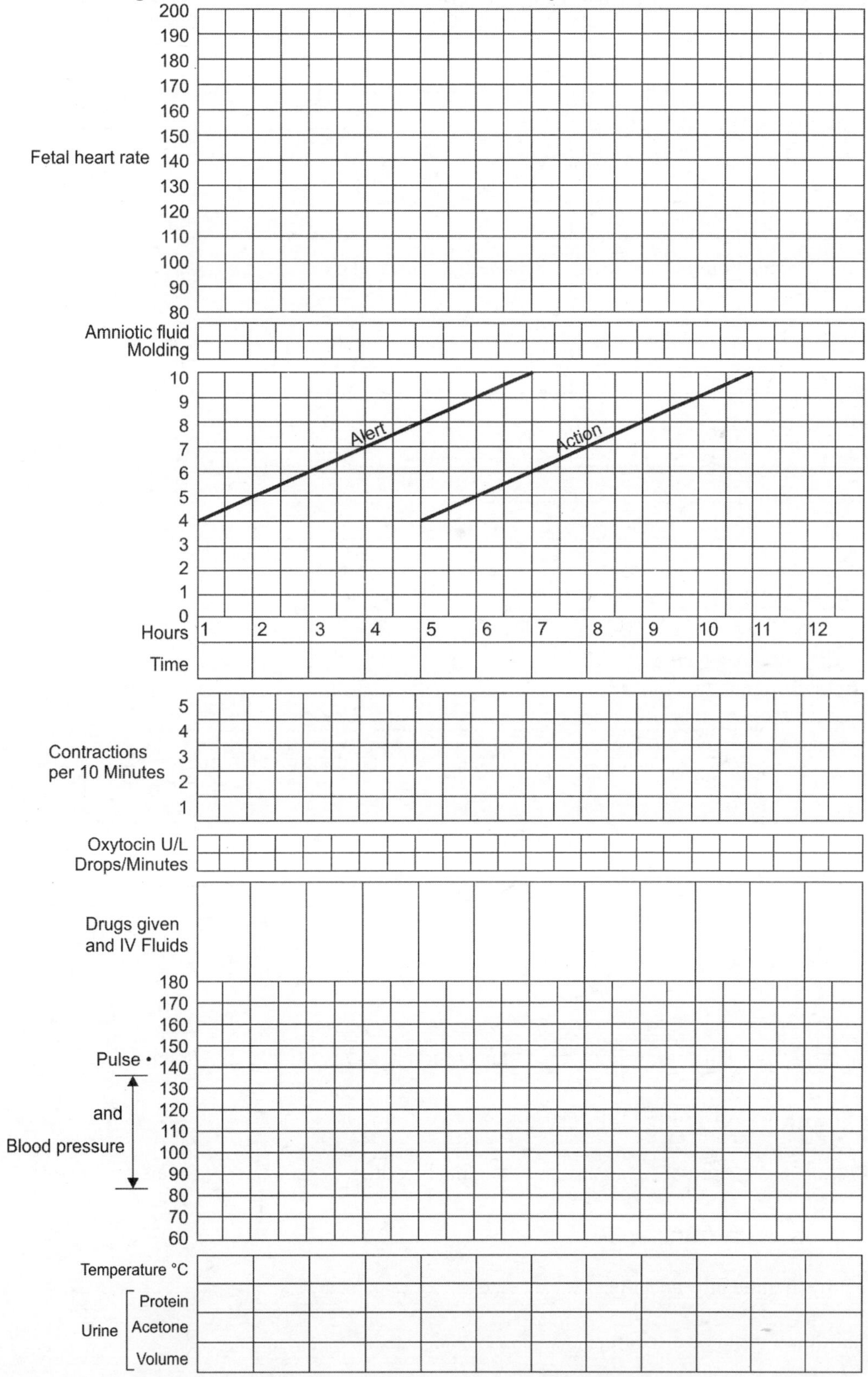

Fetal heart rate: 200, 190, 180, 170, 160, 150, 140, 130, 120, 110, 100, 90, 80

Amniotic fluid

Molding

Cervical dilatation: 10, 9, 8, 7, 6, 5, 4, 3, 2, 1, 0

Alert

Action

Hours	1	2	3	4	5	6	7	8	9	10	11	12
Time												

Contractions per 10 Minutes: 5, 4, 3, 2, 1

Oxytocin U/L

Drops/Minutes

Drugs given and IV Fluids

Pulse • and Blood pressure: 180, 170, 160, 150, 140, 130, 120, 110, 100, 90, 80, 70, 60

Temperature °C

Urine: Protein, Acetone, Volume

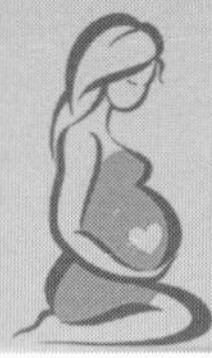

Delivery Note

Labor Progress Note Date and Time of Onset of Pain

Onset of true labor: On .... At: ....

Date and time of full cervix dilatation: .... Effacement: ....

Membrane ruptured (spontaneous/artificial/PROM) on .... At ....

Total duration of: 1st stage .... Hrs .... Min ....

2nd stage .... Hrs .... Min ....

3rd stage .... Hrs .... Min ....

Total hours = ... Hrs .... Min ....

Baby at Birth

Mode of delivery: .... Score at one minute ....

Baby born on: .... At: .... Sex: ....

Apgar scoring: .... Score at five minute .... Anus patent: ....

Initiation of breastfeeding: ....

Drug administration: ....

Delivery of Placenta and Membrane

Delivery of placenta on: .... At: .... Cord insertion: ....

Spontaneous/helped/manually removed .... Examination of placenta: Complete/Incomplete ....

Weight of placenta: ....

Cord length: .... Examination of membrane: ....

Blood Loss

Before delivery of placenta : ....

During delivery of placenta : ....

After delivery of placenta : ....

Perineum

Intact : .... Episiotomy : .... Laceration : .... Repair : ....

Condition of Mother Following Delivery

Pulse: .... BP: .... Uterus: .... Vaginal bleeding: .... Breastfeeding initiated at: ....

Condition of Mother on Transfer

Healthy/unhealthy (if unhealthy specify): ....

Condition of baby on transfer or discharge: ....

Nursing Care Plan

S.No.	Assessment	Nursing Diagnosis	Goal/Expected Out Come	Nursing Intervention	Rational	Implementation	Evaluation

Signature of Sister in Charge

Signature of Supervisor

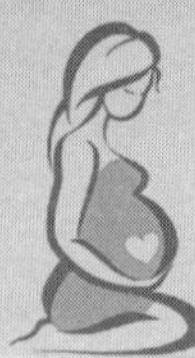

Conducted Normal Delivery (Case No. 16)

Client's Profile

Name : .... Religion : .... W/o : ....

Age : .... Education : .... Parity : ....

Hospital name : .... Occupation : .... LMP : ....

Date of booking : .... Income per month : .... EDD ....

Reg. No : .... Marriage duration : .... Period of gestation ....

Address : ....

....

Date and time of admission : ....

Date and time of discharge or transfer : ....

Admission Note

General Examinations

i. Temperature: ....

iii. Respiration: ....

ii. Pulse: ....

iv. BP: ....

Hydration: ....

Anemia: (Present/absent) ....

Labor pain: (Present/absent)..................................

Edema: (Generalized/ankle edema) ....

Abdominal Examination/Obstetrical Examination by Palpation

Height of uterus: .... cm Lie: .... Superficial grip: ....

Gestational weeks: .... Presentation: .... Deep pelvic grip: ....

Abdominal girth: ....cm Position of fetus: .... FHR: ....

Scar: .... Lateral grip: ....

Time/date of onset of contraction : ....

Uterine contraction: Present/absent/well contracted : ....

Investigation

Date	Hemoglobin	Blood Group/ Sugar	Urine		Bowel	Bladder	Any Other
			Albumin	Sugar			

Vaginal Examination

S.No	Date and time	Finding	Remark

Previous Obstetrical History

S.No	Year	Term/ preterm	Abortion/ stillbirth	Nature of delivery	Child		Immunization	Growth and development	Nature of puerperium	Remark
					Alive	Sex/ weight				

Admission History

Pregnancy complaints	
Menstrual history	
Medical history	
Surgical history	

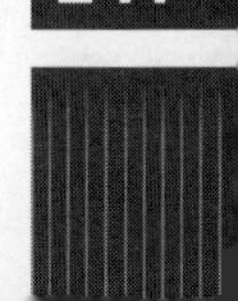

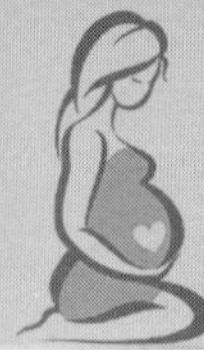

Old Pattern Partograph

Parity: *Reg No:* *Date and Time of Admission:* *Date and Time of ROM:*

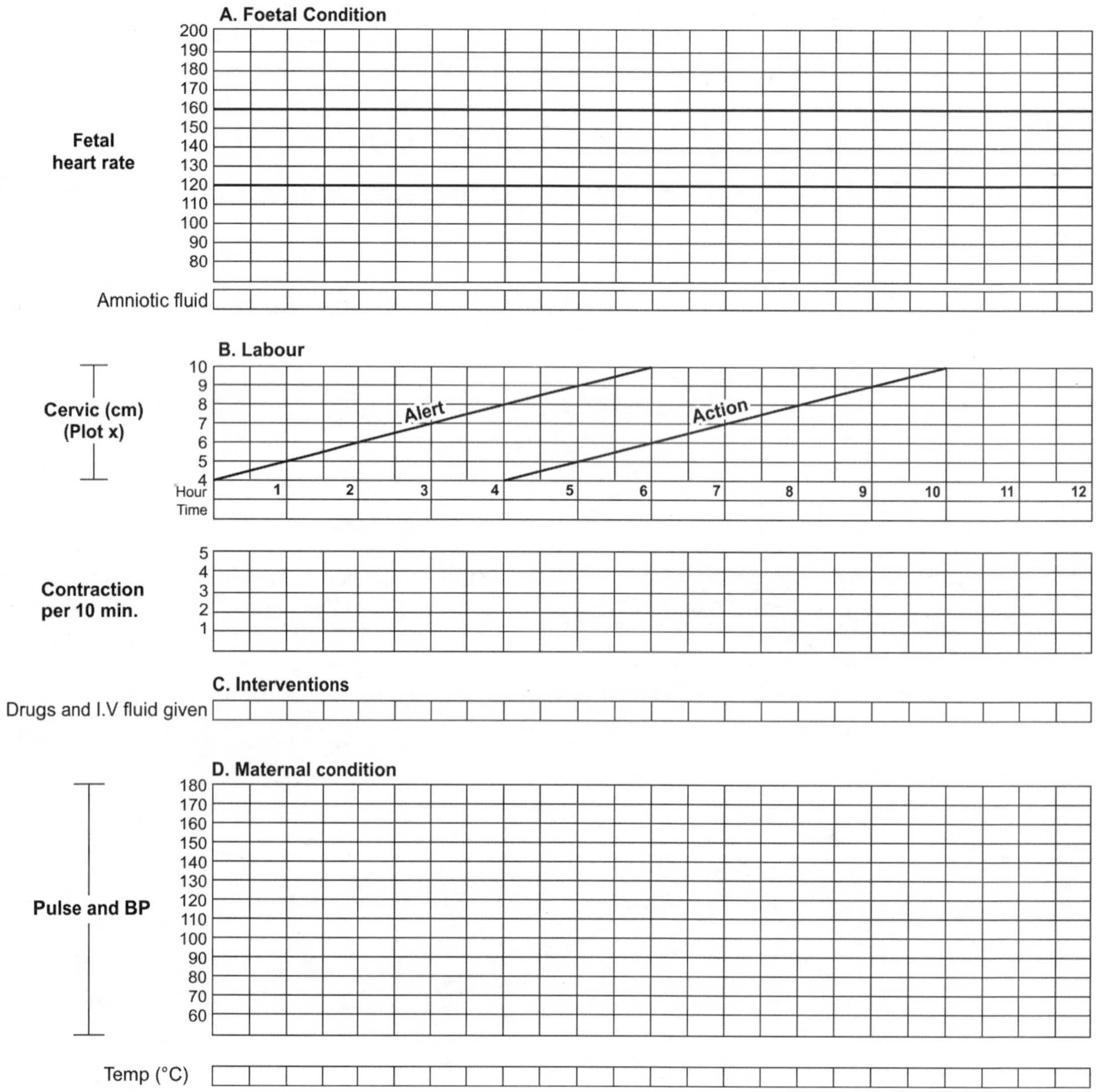

A. Foetal Condition

Fetal heart rate

200
190
180
170
160
150
140
130
120
110
100
90
80

Amniotic fluid

B. Labour

Cervic (cm) (Plot x)

10
9
8
7
6
5
4

Alert

Action

Hour 1 2 3 4 5 6 7 8 9 10 11 12

Time

Contraction per 10 min.

5
4
3
2
1

C. Interventions

Drugs and I.V fluid given

D. Maternal condition

Pulse and BP

180
170
160
150
140
130
120
110
100
90
80
70
60

Temp (°C)

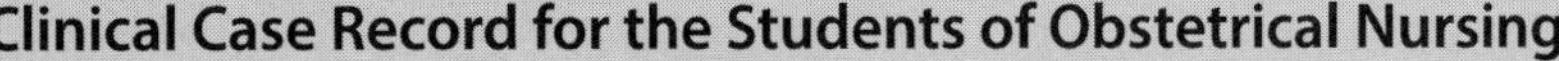

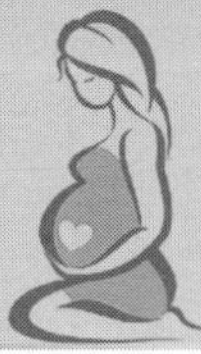

WHO Modified Partograph

Parity: *Reg No:* *Date and Time of Admission:* *Date and Time of ROM:*

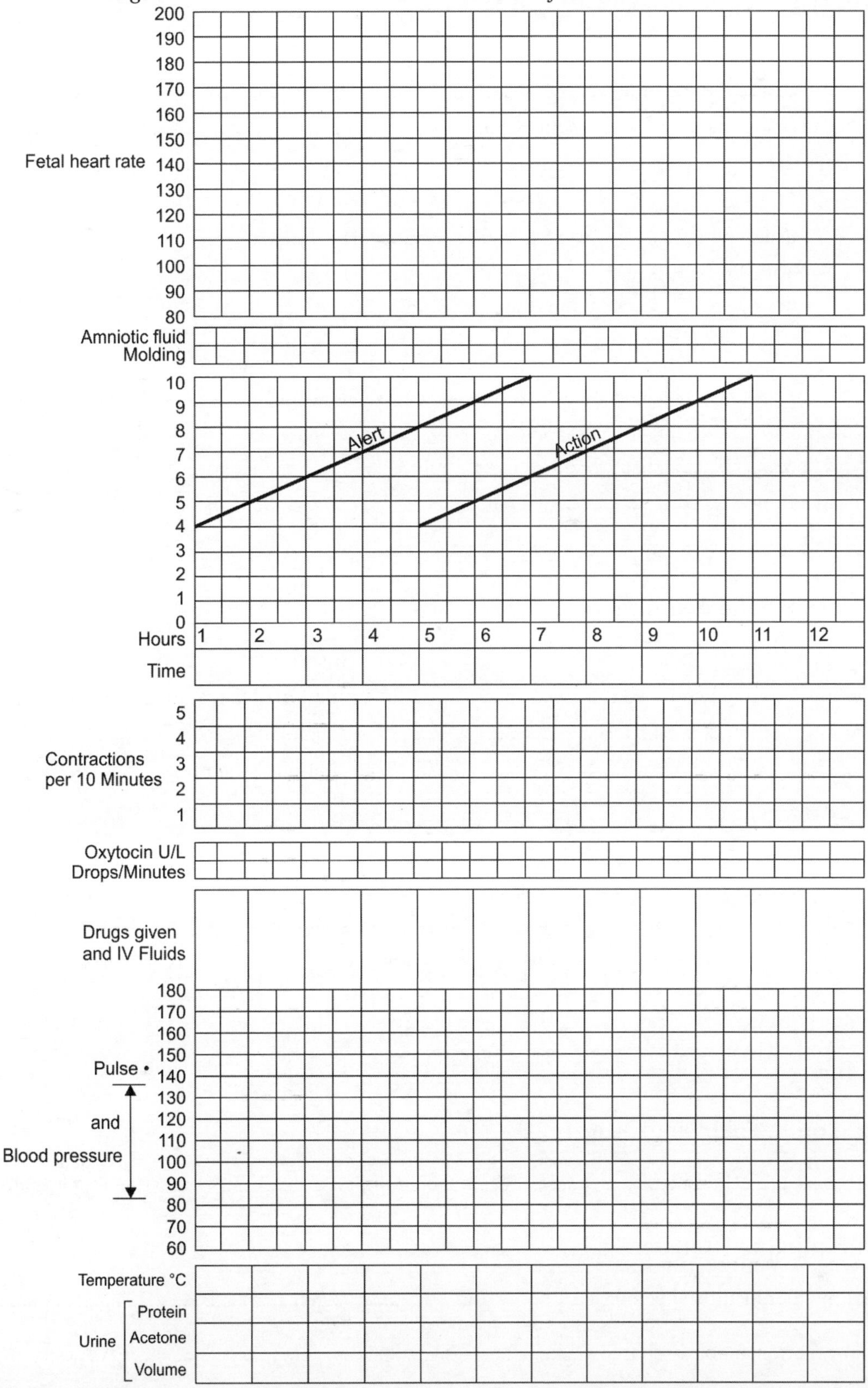

Fetal heart rate: 200, 190, 180, 170, 160, 150, 140, 130, 120, 110, 100, 90, 80

Amniotic fluid

Molding

10, 9, 8, 7, 6, 5, 4, 3, 2, 1, 0

Alert

Action

Hours	1	2	3	4	5	6	7	8	9	10	11	12
Time												

Contractions per 10 Minutes: 5, 4, 3, 2, 1

Oxytocin U/L

Drops/Minutes

Drugs given and IV Fluids

Pulse • and Blood pressure: 180, 170, 160, 150, 140, 130, 120, 110, 100, 90, 80, 70, 60

Temperature °C

Urine: Protein, Acetone, Volume

Delivery Note

Labor Progress Note Date and Time of Onset of Pain

Onset of true labor: On .... At: ....

Date and time of full cervix dilatation: .... Effacement: ....

Membrane ruptured (spontaneous/artificial/PROM) on .... At ....

Total duration of: 1st stage .... Hrs .... Min ....

2nd stage .... Hrs .... Min ....

3rd stage .... Hrs .... Min ....

Total hours = ... Hrs .... Min ....

Baby at Birth

Mode of delivery: .... Score at one minute ....

Baby born on:............................. At: .... Sex: ....

Apgar scoring: .... Score at five minute............................. Anus patent: ....

Initiation of breastfeeding: ....

Drug administration: ....

Delivery of Placenta and Membrane

Delivery of placenta on: .... At:............................. Cord insertion: ....

Spontaneous/helped/manually removed .... Examination of placenta: Complete/Incomplete ....

Weight of placenta:...

Cord length: .... Examination of membrane: ....

Blood Loss

Before delivery of placenta : ....

During delivery of placenta : ....

After delivery of placenta : ....

Perineum

Intact : .... Episiotomy : .... Laceration : .... Repair : ....

Condition of Mother Following Delivery

Pulse: .... BP: .... Uterus: .... Vaginal bleeding: .... Breastfeeding initiated at: ....

Condition of Mother on Transfer

Healthy/unhealthy (if unhealthy specify): ....

Condition of baby on transfer or discharge: ....

Nursing Care Plan

S.No.		Assessment	Nursing Diagnosis	Goal/Expected Out Come	Nursing Intervention	Rational	Implementation	Evaluation

Signature of Sister in Charge

Signature of Supervisor

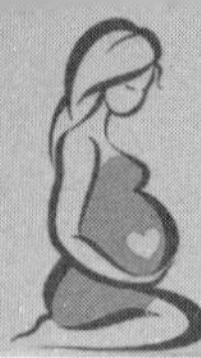

Conducted Normal Delivery (Case No. 17)

Client's Profile

Name : .... Religion : .... W/o : ....

Age : .... Education : .... Parity : ....

Hospital name : .... Occupation : .... LMP : ....

Date of booking : .... Income per month : .... EDD ....

Reg. No : .... Marriage duration : .... Period of gestation ....

Address : ....

....

Date and time of admission : ....

Date and time of discharge or transfer : ....

Admission Note

General Examinations

i. Temperature: .... iii. Respiration: ....

ii. Pulse: .... iv. BP: ....

Hydration: .... Anemia: (Present/absent) ....

Labor pain: (Present/absent)................................. Edema: (Generalized/ankle edema) ....

Abdominal Examination/Obstetrical Examination by Palpation

Height of uterus: .... cm Lie: .... Superficial grip: ....

Gestational weeks: .... Presentation: .... Deep pelvic grip: ....

Abdominal girth: ....cm Position of fetus: .... FHR: ....

Scar: .... Lateral grip: ....

Time/date of onset of contraction : ....

Uterine contraction: Present/absent/well contracted : ....

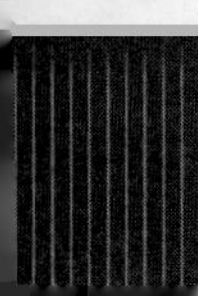

Investigation

Date	Hemoglobin	Blood Group/ Sugar	Urine		Bowel	Bladder	Any Other
			Albumin	Sugar			

Vaginal Examination

S.No	Date and time	Finding	Remark

Previous Obstetrical History

S.No	Year	Term/ preterm	Abortion/ stillbirth	Nature of delivery	Child		Immunization	Growth and development	Nature of puerperium	Remark
					Alive	Sex/ weight				

Admission History

Pregnancy complaints	
Menstrual history	
Medical history	
Surgical history	

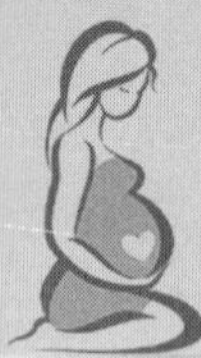

Old Pattern Partograph

Parity: *Reg No:* *Date and Time of Admission:* *Date and Time of ROM:*

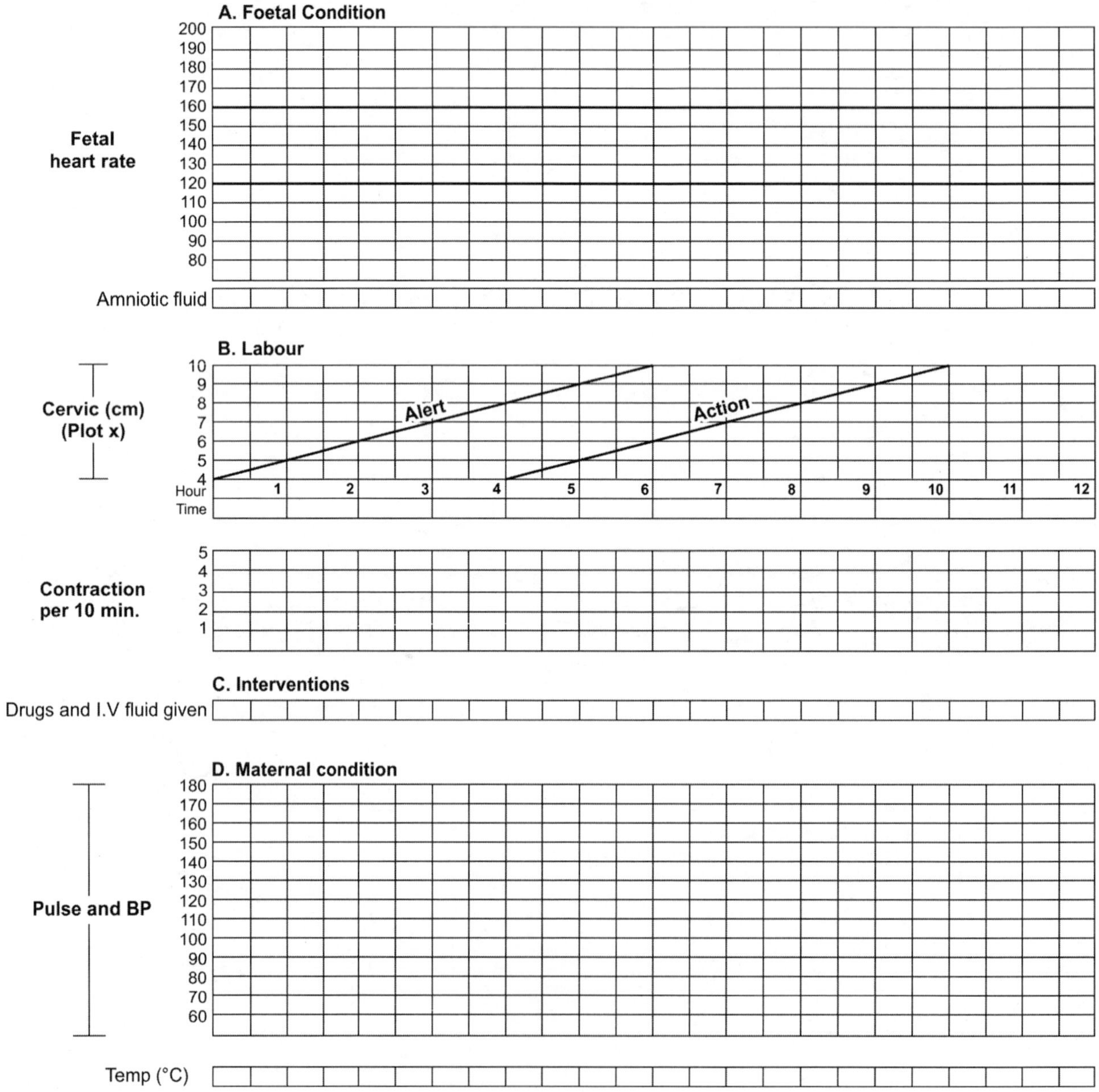

A. Foetal Condition

Fetal heart rate: 200, 190, 180, 170, 160, 150, 140, 130, 120, 110, 100, 90, 80

Amniotic fluid

B. Labour

Cervic (cm) (Plot x): 10, 9, 8, 7, 6, 5, 4

Alert

Action

Hour: 1, 2, 3, 4, 5, 6, 7, 8, 9, 10, 11, 12

Time

Contraction per 10 min.: 5, 4, 3, 2, 1

C. Interventions

Drugs and I.V fluid given

D. Maternal condition

Pulse and BP: 180, 170, 160, 150, 140, 130, 120, 110, 100, 90, 80, 70, 60

Temp (°C)

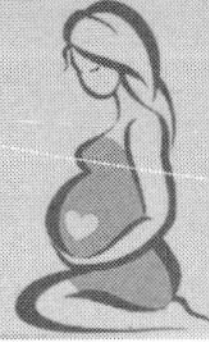

WHO Modified Partograph

Parity: *Reg No:* *Date and Time of Admission:* *Date and Time of ROM:*

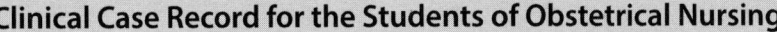

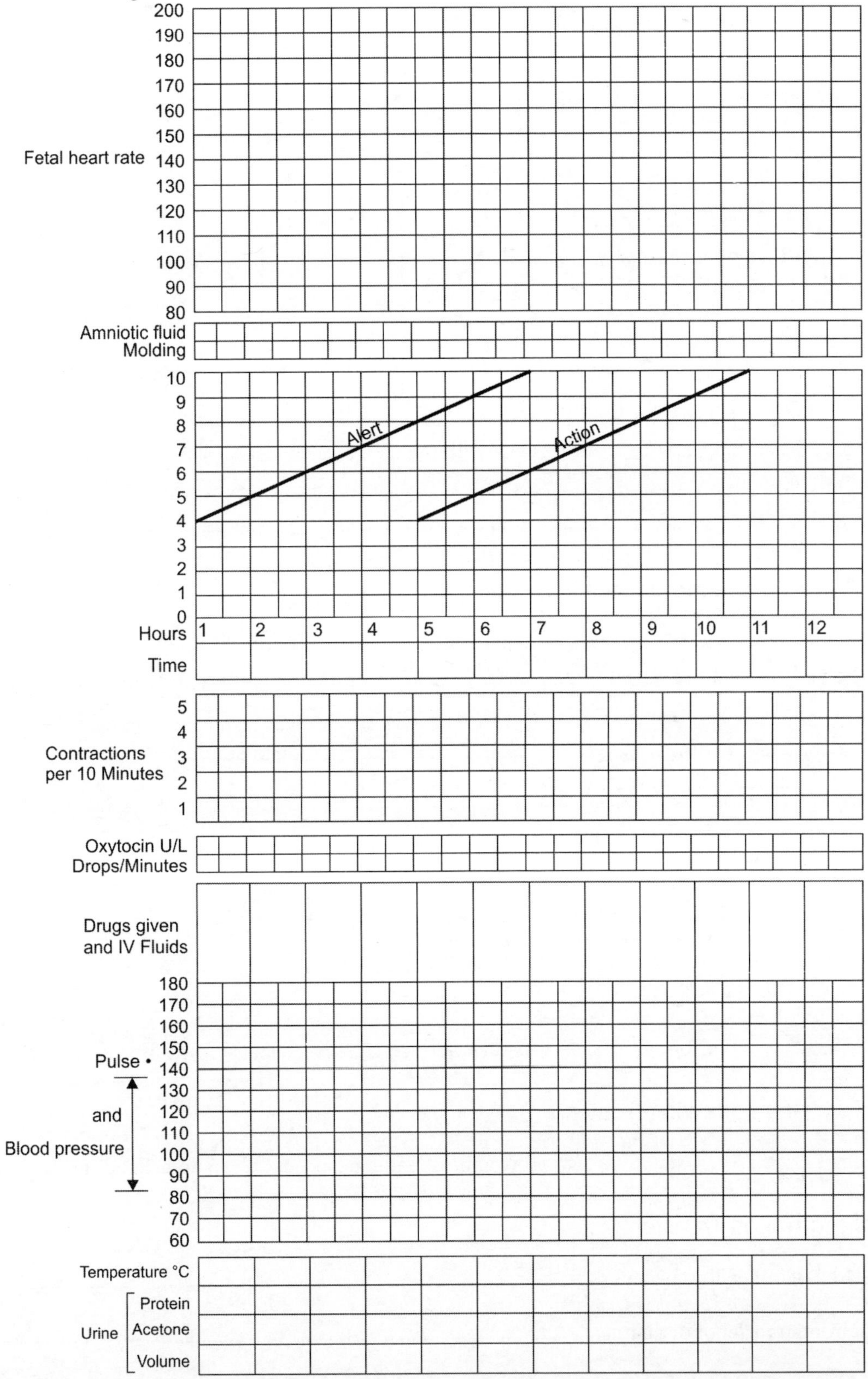

Fetal heart rate: 200, 190, 180, 170, 160, 150, 140, 130, 120, 110, 100, 90, 80

Amniotic fluid

Molding

10, 9, 8, 7, 6, 5, 4, 3, 2, 1, 0

Hours	1	2	3	4	5	6	7	8	9	10	11	12
Time												

Contractions per 10 Minutes: 5, 4, 3, 2, 1

Oxytocin U/L

Drops/Minutes

Drugs given and IV Fluids

Pulse • and Blood pressure: 180, 170, 160, 150, 140, 130, 120, 110, 100, 90, 80, 70, 60

Temperature °C

Urine: Protein, Acetone, Volume

Delivery Note

Labor Progress Note Date and Time of Onset of Pain

Onset of true labor: On .... At: ....

Date and time of full cervix dilatation: .... Effacement: ....

Membrane ruptured (spontaneous/artificial/PROM) on .... At ....

Total duration of: 1st stage .... Hrs .... Min ....

2nd stage .... Hrs .... Min ....

3rd stage .... Hrs .... Min ....

Total hours = ... Hrs .... Min ....

Baby at Birth

Mode of delivery: .... Score at one minute ....

Baby born on:.................................. At: .... Sex: ....

Apgar scoring: .... Score at five minute.................................. Anus patent: ....

Initiation of breastfeeding: ....

Drug administration: ....

Delivery of Placenta and Membrane

Delivery of placenta on:.......................... At:.......................... Cord insertion: ....

Spontaneous/helped/manually removed .... Examination of placenta: Complete/Incomplete ....

Weight of placenta:..

Cord length: .... Examination of membrane: ....

Blood Loss

Before delivery of placenta : ....

During delivery of placenta : ....

After delivery of placenta : ....

Perineum

Intact : .... Episiotomy :............. Laceration :.............................. Repair : ....

Condition of Mother Following Delivery

Pulse: .... BP: .... Uterus: .... Vaginal bleeding: .... Breastfeeding initiated at: ....

Condition of Mother on Transfer

Healthy/unhealthy (if unhealthy specify): ....

Condition of baby on transfer or discharge: ....

Nursing Care Plan

S.No.	Assessment	Nursing Diagnosis	Goal/Expected Out Come	Nursing Intervention	Rational	Implementation	Evaluation

Signature of Sister in Charge

Signature of Supervisor

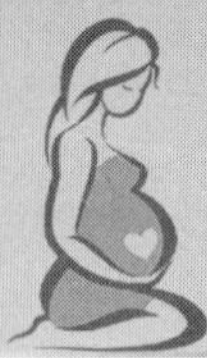

Conducted Normal Delivery (Case No. 18)

Client's Profile

Name : .... Religion : .... W/o : ....

Age : .... Education : .... Parity : ....

Hospital name : .... Occupation : .... LMP : ....

Date of booking : .... Income per month : .... EDD.................................

Reg. No : .... Marriage duration : .... Period of gestation ....

Address : ....

....

Date and time of admission : ....

Date and time of discharge or transfer : ....

Admission Note

General Examinations

i. Temperature: ....

ii. Pulse: ....

iii. Respiration: ....

iv. BP: ....

Hydration: ....

Anemia: (Present/absent) ....

Labor pain: (Present/absent)..................................

Edema: (Generalized/ankle edema) ....

Abdominal Examination/Obstetrical Examination by Palpation

Height of uterus: .... cm Lie: .... Superficial grip: ....

Gestational weeks: .... Presentation: .... Deep pelvic grip: ....

Abdominal girth: ....cm Position of fetus: .... FHR: ....

Scar: .... Lateral grip: ....

Time/date of onset of contraction : ....

Uterine contraction: Present/absent/well contracted : ....

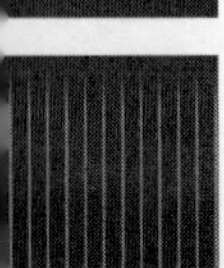

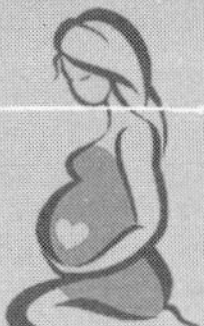

Investigation

Date	Hemoglobin	Blood Group/ Sugar	Urine		Bowel	Bladder	Any Other
			Albumin	Sugar			

Vaginal Examination

S.No	Date and time	Finding	Remark

Previous Obstetrical History

S.No	Year	Term/ preterm	Abortion/ stillbirth	Nature of delivery	Child		Immunization	Growth and development	Nature of puerperium	Remark
					Alive	Sex/ weight				

Admission History

Pregnancy complaints	
Menstrual history	
Medical history	
Surgical history	

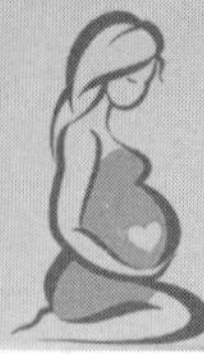

Old Pattern Partograph

Parity: *Reg No:* *Date and Time of Admission:* *Date and Time of ROM:*

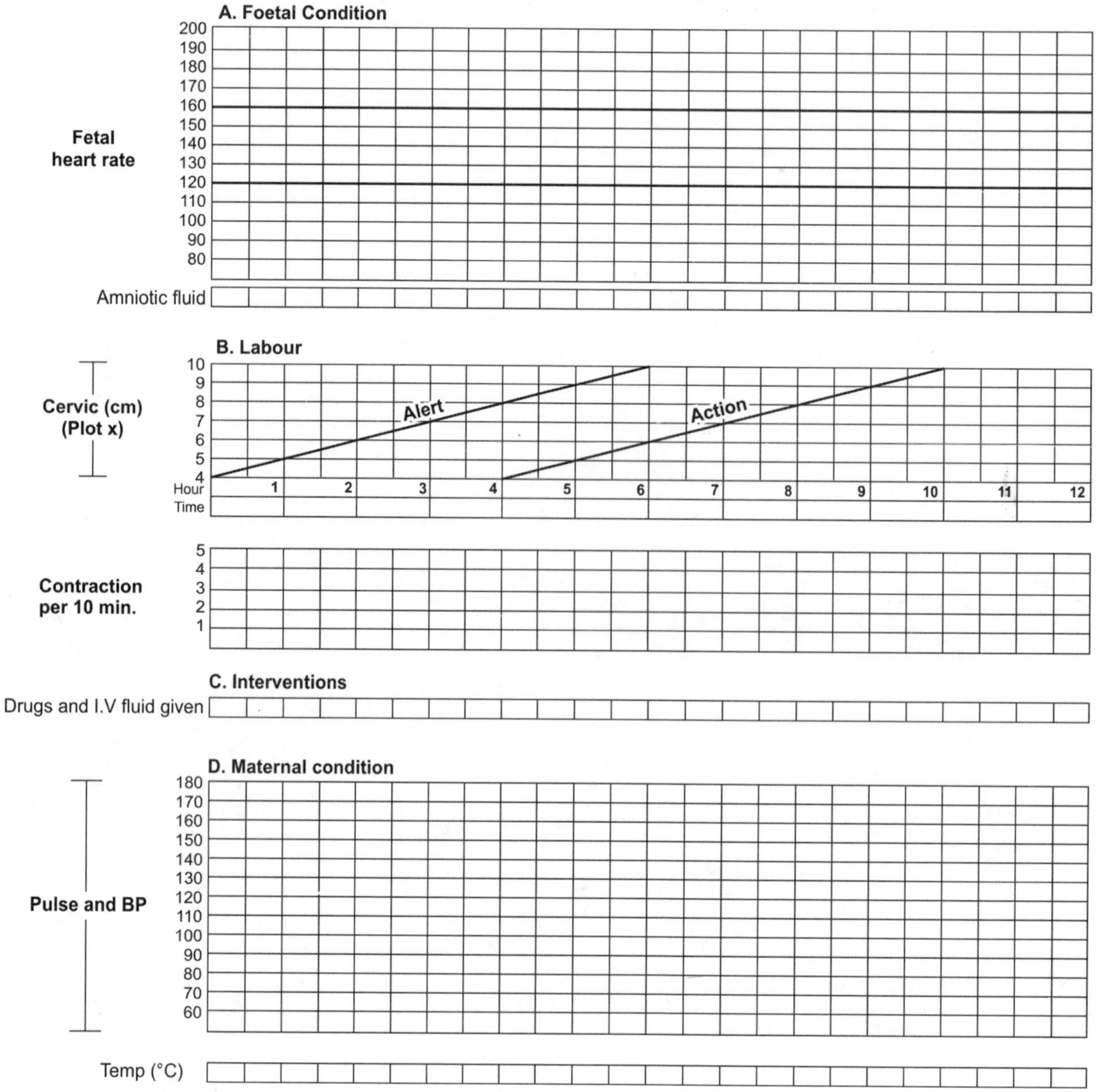

A. Foetal Condition

Fetal heart rate

200
190
180
170
160
150
140
130
120
110
100
90
80

Amniotic fluid

B. Labour

Cervic (cm) (Plot x)

10
9
8
7
6
5
4

Alert

Action

Hour 1 2 3 4 5 6 7 8 9 10 11 12

Time

Contraction per 10 min.

5
4
3
2
1

C. Interventions

Drugs and I.V fluid given

D. Maternal condition

Pulse and BP

180
170
160
150
140
130
120
110
100
90
80
70
60

Temp (°C)

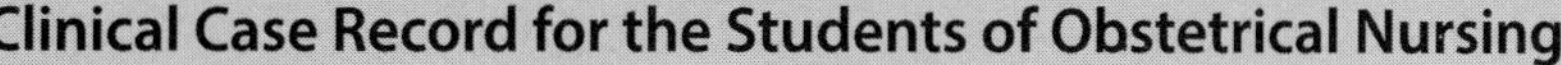

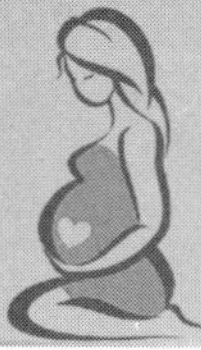

WHO Modified Partograph

Parity: *Reg No:* *Date and Time of Admission:* *Date and Time of ROM:*

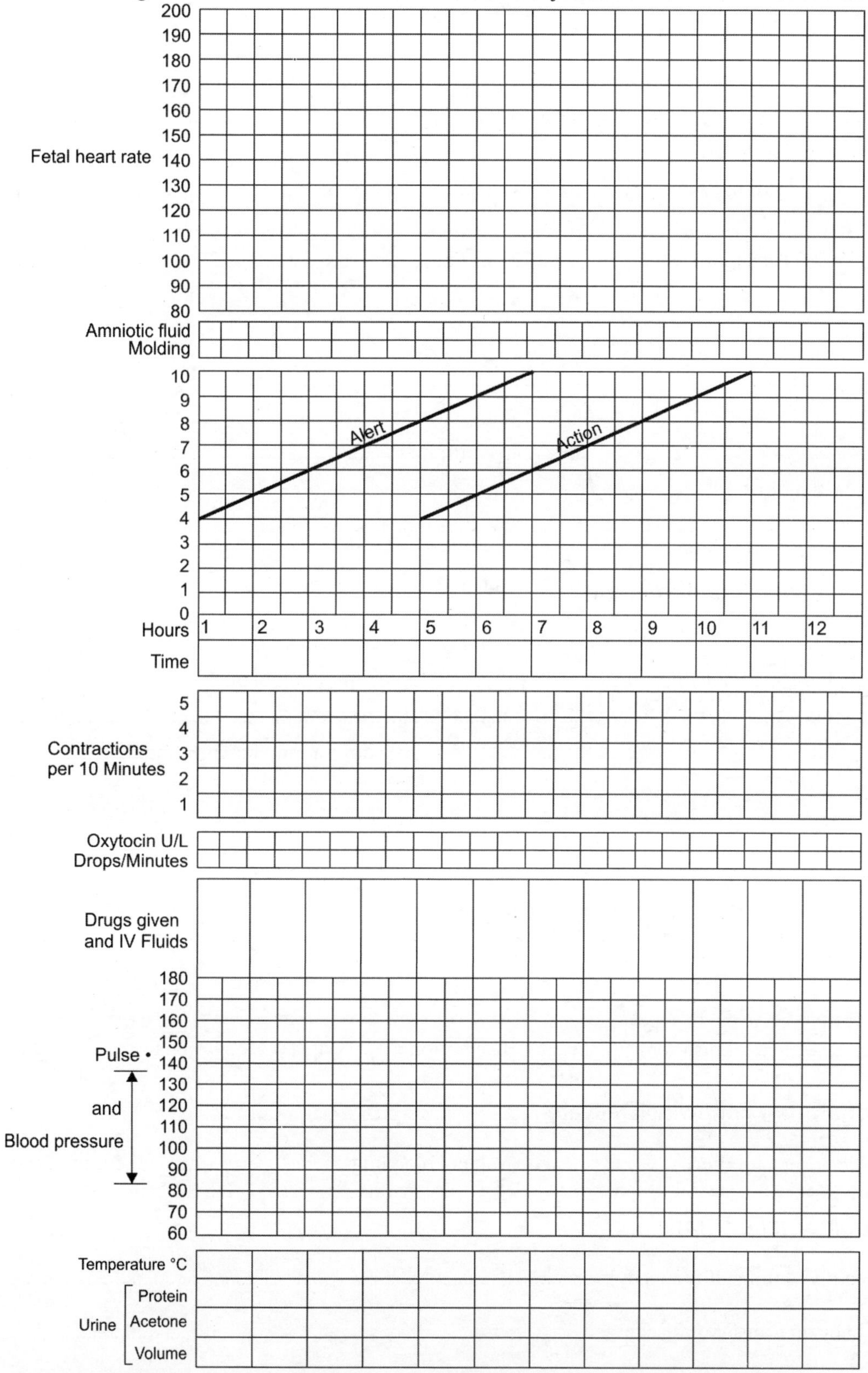

Fetal heart rate
200
190
180
170
160
150
140
130
120
110
100
90
80

Amniotic fluid
Molding

10
9
8
7
6
5
4
3
2
1
0

Alert
Action

Hours 1 2 3 4 5 6 7 8 9 10 11 12

Time

Contractions per 10 Minutes
5
4
3
2
1

Oxytocin U/L
Drops/Minutes

Drugs given and IV Fluids

Pulse •
and
Blood pressure
180
170
160
150
140
130
120
110
100
90
80
70
60

Temperature °C

Urine
Protein
Acetone
Volume

Delivery Note

Labor Progress Note Date and Time of Onset of Pain

Onset of true labor: On .... At: ....

Date and time of full cervix dilatation: .... Effacement: ....

Membrane ruptured (spontaneous/artificial/PROM) on .... At ....

Total duration of: 1st stage .... Hrs .... Min ....

2nd stage .... Hrs .... Min ....

3rd stage .... Hrs .... Min ....

Total hours = ... Hrs .... Min ....

Baby at Birth

Mode of delivery: .... Score at one minute ....

Baby born on:.. At: .... Sex: ....

Apgar scoring: .... Score at five minute................................ Anus patent: ....

Initiation of breastfeeding: ....

Drug administration: ....

Delivery of Placenta and Membrane

Delivery of placenta on: .... At:........................... Cord insertion: ....

Spontaneous/helped/manually removed .... Examination of placenta: Complete/Incomplete ....

Weight of placenta:...

Cord length: .... Examination of membrane: ....

Blood Loss

Before delivery of placenta : ....

During delivery of placenta : ....

After delivery of placenta : ....

Perineum

Intact : .... Episiotomy : .... Laceration : .... Repair : ....

Condition of Mother Following Delivery

Pulse: .... BP: .... Uterus: .... Vaginal bleeding: .... Breastfeeding initiated at: ....

Condition of Mother on Transfer

Healthy/unhealthy (if unhealthy specify): ....

Condition of baby on transfer or discharge: ....

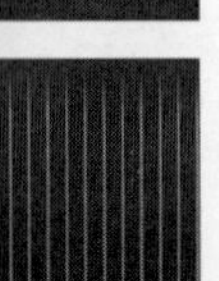

Nursing Care Plan

S.No.	Assessment	Nursing Diagnosis	Goal/Expected Out Come	Nursing Intervention	Rational	Implementation	Evaluation

Signature of Sister in Charge

Signature of Supervisor

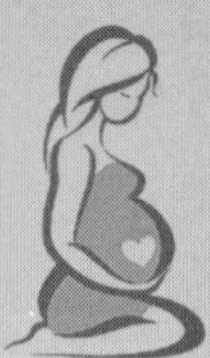

Conducted Normal Delivery (Case No. 19)

Client's Profile

Name : .... Religion : .... W/o : ....

Age : .... Education : .... Parity : ....

Hospital name : .... Occupation : .... LMP : ....

Date of booking : .... Income per month : .... EDD..................................

Reg. No : .... Marriage duration : .... Period of gestation ....

Address : ....

....

Date and time of admission : ....

Date and time of discharge or transfer : ....

Admission Note

General Examinations

i. Temperature: .... iii. Respiration: ....

ii. Pulse: .... iv. BP: ....

Hydration: .... Anemia: (Present/absent) ....

Labor pain: (Present/absent)................................. Edema: (Generalized/ankle edema) ....

Abdominal Examination/Obstetrical Examination by Palpation

Height of uterus: .... cm Lie: .... Superficial grip: ....

Gestational weeks: .... Presentation: .... Deep pelvic grip: ....

Abdominal girth: ....cm Position of fetus: .... FHR: ....

Scar: .... Lateral grip: ....

Time/date of onset of contraction : ....

Uterine contraction: Present/absent/well contracted : ....

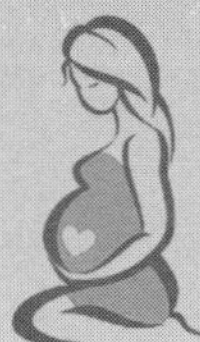

Investigation

Date	Hemoglobin	Blood Group/ Sugar	Urine		Bowel	Bladder	Any Other
			Albumin	Sugar			

Vaginal Examination

S.No	Date and time	Finding	Remark

Previous Obstetrical History

S.No	Year	Term/ preterm	Abortion/ stillbirth	Nature of delivery	Child		Immunization	Growth and development	Nature of puerperium	Remark
					Alive	Sex/ weight				

Admission History

Pregnancy complaints	
Menstrual history	
Medical history	
Surgical history	

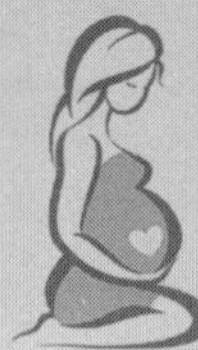

Old Pattern Partograph

Parity: *Reg No:* *Date and Time of Admission:* *Date and Time of ROM:*

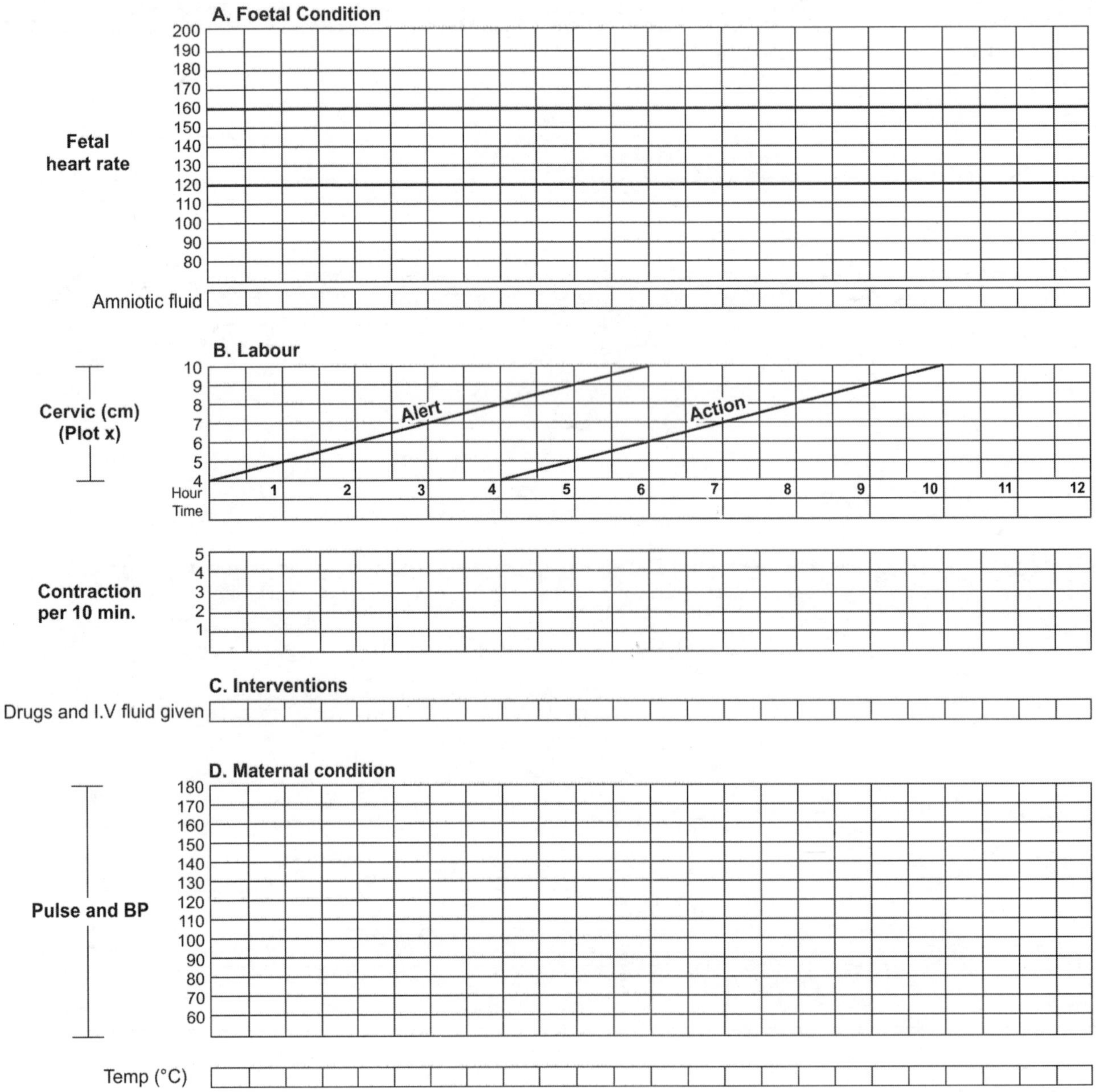

A. Foetal Condition

Fetal heart rate

200
190
180
170
160
150
140
130
120
110
100
90
80

Amniotic fluid

B. Labour

Cervic (cm) (Plot x)

10
9
8
7
6
5
4

Alert

Action

Hour 1 2 3 4 5 6 7 8 9 10 11 12

Time

Contraction per 10 min.

5
4
3
2
1

C. Interventions

Drugs and I.V fluid given

D. Maternal condition

Pulse and BP

180
170
160
150
140
130
120
110
100
90
80
70
60

Temp (°C)

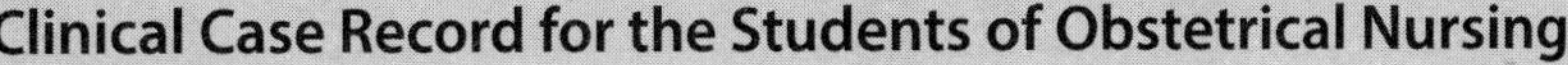

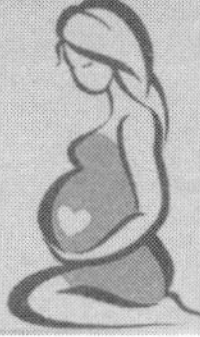

WHO Modified Partograph

Parity: *Reg No:* *Date and Time of Admission:* *Date and Time of ROM:*

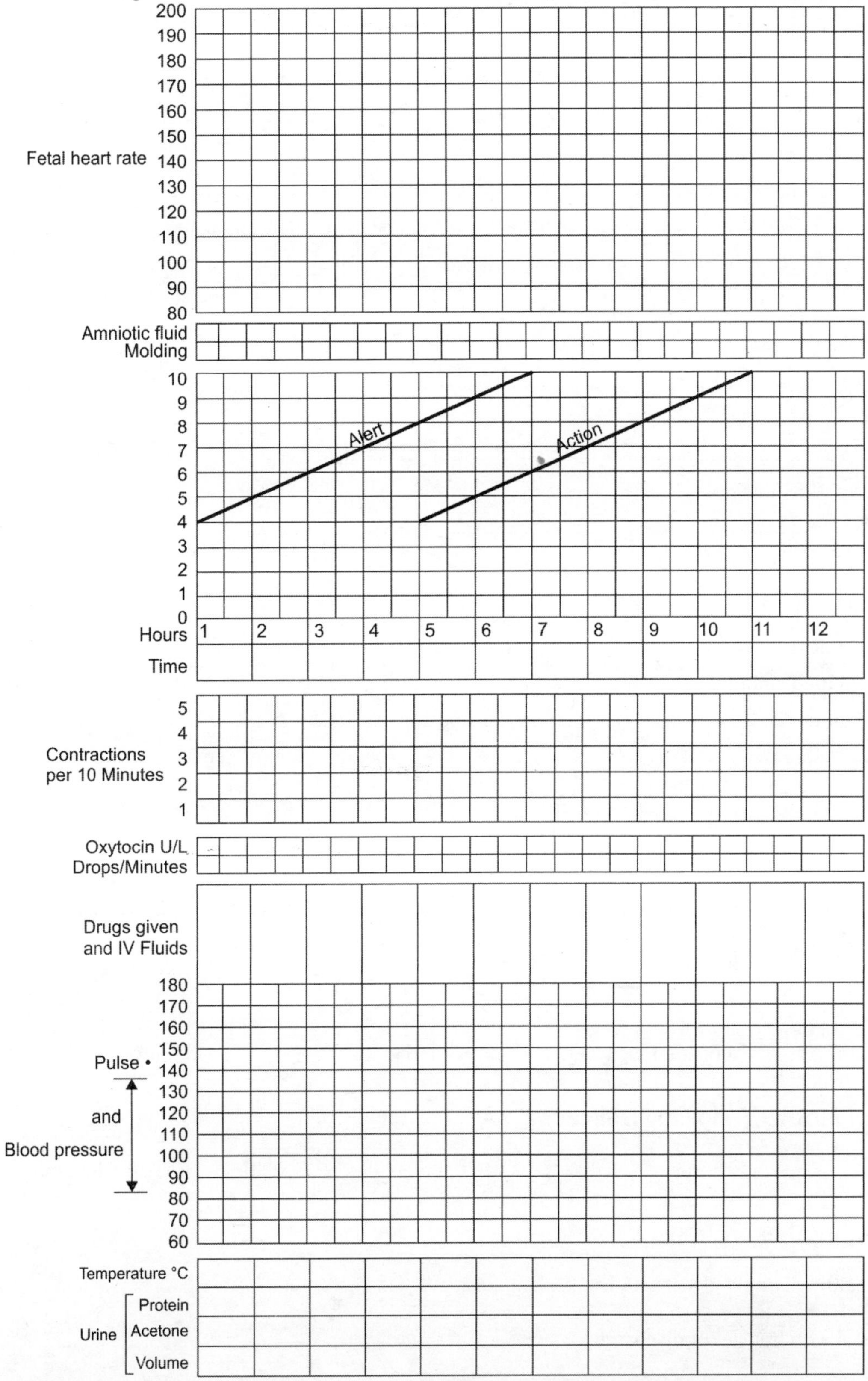

Fetal heart rate: 200, 190, 180, 170, 160, 150, 140, 130, 120, 110, 100, 90, 80

Amniotic fluid

Molding

Cervical dilatation: 10, 9, 8, 7, 6, 5, 4, 3, 2, 1, 0

Hours: 1, 2, 3, 4, 5, 6, 7, 8, 9, 10, 11, 12

Time

Contractions per 10 Minutes: 5, 4, 3, 2, 1

Oxytocin U/L

Drops/Minutes

Drugs given and IV Fluids

Pulse • and Blood pressure: 180, 170, 160, 150, 140, 130, 120, 110, 100, 90, 80, 70, 60

Temperature °C

Urine: Protein, Acetone, Volume

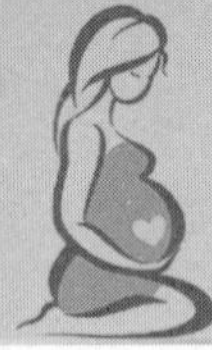

Delivery Note

Labor Progress Note Date and Time of Onset of Pain

Onset of true labor: On .... At: ....

Date and time of full cervix dilatation: .... Effacement: ....

Membrane ruptured (spontaneous/artificial/PROM) on .... At ....

Total duration of: 1st stage .... Hrs .... Min ....

2nd stage .... Hrs .... Min ....

3rd stage .... Hrs .... Min ....

Total hours = ... Hrs .... Min ....

Baby at Birth

Mode of delivery: .... Score at one minute ....

Baby born on:.............................. At: .... Sex: ....

Apgar scoring: .... Score at five minute.............................. Anus patent: ....

Initiation of breastfeeding: ....

Drug administration: ....

Delivery of Placenta and Membrane

Delivery of placenta on: .... At:........................ Cord insertion: ....

Spontaneous/helped/manually removed .... Examination of placenta: Complete/Incomplete ....

Weight of placenta:..

Cord length: .... Examination of membrane: ....

Blood Loss

Before delivery of placenta : ....

During delivery of placenta : ....

After delivery of placenta : ....

Perineum

Intact : .... Episiotomy :............ Laceration :.............................. Repair : ....

Condition of Mother Following Delivery

Pulse: ...... BP: .... Uterus: .... Vaginal bleeding: .... Breastfeeding initiated at: ....

Condition of Mother on Transfer

Healthy/unhealthy (if unhealthy specify): ....

Condition of baby on transfer or discharge: ....

Nursing Care Plan

S.No.	Assessment	Nursing Diagnosis	Goal/Expected Out Come	Nursing Intervention	Rational	Implementation	Evaluation

Signature of Sister in Charge

Signature of Supervisor

Conducted Normal Delivery (Case No. 20)

Client's Profile

Name : .... Religion : .... W/o : ....

Age : .... Education : .... Parity : ....

Hospital name : .... Occupation : .... LMP : ....

Date of booking : .... Income per month : .... EDD.................................

Reg. No : .... Marriage duration : .... Period of gestation ....

Address : ....

....

Date and time of admission : ....

Date and time of discharge or transfer : ....

Admission Note

General Examinations

i. Temperature: ....

ii. Pulse: ....

iii. Respiration: ....

iv. BP: ....

Hydration: ....

Labor pain: (Present/absent)...................................

Anemia: (Present/absent) ....

Edema: (Generalized/ankle edema) ....

Abdominal Examination/Obstetrical Examination by Palpation

Height of uterus: .... cm Lie: .... Superficial grip: ....

Gestational weeks: .... Presentation: .... Deep pelvic grip: ....

Abdominal girth: ....cm Position of fetus: .... FHR: ....

Scar: .... Lateral grip: ....

Time/date of onset of contraction : ....

Uterine contraction: Present/absent/well contracted : ....

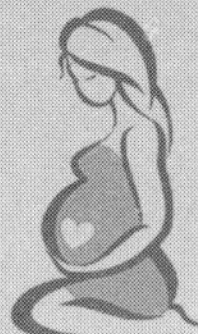

Investigation

Date	Hemoglobin	Blood Group/ Sugar	Urine		Bowel	Bladder	Any Other
			Albumin	Sugar			

Vaginal Examination

S.No	Date and time	Finding	Remark

Previous Obstetrical History

S.No	Year	Term/ preterm	Abortion/ stillbirth	Nature of delivery	Child		Immunization	Growth and development	Nature of puerperium	Remark
					Alive	Sex/ weight				

Admission History

Pregnancy complaints	
Menstrual history	
Medical history	
Surgical history	

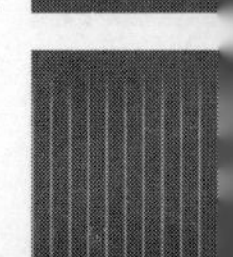

Old Pattern Partograph

Parity: *Reg No:* *Date and Time of Admission:* *Date and Time of ROM:*

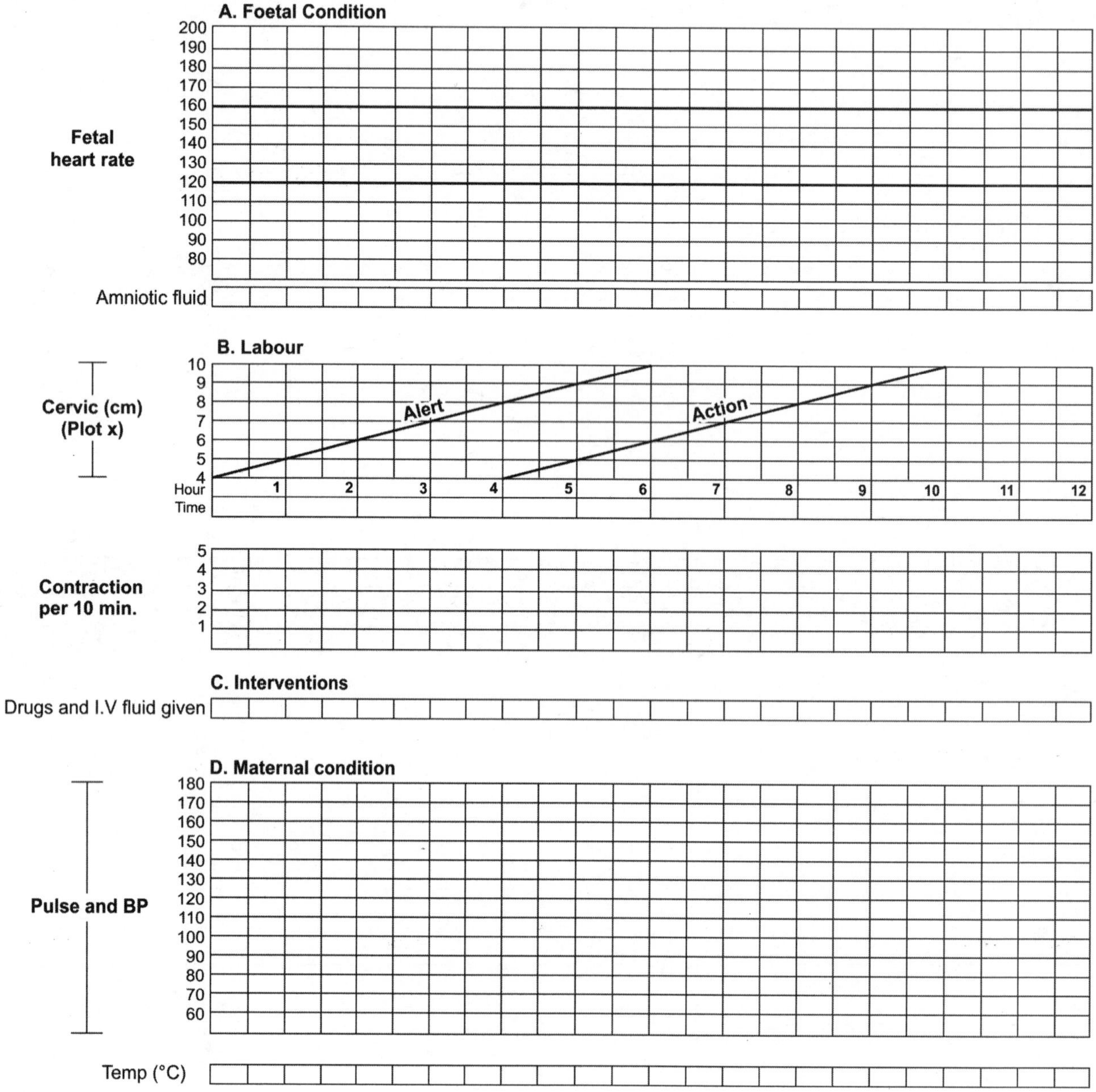

A. Foetal Condition

Fetal heart rate

200
190
180
170
160
150
140
130
120
110
100
90
80

Amniotic fluid

B. Labour

Cervic (cm) (Plot x)

10
9
8
7
6
5
4

Alert

Action

Hour	1	2	3	4	5	6	7	8	9	10	11	12
Time												

Contraction per 10 min.

5
4
3
2
1

C. Interventions

Drugs and I.V fluid given

D. Maternal condition

Pulse and BP

180
170
160
150
140
130
120
110
100
90
80
70
60

Temp (°C)

WHO Modified Partograph

Parity: *Reg No:* *Date and Time of Admission:* *Date and Time of ROM:*

Fetal heart rate: 200, 190, 180, 170, 160, 150, 140, 130, 120, 110, 100, 90, 80

Amniotic fluid

Molding

10, 9, 8, 7, 6, 5, 4, 3, 2, 1, 0

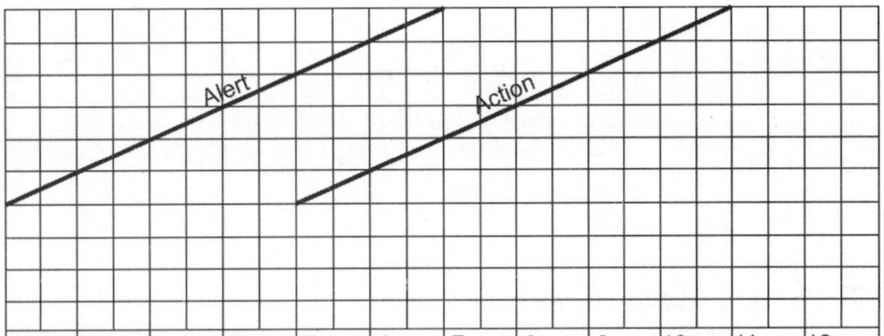

Alert

Action

Hours	1	2	3	4	5	6	7	8	9	10	11	12
Time												

Contractions per 10 Minutes: 5, 4, 3, 2, 1

Oxytocin U/L

Drops/Minutes

Drugs given and IV Fluids

Pulse • and Blood pressure: 180, 170, 160, 150, 140, 130, 120, 110, 100, 90, 80, 70, 60

Temperature °C

Urine: Protein, Acetone, Volume

Delivery Note

Labor Progress Note Date and Time of Onset of Pain

Onset of true labor: On .... At: ....

Date and time of full cervix dilatation: .... Effacement: ....

Membrane ruptured (spontaneous/artificial/PROM) on .... At ....

Total duration of: 1st stage .... Hrs .... Min ....

2nd stage .... Hrs .... Min ....

3rd stage .... Hrs .... Min ....

Total hours = ... Hrs .... Min ....

Baby at Birth

Mode of delivery: .... Score at one minute ....

Baby born on:.................... At: .... Sex: ....

Apgar scoring: .... Score at five minute.................... Anus patent: ....

Initiation of breastfeeding: ....

Drug administration: ....

Delivery of Placenta and Membrane

Delivery of placenta on: .... At:.................... Cord insertion: ....

Spontaneous/helped/manually removed .... Examination of placenta: Complete/Incomplete ....

Weight of placenta:..

Cord length: .... Examination of membrane: ....

Blood Loss

Before delivery of placenta : ....

During delivery of placenta : ....

After delivery of placenta : ....

Perineum

Intact : .... Episiotomy :............. Laceration :.................... Repair : ....

Condition of Mother Following Delivery

Pulse: .... BP: .... Uterus: .... Vaginal bleeding: .... Breastfeeding initiated at: ....

Condition of Mother on Transfer

Healthy/unhealthy (if unhealthy specify): ....

Condition of baby on transfer or discharge: ....

Nursing Care Plan

S.No.	Assessment	Nursing Diagnosis	Goal/Expected Out Come	Nursing Intervention	Rational	Implementation	Evaluation

Signature of Sister in Charge

Signature of Supervisor

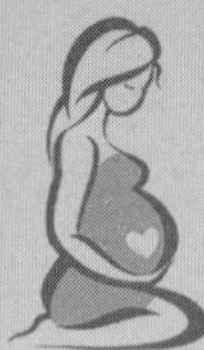

Postnatal Assessment (Case No. 1)

Client's Profile

Name : .... Occupation : ....

Age : .... Income per month : ....

Hospital name : .... W/o : ....

Date of booking : .... Period of gestation : ....

Reg. No : .... Religion : ....

Address : ....

Education : ....

Menstrual History

Age at menarche : ....year of age

Cycle of : .... days

Period duration of : .... days

Blood flow: Average/scanty/heavy ....

Dysmenorrhea: ....

Obstetric History

S.No.	Year	Term/ preterm	Abortion/ stillbirth	Nature of delivery	Child		Immunization	Growth and development	Nature of puerperium	Remark
					Alive	Sex/ weight				

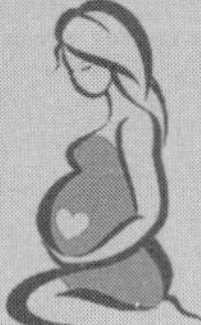

Personal History

Allergies to drug : .... Body built : ....

Habit : Smoking/alcohol/betel chewing/any drug addiction

Hobbies : ....

Dietary habits : Veg/nonvegetarian,...................... Diet per day : 2/3/4/5/6

Immunization status : TT: 1st dose .... 2nd dose ....

Present and Past Medical History

High BP/diabetes/breathlessness on exertion/palpitation/tuberculosis/asthma/renal disease/convulsion/jaundice/malaria/RTI/STI/HIV/AIDS/no any/if any other specify ....

Family History

Family History of :

Systemic Illness : High BP/Diabetes/Tuberculosis/No Any

Blood Disorder : Thalassemia/Repeated blood transfusion

Delivery of : Twins/Congenital abnormalities

Notes on Admission for Labor

Present pregnancy : Full term/pre term .... Period of gestation : ....

Presentation of fetus : .... FHS : ....

Labor Notes

Membrane ruptured on : .... at: ....

Length of labor : ....

1st stage : .... 2nd stage : ....

3rd stage : .... **Total hours** **: ....**

Maternal Condition on Shifting

Date and time of shifting (in postnatal ward) : ....

Newborn general condition on shifting : ....

Newborn date and time of shifting (in postnatal ward) : ....

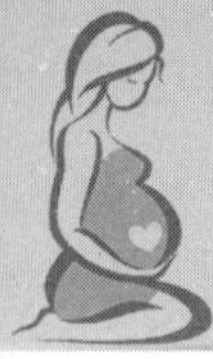

Postnatal Assessment for Mother and Baby

Mother

Postnatal day	1	2	3	4	5	6
Date						
Time						
Vital sign						
Temperature						
Pulse						
Respiration						
BP						
Fundal height						
Uterus						
Lochia						
Perineal care/episiotomy (REEDA)						
Breast						
Bowel/stool						
Bladder/urine						

Baby

Postnatal day	1	2	3	4	5	6
Date						
Time						
Vital sign						
Temperature						
Pulse						
Respiration						
Urine (time/day)						
Stool (time/day)						
Eye care						
Cord care						
Fontanels (Normal/Absent)						
Reflexes						
Activity						
Breastfeeding						
Anthropometric measurement						
Length (cm)						
Head circumference (cm)						
Chest (cm)						
Abdominal (cm)						
Weight (kg)						

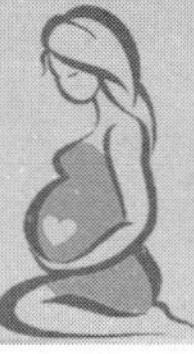

Chief Complaints

....

....

....

....

Condition of Mother at Discharge

....

....

....

....

Condition of Newborn at Discharge

....

....

....

....

Health Education (Diet, Family Planning/Follow-up)

....

....

....

....

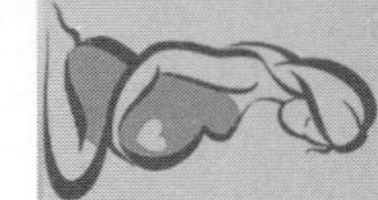
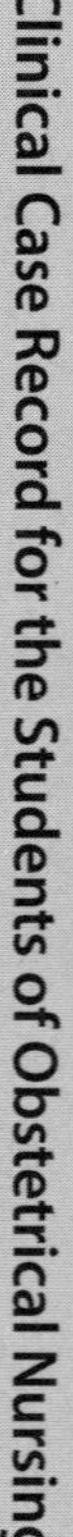

Nursing Care Plan

S.No.	Assessment	Nursing Diagnosis	Goal/Expected Out Come	Nursing Intervention	Rational	Implementation	Evaluation

Signature of Sister in Charge ____________________

Signature of Supervisor ____________________

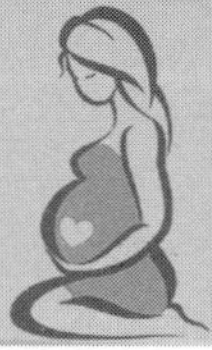

Postnatal Assessment (Case No. 2)

Client's Profile

Name : .... Occupation : ....

Age : .... Income per month : ....

Hospital name : .... W/o : ....

Date of booking : .... Period of gestation : ....

Reg. No : .... Religion : ....

Address : ....

Education : ....

Menstrual History

Age at menarche : ....year of age

Cycle of : .... days

Period duration of : .... days

Blood flow: Average/scanty/heavy ....

Dysmenorrhea: ....

Obstetric History

S.No.	Year	Term/ preterm	Abortion/ stillbirth	Nature of delivery	Child		Immunization	Growth and development	Nature of puerperium	Remark
					Alive	Sex/ weight				

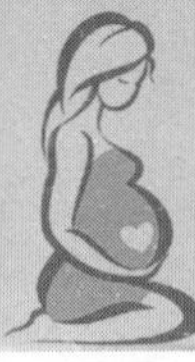

Personal History

Allergies to drug : .... Body built : ....

Habit : Smoking/alcohol/betel chewing/any drug addiction

Hobbies : ....

Dietary habits : Veg/nonvegetarian,........................ Diet per day : 2/3/4/5/6

Immunization status : TT: 1st dose .... 2nd dose ....

Present and Past Medical History

High BP/diabetes/breathlessness on exertion/palpitation/tuberculosis/asthma/renal disease/convulsion/jaundice/malaria/RTI/STI/HIV/AIDS/no any/if any other specify ....

Family History

Family History of :

Systemic Illness : High BP/Diabetes/Tuberculosis/No Any

Blood Disorder : Thalassemia/Repeated blood transfusion

Delivery of : Twins/Congenital abnormalities

Notes on Admission for Labor

Present pregnancy : Full term/pre term .... Period of gestation : ....

Presentation of fetus : .... FHS : ....

Labor Notes

Membrane ruptured on : .... at: ....

Length of labor : ....

1st stage : .... 2nd stage : ....

3rd stage : .... **Total hours** **: ....**

Maternal Condition on Shifting

Date and time of shifting (in postnatal ward) : ....

Newborn general condition on shifting : ....

Newborn date and time of shifting (in postnatal ward) : ....

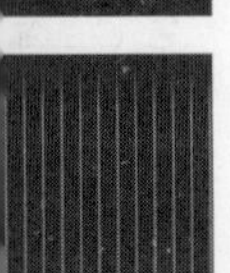

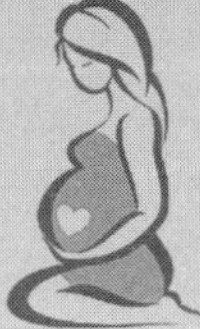

Postnatal Assessment for Mother and Baby

Mother

Postnatal day	1	2	3	4	5	6
Date						
Time						
Vital sign						
Temperature						
Pulse						
Respiration						
BP						
Fundal height						
Uterus						
Lochia						
Perineal care/episiotomy (REEDA)						
Breast						
Bowel/stool						
Bladder/urine						

Baby

Postnatal day	1	2	3	4	5	6
Date						
Time						
Vital sign						
Temperature						
Pulse						
Respiration						
Urine (time/day)						
Stool (time/day)						
Eye care						
Cord care						
Fontanels (Normal/Absent)						
Reflexes						
Activity						
Breastfeeding						
Anthropometric measurement						
Length (cm)						
Head circumference (cm)						
Chest (cm)						
Abdominal (cm)						
Weight (kg)						

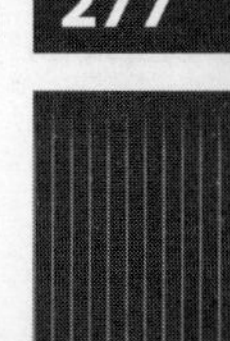

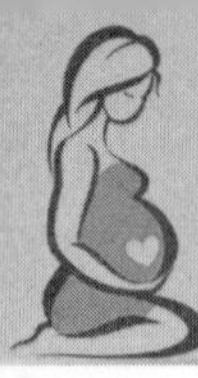

Chief Complaints

....

....

....

....

Condition of Mother at Discharge

....

....

....

....

Condition of Newborn at Discharge

....

....

....

....

Health Education (Diet, Family Planning/Follow-up)

....

....

....

....

Nursing Care Plan

S.No.	Assessment	Nursing Diagnosis	Goal/Expected Out Come	Nursing Intervention	Rational	Implementation	Evaluation

Signature of Sister in Charge

Signature of Supervisor

Postnatal Assessment (Case No. 3)

Client's Profile

Name : .... Occupation : ....

Age : .... Income per month : ....

Hospital name : .... W/o : ....

Date of booking : .... Period of gestation : ....

Reg. No : .... Religion : ....

Address : ....

Education : ....

Menstrual History

Age at menarche : ....year of age

Cycle of : .... days

Period duration of : .... days

Blood flow: Average/scanty/heavy ....

Dysmenorrhea: ....

Obstetric History

S.No.	Year	Term/ preterm	Abortion/ stillbirth	Nature of delivery	Child		Immunization	Growth and development	Nature of puerperium	Remark
					Alive	Sex/ weight				

Personal History

Allergies to drug : .... Body built : ....

Habit : Smoking/alcohol/betel chewing/any drug addiction

Hobbies : ....

Dietary habits : Veg/nonvegetarian,...................... Diet per day : 2/3/4/5/6

Immunization status : TT: 1st dose .... 2nd dose ....

Present and Past Medical History

High BP/diabetes/breathlessness on exertion/palpitation/tuberculosis/asthma/renal disease/convulsion/jaundice/malaria/RTI/STI/HIV/AIDS/no any/if any other specify ....

Family History

Family History of :

Systemic Illness : High BP/Diabetes/Tuberculosis/No Any

Blood Disorder : Thalassemia/Repeated blood transfusion

Delivery of : Twins/Congenital abnormalities

Notes on Admission for Labor

Present pregnancy : Full term/pre term .... Period of gestation : ....

Presentation of fetus : .... FHS : ....

Labor Notes

Membrane ruptured on : .... at: ....

Length of labor : ....

1st stage : .... 2nd stage : ....

3rd stage : .... **Total hours** : **...**

Maternal Condition on Shifting

Date and time of shifting (in postnatal ward) : ....

Newborn general condition on shifting : ....

Newborn date and time of shifting (in postnatal ward) : ....

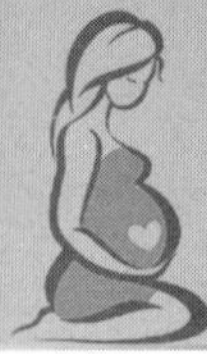

Postnatal Assessment for Mother and Baby

Mother

Postnatal day	1	2	3	4	5	6
Date						
Time						
Vital sign						
Temperature						
Pulse						
Respiration						
BP						
Fundal height						
Uterus						
Lochia						
Perineal care/episiotomy (REEDA)						
Breast						
Bowel/stool						
Bladder/urine						

Baby

Postnatal day	1	2	3	4	5	6
Date						
Time						
Vital sign						
Temperature						
Pulse						
Respiration						
Urine (time/day)						
Stool (time/day)						
Eye care						
Cord care						
Fontanels (Normal/Absent)						
Reflexes						
Activity						
Breastfeeding						
Anthropometric measurement						
Length (cm)						
Head circumference (cm)						
Chest (cm)						
Abdominal (cm)						
Weight (kg)						

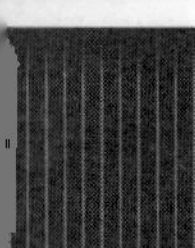

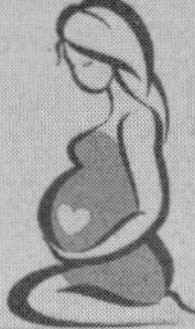

Chief Complaints

....

....

....

....

Condition of Mother at Discharge

....

....

....

....

Condition of Newborn at Discharge

....

....

....

....

Health Education (Diet, Family Planning/Follow-up)

....

....

....

....

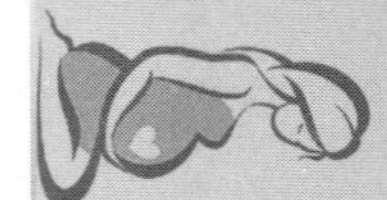

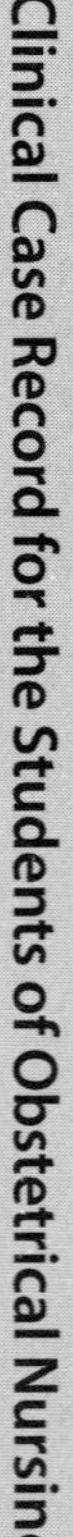

Nursing Care Plan

S.No.	Assessment	Nursing Diagnosis	Goal/Expected Out Come	Nursing Intervention	Rational	Implementation	Evaluation

Signature of Sister in Charge

Signature of Supervisor

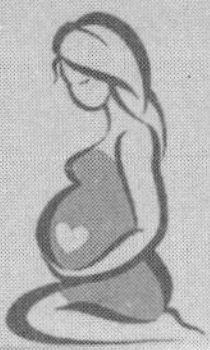

Postnatal Assessment (Case No. 4)

Client's Profile

Name : .... Occupation : ....

Age : .... Income per month : ....

Hospital name : .... W/o : ....

Date of booking : .... Period of gestation : ....

Reg. No : .... Religion : ....

Address : ....

Education : ....

Menstrual History

Age at menarche : ....year of age

Cycle of : .... days

Period duration of : .... days

Blood flow: Average/scanty/heavy ....

Dysmenorrhea: ....

Obstetric History

S.No.	Year	Term/ preterm	Abortion/ stillbirth	Nature of delivery	Child		Immunization	Growth and development	Nature of puerperium	Remark
					Alive	Sex/ weight				

Personal History

Allergies to drug : .... Body built : ....

Habit : Smoking/alcohol/betel chewing/any drug addiction

Hobbies : ....

Dietary habits : Veg/nonvegetarian,...................... Diet per day : 2/3/4/5/6

Immunization status : TT: 1st dose .... 2nd dose ....

Present and Past Medical History

High BP/diabetes/breathlessness on exertion/palpitation/tuberculosis/asthma/renal disease/convulsion/jaundice/malaria/RTI/STI/HIV/AIDS/no any/if any other specify ....

Family History

Family History of :

Systemic Illness : High BP/Diabetes/Tuberculosis/No Any

Blood Disorder : Thalassemia/Repeated blood transfusion

Delivery of : Twins/Congenital abnormalities

Notes on Admission for Labor

Present pregnancy : Full term/pre term .... Period of gestation : ....

Presentation of fetus : .... FHS : ....

Labor Notes

Membrane ruptured on : .... at: ....

Length of labor : ....

1st stage : .... 2nd stage : ....

3rd stage : .... **Total hours** : **..**

Maternal Condition on Shifting

Date and time of shifting (in postnatal ward) : ....

Newborn general condition on shifting : ....

Newborn date and time of shifting (in postnatal ward) : ....

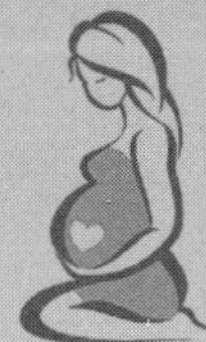

Postnatal Assessment for Mother and Baby

Mother

Postnatal day	1	2	3	4	5	6
Date						
Time						
Vital sign						
Temperature						
Pulse						
Respiration						
BP						
Fundal height						
Uterus						
Lochia						
Perineal care/episiotomy (REEDA)						
Breast						
Bowel/stool						
Bladder/urine						

Baby

Postnatal day	1	2	3	4	5	6
Date						
Time						
Vital sign						
Temperature						
Pulse						
Respiration						
Urine (time/day)						
Stool (time/day)						
Eye care						
Cord care						
Fontanels (Normal/Absent)						
Reflexes						
Activity						
Breastfeeding						
Anthropometric measurement						
Length (cm)						
Head circumference (cm)						
Chest (cm)						
Abdominal (cm)						
Weight (kg)						

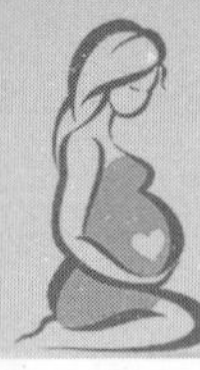

Chief Complaints

....

....

....

....

Condition of Mother at Discharge

....

....

....

....

Condition of Newborn at Discharge

....

....

....

....

Health Education (Diet, Family Planning/Follow-up)

....

....

....

....

Nursing Care Plan

S.No.	Assessment	Nursing Diagnosis	Goal/Expected Out Come	Nursing Intervention	Rational	Implementation	Evaluation

Signature of Sister in Charge

Signature of Supervisor

Postnatal Assessment (Case No. 5)

Client's Profile

Name : .... Occupation : ....

Age : .... Income per month : ....

Hospital name : .... W/o : ....

Date of booking : .... Period of gestation : ....

Reg. No : .... Religion : ....

Address : ....

Education : ....

Menstrual History

Age at menarche : ....year of age

Cycle of : .... days

Period duration of : .... days

Blood flow: Average/scanty/heavy ....

Dysmenorrhea: ....

Obstetric History

S.No.	Year	Term/ preterm	Abortion/ stillbirth	Nature of delivery	Child		Immunization	Growth and development	Nature of puerperium	Remark
					Alive	Sex/ weight				

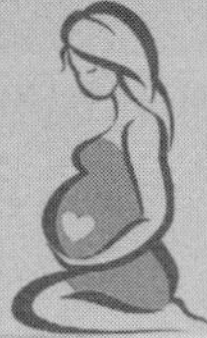

Personal History

Allergies to drug : .... Body built : ....

Habit : Smoking/alcohol/betel chewing/any drug addiction

Hobbies : ....

Dietary habits : Veg/nonvegetarian,........................ Diet per day : 2/3/4/5/6

Immunization status : TT: 1st dose .... 2nd dose ....

Present and Past Medical History

High BP/diabetes/breathlessness on exertion/palpitation/tuberculosis/asthma/renal disease/convulsion/jaundice/ malaria/RTI/STI/HIV/AIDS/no any/if any other specify ....

Family History

Family History of :

Systemic Illness : High BP/Diabetes/Tuberculosis/No Any

Blood Disorder : Thalassemia/Repeated blood transfusion

Delivery of : Twins/Congenital abnormalities

Notes on Admission for Labor

Present pregnancy : Full term/pre term .... Period of gestation : ....

Presentation of fetus : .... FHS : ....

Labor Notes

Membrane ruptured on : .... at: ....

Length of labor : ....

1st stage : .... 2nd stage : ....

3rd stage : .... **Total hours** : **..**

Maternal Condition on Shifting

Date and time of shifting (in postnatal ward) : ....

Newborn general condition on shifting : ....

Newborn date and time of shifting (in postnatal ward) : ....

Postnatal Assessment for Mother and Baby

Mother

Postnatal day	1	2	3	4	5	6
Date						
Time						
Vital sign						
Temperature						
Pulse						
Respiration						
BP						
Fundal height						
Uterus						
Lochia						
Perineal care/episiotomy (REEDA)						
Breast						
Bowel/stool						
Bladder/urine						

Baby

Postnatal day	1	2	3	4	5	6
Date						
Time						
Vital sign						
Temperature						
Pulse						
Respiration						
Urine (time/day)						
Stool (time/day)						
Eye care						
Cord care						
Fontanels (Normal/Absent)						
Reflexes						
Activity						
Breastfeeding						
Anthropometric measurement						
Length (cm)						
Head circumference (cm)						
Chest (cm)						
Abdominal (cm)						
Weight (kg)						

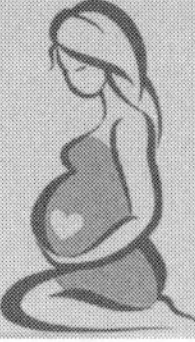

Chief Complaints

....

....

....

....

Condition of Mother at Discharge

....

....

....

....

Condition of Newborn at Discharge

....

....

....

....

Health Education (Diet, Family Planning/Follow-up)

....

....

....

....

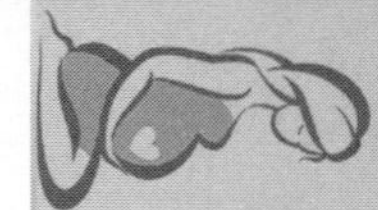
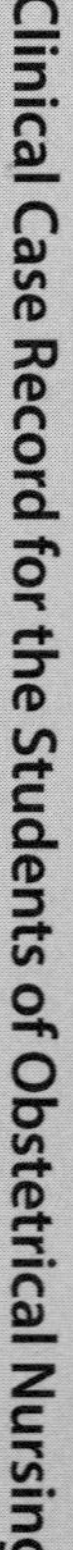

Nursing Care Plan

S.No.	Assessment	Nursing Diagnosis	Goal/Expected Out Come	Nursing Intervention	Rational	Implementation	Evaluation

Signature of Sister in Charge ____________________

Signature of Supervisor ____________________

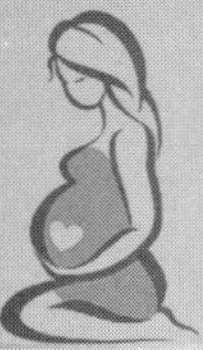

Postnatal Assessment (Case No. 6)

Client's Profile

Name : .... Occupation : ....

Age : .... Income per month : ....

Hospital name : .... W/o : ....

Date of booking : .... Period of gestation : ....

Reg. No : .... Religion : ....

Address : ....

Education : ....

Menstrual History

Age at menarche : ....year of age

Cycle of : .... days

Period duration of : .... days

Blood flow: Average/scanty/heavy ....

Dysmenorrhea: ....

Obstetric History

S.No.	Year	Term/ preterm	Abortion/ stillbirth	Nature of delivery	Child		Immunization	Growth and development	Nature of puerperium	Remark
					Alive	Sex/ weight				

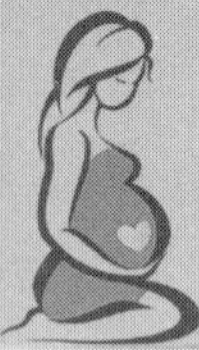

Personal History

Allergies to drug : .... Body built : ....

Habit : Smoking/alcohol/betel chewing/any drug addiction

Hobbies : ....

Dietary habits : Veg/nonvegetarian,........................ Diet per day : 2/3/4/5/6

Immunization status : TT: 1st dose .... 2nd dose ....

Present and Past Medical History

High BP/diabetes/breathlessness on exertion/palpitation/tuberculosis/asthma/renal disease/convulsion/jaundice/malaria/RTI/STI/HIV/AIDS/no any/if any other specify ....

Family History

Family History of :

Systemic Illness : High BP/Diabetes/Tuberculosis/No Any

Blood Disorder : Thalassemia/Repeated blood transfusion

Delivery of : Twins/Congenital abnormalities

Notes on Admission for Labor

Present pregnancy : Full term/pre term .... Period of gestation : ....

Presentation of fetus : .... FHS : ....

Labor Notes

Membrane ruptured on : .... at: ....

Length of labor : ....

1st stage : .... 2nd stage : ....

3rd stage : .... **Total hours** : **..**

Maternal Condition on Shifting

Date and time of shifting (in postnatal ward) : ....

Newborn general condition on shifting : ....

Newborn date and time of shifting (in postnatal ward) : ....

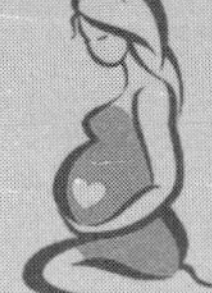

Postnatal Assessment for Mother and Baby

Mother

Postnatal day	1	2	3	4	5	6
Date						
Time						
Vital sign						
Temperature						
Pulse						
Respiration						
BP						
Fundal height						
Uterus						
Lochia						
Perineal care/episiotomy (REEDA)						
Breast						
Bowel/stool						
Bladder/urine						

Baby

Postnatal day	1	2	3	4	5	6
Date						
Time						
Vital sign						
Temperature						
Pulse						
Respiration						
Urine (time/day)						
Stool (time/day)						
Eye care						
Cord care						
Fontanels (Normal/Absent)						
Reflexes						
Activity						
Breastfeeding						
Anthropometric measurement						
Length (cm)						
Head circumference (cm)						
Chest (cm)						
Abdominal (cm)						
Weight (kg)						

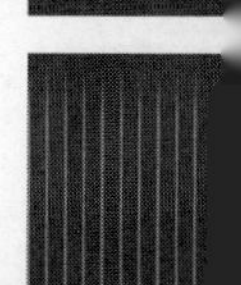

Chief Complaints

....

....

....

....

Condition of Mother at Discharge

....

....

....

....

Condition of Newborn at Discharge

....

....

....

....

Health Education (Diet, Family Planning/Follow-up)

....

....

....

....

Nursing Care Plan

S.No.	Assessment	Nursing Diagnosis	Goal/Expected Out Come	Nursing Intervention	Rational	Implementation	Evaluation

Signature of Sister in Charge

Signature of Supervisor

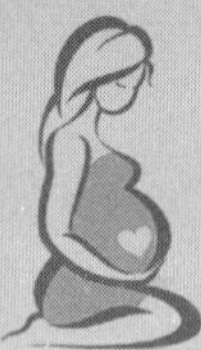

Postnatal Assessment (Case No. 7)

Client's Profile

Name : .... Occupation : ....

Age : .... Income per month : ....

Hospital name : .... W/o : ....

Date of booking : .... Period of gestation : ....

Reg. No : .... Religion : ....

Address : ....

Education : ....

Menstrual History

Age at menarche : ....year of age

Cycle of : .... days

Period duration of : .... days

Blood flow: Average/scanty/heavy ....

Dysmenorrhea: ....

Obstetric History

S.No.	Year	Term/ preterm	Abortion/ stillbirth	Nature of delivery	Child		Immunization	Growth and development	Nature of puerperium	Remark
					Alive	Sex/ weight				

Personal History

Allergies to drug : .... Body built : ....

Habit : Smoking/alcohol/betel chewing/any drug addiction

Hobbies : ....

Dietary habits : Veg/nonvegetarian,......................... Diet per day : 2/3/4/5/6

Immunization status : TT: 1st dose .... 2nd dose ....

Present and Past Medical History

High BP/diabetes/breathlessness on exertion/palpitation/tuberculosis/asthma/renal disease/convulsion/jaundice/malaria/RTI/STI/HIV/AIDS/no any/if any other specify ....

Family History

Family History of :

Systemic Illness : High BP/Diabetes/Tuberculosis/No Any

Blood Disorder : Thalassemia/Repeated blood transfusion

Delivery of : Twins/Congenital abnormalities

Notes on Admission for Labor

Present pregnancy : Full term/pre term .... Period of gestation : ....

Presentation of fetus : .... FHS : ....

Labor Notes

Membrane ruptured on : .... at: ....

Length of labor : ....

1st stage : .... 2nd stage : ....

3rd stage : .... **Total hours** : ....

Maternal Condition on Shifting

Date and time of shifting (in postnatal ward) : ....

Newborn general condition on shifting : ....

Newborn date and time of shifting (in postnatal ward) : ....

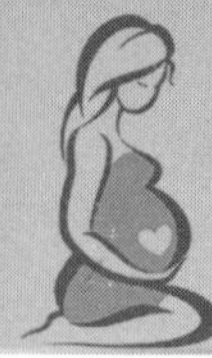

Postnatal Assessment for Mother and Baby

Mother

Postnatal day	1	2	3	4	5	6
Date						
Time						
Vital sign						
Temperature						
Pulse						
Respiration						
BP						
Fundal height						
Uterus						
Lochia						
Perineal care/episiotomy (REEDA)						
Breast						
Bowel/stool						
Bladder/urine						

Baby

Postnatal day	1	2	3	4	5	6
Date						
Time						
Vital sign						
Temperature						
Pulse						
Respiration						
Urine (time/day)						
Stool (time/day)						
Eye care						
Cord care						
Fontanels (Normal/Absent)						
Reflexes						
Activity						
Breastfeeding						
Anthropometric measurement						
Length (cm)						
Head circumference (cm)						
Chest (cm)						
Abdominal (cm)						
Weight (kg)						

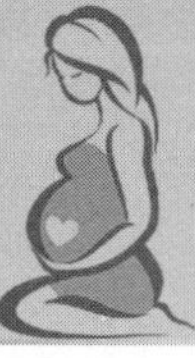

Chief Complaints

....

....

....

....

Condition of Mother at Discharge

....

....

....

....

Condition of Newborn at Discharge

....

....

....

....

Health Education (Diet, Family Planning/Follow-up)

....

....

....

....

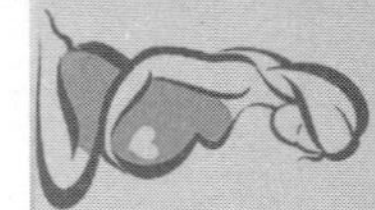

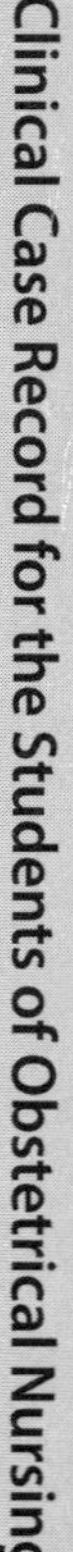

Nursing Care Plan

S.No.	Assessment	Nursing Diagnosis	Goal/Expected Out Come	Nursing Intervention	Rational	Implementation	Evaluation

Signature of Sister in Charge ____________________

Signature of Supervisor ____________________

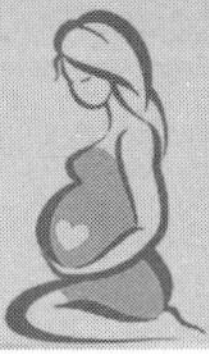

Postnatal Assessment (Case No. 8)

Client's Profile

Name : .... Occupation : ....

Age : .... Income per month : ....

Hospital name : .... W/o : ....

Date of booking : .... Period of gestation : ....

Reg. No : .... Religion : ....

Address : ....

Education : ....

Menstrual History

Age at menarche : ....year of age

Cycle of : .... days

Period duration of : .... days

Blood flow: Average/scanty/heavy ....

Dysmenorrhea: ....

Obstetric History

S.No.	Year	Term/ preterm	Abortion/ stillbirth	Nature of delivery	Child		Immunization	Growth and development	Nature of puerperium	Remark
					Alive	Sex/ weight				

Personal History

Allergies to drug : .... Body built : ....

Habit : Smoking/alcohol/betel chewing/any drug addiction

Hobbies : ....

Dietary habits : Veg/nonvegetarian,........................ Diet per day : 2/3/4/5/6

Immunization status : TT: 1st dose .... 2nd dose ....

Present and Past Medical History

High BP/diabetes/breathlessness on exertion/palpitation/tuberculosis/asthma/renal disease/convulsion/jaundice/malaria/RTI/STI/HIV/AIDS/no any/if any other specify ....

Family History

Family History of :

Systemic Illness : High BP/Diabetes/Tuberculosis/No Any

Blood Disorder : Thalassemia/Repeated blood transfusion

Delivery of : Twins/Congenital abnormalities

Notes on Admission for Labor

Present pregnancy : Full term/pre term .... Period of gestation : ....

Presentation of fetus : .... FHS : ....

Labor Notes

Membrane ruptured on : .... at: ....

Length of labor : ....

1st stage : .... 2nd stage : ....

3rd stage : .... **Total hours** : ....

Maternal Condition on Shifting

Date and time of shifting (in postnatal ward) : ....

Newborn general condition on shifting : ....

Newborn date and time of shifting (in postnatal ward) : ....

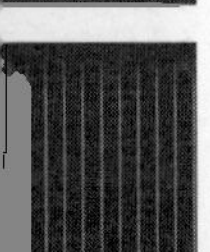

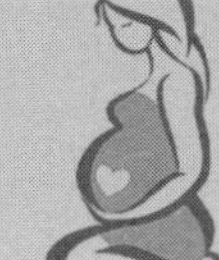

Postnatal Assessment for Mother and Baby

Mother

Postnatal day	1	2	3	4	5	6
Date						
Time						
Vital sign						
Temperature						
Pulse						
Respiration						
BP						
Fundal height						
Uterus						
Lochia						
Perineal care/episiotomy (REEDA)						
Breast						
Bowel/stool						
Bladder/urine						

Baby

Postnatal day	1	2	3	4	5	6
Date						
Time						
Vital sign						
Temperature						
Pulse						
Respiration						
Urine (time/day)						
Stool (time/day)						
Eye care						
Cord care						
Fontanels (Normal/Absent)						
Reflexes						
Activity						
Breastfeeding						
Anthropometric measurement						
Length (cm)						
Head circumference (cm)						
Chest (cm)						
Abdominal (cm)						
Weight (kg)						

Chief Complaints

....

....

....

....

Condition of Mother at Discharge

....

....

....

....

Condition of Newborn at Discharge

....

....

....

....

Health Education (Diet, Family Planning/Follow-up)

....

....

....

....

Nursing Care Plan

S.No.	Assessment	Nursing Diagnosis	Goal/Expected Out Come	Nursing Intervention	Rational	Implementation	Evaluation

Signature of Sister in Charge

Signature of Supervisor

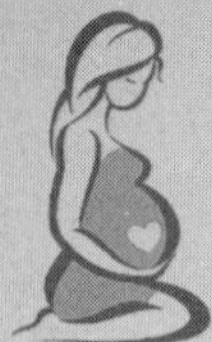

Postnatal Assessment (Case No. 9)

Client's Profile

Name : ....

Occupation : ....

Age : ....

Income per month : ....

Hospital name : ....

W/o : ....

Date of booking : ....

Period of gestation : ....

Reg. No : ....

Religion : ....

Address : ....

Education : ....

Menstrual History

Age at menarche : ....year of age

Cycle of : .... days

Period duration of : .... days

Blood flow: Average/scanty/heavy ....

Dysmenorrhea: ....

Obstetric History

S.No.	Year	Term/ preterm	Abortion/ stillbirth	Nature of delivery	Child		Immunization	Growth and development	Nature of puerperium	Remark
					Alive	Sex/ weight				

Personal History

Allergies to drug : .... Body built : ....

Habit : Smoking/alcohol/betel chewing/any drug addiction

Hobbies : ....

Dietary habits : Veg/nonvegetarian,...................... Diet per day : 2/3/4/5/6

Immunization status : TT: 1st dose .... 2nd dose ....

Present and Past Medical History

High BP/diabetes/breathlessness on exertion/palpitation/tuberculosis/asthma/renal disease/convulsion/jaundice/malaria/RTI/STI/HIV/AIDS/no any/if any other specify ....

Family History

Family History of :

Systemic Illness : High BP/Diabetes/Tuberculosis/No Any

Blood Disorder : Thalassemia/Repeated blood transfusion

Delivery of : Twins/Congenital abnormalities

Notes on Admission for Labor

Present pregnancy : Full term/pre term .... Period of gestation : ....

Presentation of fetus : .... FHS : ....

Labor Notes

Membrane ruptured on : .... at: ....

Length of labor : ....

1st stage : .... 2nd stage : ....

3rd stage : .... **Total hours** **: ....**

Maternal Condition on Shifting

Date and time of shifting (in postnatal ward) : ....

Newborn general condition on shifting : ....

Newborn date and time of shifting (in postnatal ward) : ....

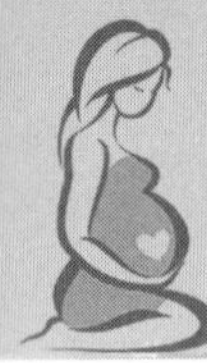

Postnatal Assessment for Mother and Baby

Mother

Postnatal day	1	2	3	4	5	6
Date						
Time						
Vital sign						
Temperature						
Pulse						
Respiration						
BP						
Fundal height						
Uterus						
Lochia						
Perineal care/episiotomy (REEDA)						
Breast						
Bowel/stool						
Bladder/urine						

Baby

Postnatal day	1	2	3	4	5	6
Date						
Time						
Vital sign						
Temperature						
Pulse						
Respiration						
Urine (time/day)						
Stool (time/day)						
Eye care						
Cord care						
Fontanels (Normal/Absent)						
Reflexes						
Activity						
Breastfeeding						
Anthropometric measurement						
Length (cm)						
Head circumference (cm)						
Chest (cm)						
Abdominal (cm)						
Weight (kg)						

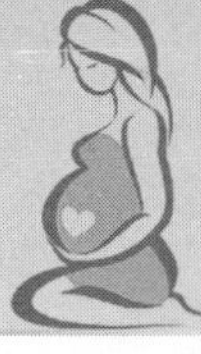

Chief Complaints

....

....

....

....

Condition of Mother at Discharge

....

....

....

....

Condition of Newborn at Discharge

....

....

....

....

Health Education (Diet, Family Planning/Follow-up)

....

....

....

....

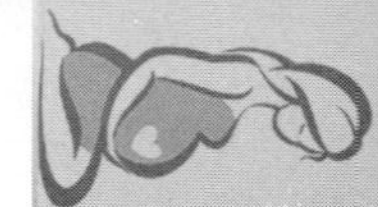

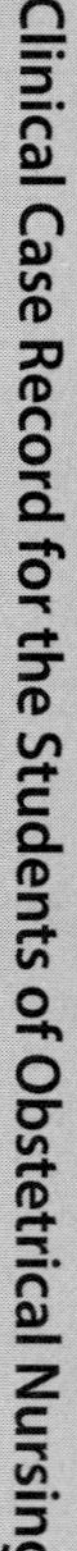

Nursing Care Plan

S.No.	Assessment	Nursing Diagnosis	Goal/Expected Out Come	Nursing Intervention	Rational	Implementation	Evaluation

Signature of Sister in Charge

Signature of Supervisor

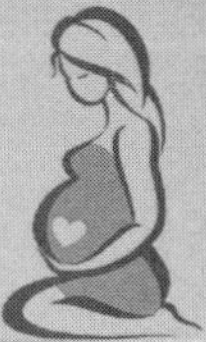

Postnatal Assessment (Case No. 10)

Client's Profile

Name : .... Occupation : ....

Age : .... Income per month : ....

Hospital name : .... W/o : ....

Date of booking : .... Period of gestation : ....

Reg. No : .... Religion : ....

Address : ....

Education : ....

Menstrual History

Age at menarche : ....year of age Blood flow: Average/scanty/heavy ....

Cycle of : .... days Dysmenorrhea: ....

Period duration of : .... days

Obstetric History

S.No.	Year	Term/ preterm	Abortion/ stillbirth	Nature of delivery	Child		Immunization	Growth and development	Nature of puerperium	Remark
					Alive	Sex/ weight				

Personal History

Allergies to drug : .... Body built : ....

Habit : Smoking/alcohol/betel chewing/any drug addiction

Hobbies : ....

Dietary habits : Veg/nonvegetarian,...................... Diet per day : 2/3/4/5/6

Immunization status : TT: 1st dose .... 2nd dose ....

Present and Past Medical History

High BP/diabetes/breathlessness on exertion/palpitation/tuberculosis/asthma/renal disease/convulsion/jaundice/malaria/RTI/STI/HIV/AIDS/no any/if any other specify ....

Family History

Family History of :

Systemic Illness : High BP/Diabetes/Tuberculosis/No Any

Blood Disorder : Thalassemia/Repeated blood transfusion

Delivery of : Twins/Congenital abnormalities

Notes on Admission for Labor

Present pregnancy : Full term/pre term .... Period of gestation : ....

Presentation of fetus : .... FHS : ....

Labor Notes

Membrane ruptured on : .... at: ....

Length of labor : ....

1st stage : .... 2nd stage : ....

3rd stage : .... **Total hours : ....**

Maternal Condition on Shifting

Date and time of shifting (in postnatal ward) : ....

Newborn general condition on shifting : ....

Newborn date and time of shifting (in postnatal ward) : ....

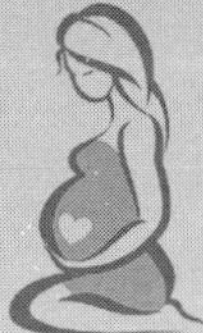

Postnatal Assessment for Mother and Baby

Mother

Postnatal day	1	2	3	4	5	6
Date						
Time						
Vital sign						
Temperature						
Pulse						
Respiration						
BP						
Fundal height						
Uterus						
Lochia						
Perineal care/episiotomy (REEDA)						
Breast						
Bowel/stool						
Bladder/urine						

Baby

Postnatal day	1	2	3	4	5	6
Date						
Time						
Vital sign						
Temperature						
Pulse						
Respiration						
Urine (time/day)						
Stool (time/day)						
Eye care						
Cord care						
Fontanels (Normal/Absent)						
Reflexes						
Activity						
Breastfeeding						
Anthropometric measurement						
Length (cm)						
Head circumference (cm)						
Chest (cm)						
Abdominal (cm)						
Weight (kg)						

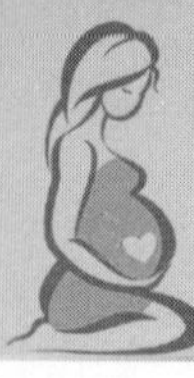

Chief Complaints

....

....

....

....

Condition of Mother at Discharge

....

....

....

....

Condition of Newborn at Discharge

....

....

....

....

Health Education (Diet, Family Planning/Follow-up)

....

....

....

....

Nursing Care Plan

S.No.	Assessment	Nursing Diagnosis	Goal/Expected Out Come	Nursing Intervention	Rational	Implementation	Evaluation

Signature of Sister in Charge ________________

Signature of Supervisor ________________

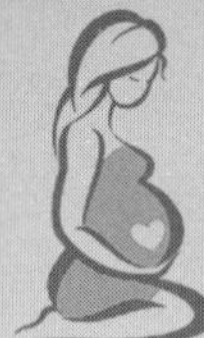

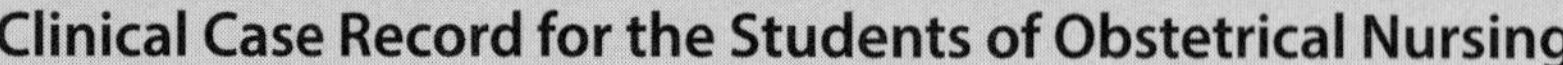

Postnatal Assessment (Case No. 11)

Client's Profile

Name : .... Occupation : ....

Age : .... Income per month : ....

Hospital name : .... W/o : ....

Date of booking : .... Period of gestation : ....

Reg. No : .... Religion : ....

Address : ....

Education : ....

Menstrual History

Age at menarche : ....year of age

Cycle of : .... days

Period duration of : .... days

Blood flow: Average/scanty/heavy ....

Dysmenorrhea: ....

Obstetric History

S.No.	Year	Term/ preterm	Abortion/ stillbirth	Nature of delivery	Child		Immunization	Growth and development	Nature of puerperium	Remark
					Alive	Sex/ weight				

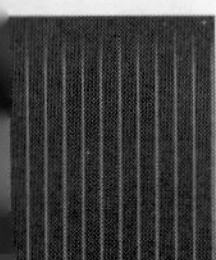

Personal History

Allergies to drug : .... Body built : ....

Habit : Smoking/alcohol/betel chewing/any drug addiction

Hobbies : ....

Dietary habits : Veg/nonvegetarian,......................... Diet per day : 2/3/4/5/6

Immunization status : TT: 1st dose .... 2nd dose ....

Present and Past Medical History

High BP/diabetes/breathlessness on exertion/palpitation/tuberculosis/asthma/renal disease/convulsion/jaundice/malaria/RTI/STI/HIV/AIDS/no any/if any other specify ....

Family History

Family History of :

Systemic Illness : High BP/Diabetes/Tuberculosis/No Any

Blood Disorder : Thalassemia/Repeated blood transfusion

Delivery of : Twins/Congenital abnormalities

Notes on Admission for Labor

Present pregnancy : Full term/pre term .... Period of gestation : ....

Presentation of fetus : .... FHS : ....

Labor Notes

Membrane ruptured on : .... at: ....

Length of labor : ....

1st stage : .... 2nd stage : ....

3rd stage : .... **Total hours** : **..**

Maternal Condition on Shifting

Date and time of shifting (in postnatal ward) : ....

Newborn general condition on shifting : ....

Newborn date and time of shifting (in postnatal ward) : ....

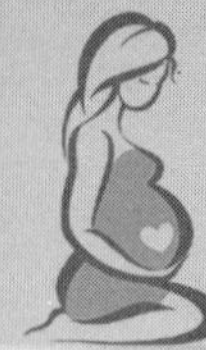

Postnatal Assessment for Mother and Baby

Mother

Postnatal day	1	2	3	4	5	6
Date						
Time						
Vital sign						
Temperature						
Pulse						
Respiration						
BP						
Fundal height						
Uterus						
Lochia						
Perineal care/episiotomy (REEDA)						
Breast						
Bowel/stool						
Bladder/urine						

Baby

Postnatal day	1	2	3	4	5	6
Date						
Time						
Vital sign						
Temperature						
Pulse						
Respiration						
Urine (time/day)						
Stool (time/day)						
Eye care						
Cord care						
Fontanels (Normal/Absent)						
Reflexes						
Activity						
Breastfeeding						
Anthropometric measurement						
Length (cm)						
Head circumference (cm)						
Chest (cm)						
Abdominal (cm)						
Weight (kg)						

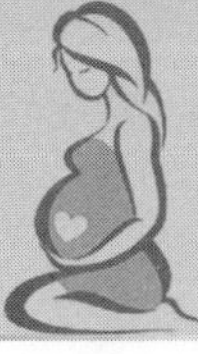

Chief Complaints

....

....

....

....

Condition of Mother at Discharge

....

....

....

....

Condition of Newborn at Discharge

....

....

....

....

Health Education (Diet, Family Planning/Follow-up)

....

....

....

....

Nursing Care Plan

S.No.	Assessment	Nursing Diagnosis	Goal/Expected Out Come	Nursing Intervention	Rational	Implementation	Evaluation

Signature of Sister in Charge ____________________

Signature of Supervisor ____________________

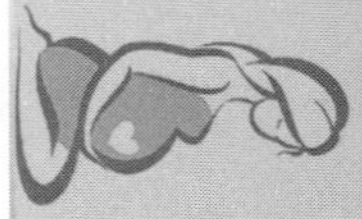

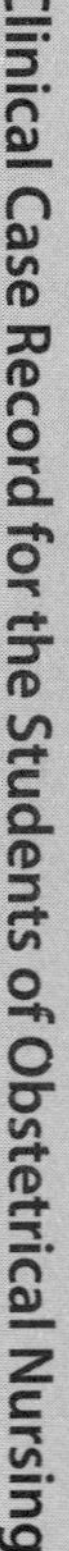

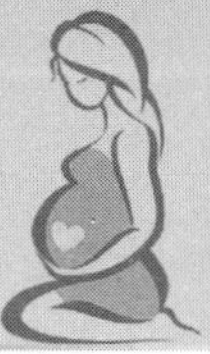

Postnatal Assessment (Case No. 12)

Client's Profile

Name : .... Occupation : ....

Age : .... Income per month : ....

Hospital name : .... W/o : ....

Date of booking : .... Period of gestation : ....

Reg. No : .... Religion : ....

Address : ....

Education : ....

Menstrual History

Age at menarche : ....year of age

Cycle of : .... days

Period duration of : .... days

Blood flow: Average/scanty/heavy ....

Dysmenorrhea: ....

Obstetric History

S.No.	Year	Term/ preterm	Abortion/ stillbirth	Nature of delivery	Child		Immunization	Growth and development	Nature of puerperium	Remark
					Alive	Sex/ weight				

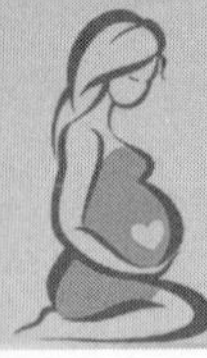

Personal History

Allergies to drug : .... Body built : ....

Habit : Smoking/alcohol/betel chewing/any drug addiction

Hobbies : ....

Dietary habits : Veg/nonvegetarian,...................... Diet per day : 2/3/4/5/6

Immunization status : TT: 1st dose .... 2nd dose ....

Present and Past Medical History

High BP/diabetes/breathlessness on exertion/palpitation/tuberculosis/asthma/renal disease/convulsion/jaundice/malaria/RTI/STI/HIV/AIDS/no any/if any other specify ....

Family History

Family History of :

Systemic Illness : High BP/Diabetes/Tuberculosis/No Any

Blood Disorder : Thalassemia/Repeated blood transfusion

Delivery of : Twins/Congenital abnormalities

Notes on Admission for Labor

Present pregnancy : Full term/pre term .... Period of gestation : ....

Presentation of fetus : .... FHS : ....

Labor Notes

Membrane ruptured on : .... at: ....

Length of labor : ....

1st stage : .... 2nd stage : ....

3rd stage : .... **Total hours** **: ....**

Maternal Condition on Shifting

Date and time of shifting (in postnatal ward) : ....

Newborn general condition on shifting : ....

Newborn date and time of shifting (in postnatal ward) : ....

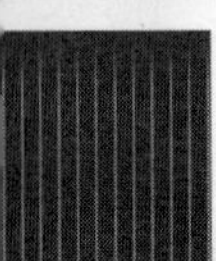

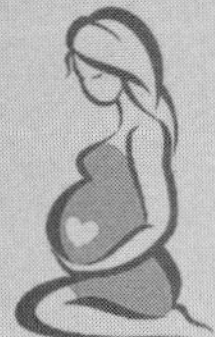

Postnatal Assessment for Mother and Baby

Mother

Postnatal day	1	2	3	4	5	6
Date						
Time						
Vital sign						
Temperature						
Pulse						
Respiration						
BP						
Fundal height						
Uterus						
Lochia						
Perineal care/episiotomy (REEDA)						
Breast						
Bowel/stool						
Bladder/urine						

Baby

Postnatal day	1	2	3	4	5	6
Date						
Time						
Vital sign						
Temperature						
Pulse						
Respiration						
Urine (time/day)						
Stool (time/day)						
Eye care						
Cord care						
Fontanels (Normal/Absent)						
Reflexes						
Activity						
Breastfeeding						
Anthropometric measurement						
Length (cm)						
Head circumference (cm)						
Chest (cm)						
Abdominal (cm)						
Weight (kg)						

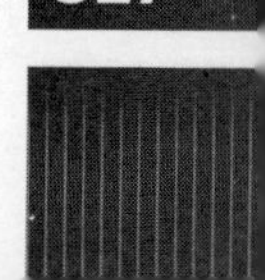

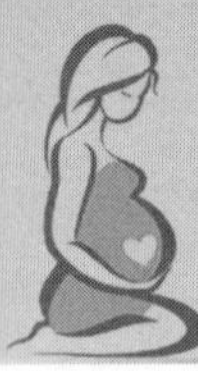

Chief Complaints

....

....

....

....

Condition of Mother at Discharge

....

....

....

....

Condition of Newborn at Discharge

....

....

....

....

Health Education (Diet, Family Planning/Follow-up)

....

....

....

....

Nursing Care Plan

S.No.	Assessment	Nursing Diagnosis	Goal/Expected Out Come	Nursing Intervention	Rational	Implementation	Evaluation

Signature of Sister in Charge

Signature of Supervisor

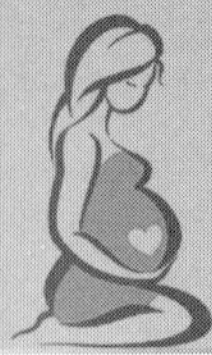

Postnatal Assessment (Case No. 13)

Client's Profile

Name : ....

Occupation : ....

Age : ....

Income per month : ....

Hospital name : ....

W/o : ....

Date of booking : ....

Period of gestation : ....

Reg. No : ....

Religion : ....

Address : ....

Education : ....

Menstrual History

Age at menarche : ....year of age

Cycle of : .... days

Period duration of : .... days

Blood flow: Average/scanty/heavy ....

Dysmenorrhea: ....

Obstetric History

S.No.	Year	Term/ preterm	Abortion/ stillbirth	Nature of delivery	Child		Immunization	Growth and development	Nature of puerperium	Remark
					Alive	Sex/ weight				

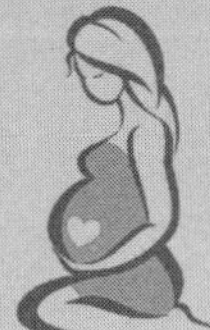

Personal History

Allergies to drug : .... Body built : ....

Habit : Smoking/alcohol/betel chewing/any drug addiction

Hobbies : ....

Dietary habits : Veg/nonvegetarian,....................... Diet per day : 2/3/4/5/6

Immunization status : TT: 1st dose .... 2nd dose ....

Present and Past Medical History

High BP/diabetes/breathlessness on exertion/palpitation/tuberculosis/asthma/renal disease/convulsion/jaundice/malaria/RTI/STI/HIV/AIDS/no any/if any other specify ....

Family History

Family History of :

Systemic Illness : High BP/Diabetes/Tuberculosis/No Any

Blood Disorder : Thalassemia/Repeated blood transfusion

Delivery of : Twins/Congenital abnormalities

Notes on Admission for Labor

Present pregnancy : Full term/pre term .... Period of gestation : ....

Presentation of fetus : .... FHS : ....

Labor Notes

Membrane ruptured on : .... at: ....

Length of labor : ....

1st stage : .... 2nd stage : ....

3rd stage : .... **Total hours** **: ....**

Maternal Condition on Shifting

Date and time of shifting (in postnatal ward) : ....

Newborn general condition on shifting : ....

Newborn date and time of shifting (in postnatal ward) : ....

Postnatal Assessment for Mother and Baby

Mother

Postnatal day	1	2	3	4	5	6
Date						
Time						
Vital sign						
Temperature						
Pulse						
Respiration						
BP						
Fundal height						
Uterus						
Lochia						
Perineal care/episiotomy (REEDA)						
Breast						
Bowel/stool						
Bladder/urine						

Baby

Postnatal day	1	2	3	4	5	6
Date						
Time						
Vital sign						
Temperature						
Pulse						
Respiration						
Urine (time/day)						
Stool (time/day)						
Eye care						
Cord care						
Fontanels (Normal/Absent)						
Reflexes						
Activity						
Breastfeeding						
Anthropometric measurement						
Length (cm)						
Head circumference (cm)						
Chest (cm)						
Abdominal (cm)						
Weight (kg)						

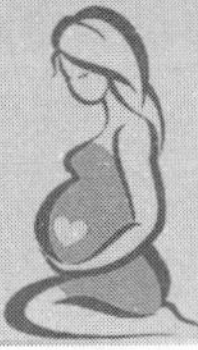

Chief Complaints

....

....

....

....

Condition of Mother at Discharge

....

....

....

....

Condition of Newborn at Discharge

....

....

....

....

Health Education (Diet, Family Planning/Follow-up)

....

....

....

....

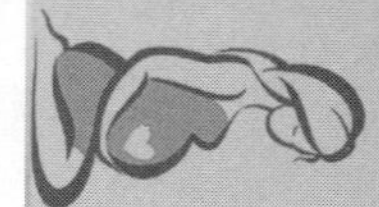

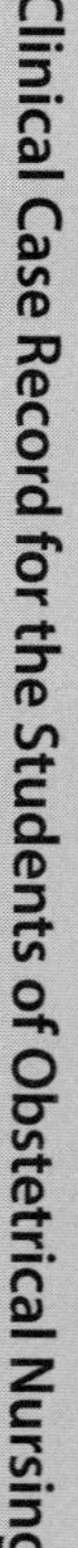

Nursing Care Plan

S.No.	Assessment	Nursing Diagnosis	Goal/Expected Out Come	Nursing Intervention	Rational	Implementation	Evaluation

Signature of Sister in Charge

Signature of Supervisor

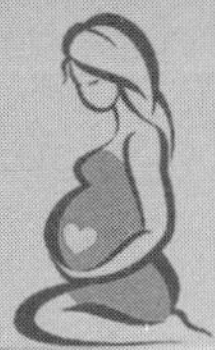

Postnatal Assessment (Case No. 14)

Client's Profile

Name : .... Occupation : ....

Age : .... Income per month : ....

Hospital name : .... W/o : ....

Date of booking : .... Period of gestation : ....

Reg. No : .... Religion : ....

Address : ....

Education : ....

Menstrual History

Age at menarche : ....year of age

Cycle of : .... days

Period duration of : .... days

Blood flow: Average/scanty/heavy ....

Dysmenorrhea: ....

Obstetric History

S.No.	Year	Term/ preterm	Abortion/ stillbirth	Nature of delivery	Child		Immunization	Growth and development	Nature of puerperium	Remark
					Alive	Sex/ weight				

Personal History

Allergies to drug : .... Body built : ....

Habit : Smoking/alcohol/betel chewing/any drug addiction

Hobbies : ....

Dietary habits : Veg/nonvegetarian,....................... Diet per day : 2/3/4/5/6

Immunization status : TT: 1st dose .... 2nd dose ....

Present and Past Medical History

High BP/diabetes/breathlessness on exertion/palpitation/tuberculosis/asthma/renal disease/convulsion/jaundice/malaria/RTI/STI/HIV/AIDS/no any/if any other specify ....

Family History

Family History of :

Systemic Illness : High BP/Diabetes/Tuberculosis/No Any

Blood Disorder : Thalassemia/Repeated blood transfusion

Delivery of : Twins/Congenital abnormalities

Notes on Admission for Labor

Present pregnancy : Full term/pre term .... Period of gestation : ....

Presentation of fetus : .... FHS : ....

Labor Notes

Membrane ruptured on : .... at: ....

Length of labor : ....

1st stage : .... 2nd stage : ....

3rd stage : .... **Total hours** **: ....**

Maternal Condition on Shifting

Date and time of shifting (in postnatal ward) : ....

Newborn general condition on shifting : ....

Newborn date and time of shifting (in postnatal ward) : ....

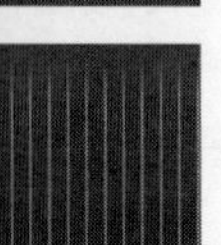

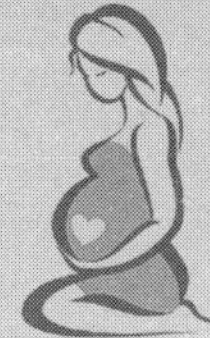

Postnatal Assessment for Mother and Baby

Mother

Postnatal day	1	2	3	4	5	6
Date						
Time						
Vital sign						
Temperature						
Pulse						
Respiration						
BP						
Fundal height						
Uterus						
Lochia						
Perineal care/episiotomy (REEDA)						
Breast						
Bowel/stool						
Bladder/urine						

Baby

Postnatal day	1	2	3	4	5	6
Date						
Time						
Vital sign						
Temperature						
Pulse						
Respiration						
Urine (time/day)						
Stool (time/day)						
Eye care						
Cord care						
Fontanels (Normal/Absent)						
Reflexes						
Activity						
Breastfeeding						
Anthropometric measurement						
Length (cm)						
Head circumference (cm)						
Chest (cm)						
Abdominal (cm)						
Weight (kg)						

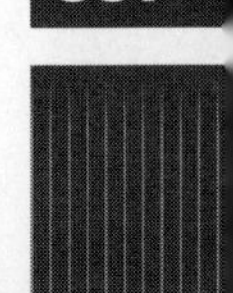

Chief Complaints

....

....

....

....

Condition of Mother at Discharge

....

....

....

....

Condition of Newborn at Discharge

....

....

....

....

Health Education (Diet, Family Planning/Follow-up)

....

....

....

....

Nursing Care Plan

S.No.	Assessment	Nursing Diagnosis	Goal/Expected Out Come	Nursing Intervention	Rational	Implementation	Evaluation

Signature of Sister in Charge

Signature of Supervisor

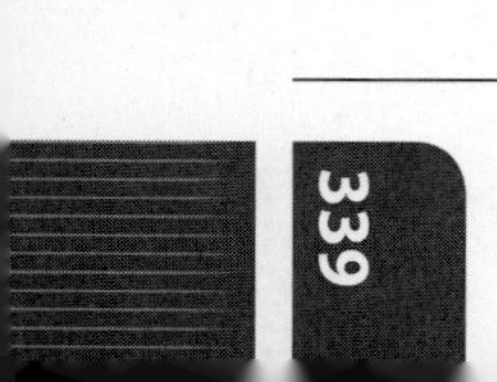

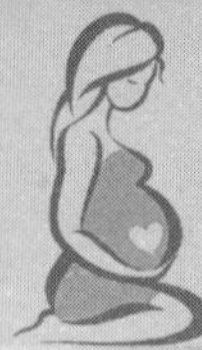

Postnatal Assessment (Case No. 15)

Client's Profile

Name : .... Occupation : ....

Age : .... Income per month : ....

Hospital name : .... W/o : ....

Date of booking : .... Period of gestation : ....

Reg. No : .... Religion : ....

Address : ....

Education : ....

Menstrual History

Age at menarche : ....year of age

Cycle of : .... days

Period duration of : .... days

Blood flow: Average/scanty/heavy ....

Dysmenorrhea: ....

Obstetric History

S.No.	Year	Term/ preterm	Abortion/ stillbirth	Nature of delivery	Child		Immunization	Growth and development	Nature of puerperium	Remark
					Alive	Sex/ weight				

Personal History

Allergies to drug : .... Body built : ....

Habit : Smoking/alcohol/betel chewing/any drug addiction

Hobbies : ....

Dietary habits : Veg/nonvegetarian,........................ Diet per day : 2/3/4/5/6

Immunization status : TT: 1st dose .... 2nd dose ....

Present and Past Medical History

High BP/diabetes/breathlessness on exertion/palpitation/tuberculosis/asthma/renal disease/convulsion/jaundice/malaria/RTI/STI/HIV/AIDS/no any/if any other specify ....

Family History

Family History of :

Systemic Illness : High BP/Diabetes/Tuberculosis/No Any

Blood Disorder : Thalassemia/Repeated blood transfusion

Delivery of : Twins/Congenital abnormalities

Notes on Admission for Labor

Present pregnancy : Full term/pre term .... Period of gestation : ....

Presentation of fetus : .... FHS : ....

Labor Notes

Membrane ruptured on : .... at: ....

Length of labor : ....

1st stage : .... 2nd stage : ....

3rd stage : .... **Total hours** **: ....**

Maternal Condition on Shifting

Date and time of shifting (in postnatal ward) : ....

Newborn general condition on shifting : ....

Newborn date and time of shifting (in postnatal ward) : ....

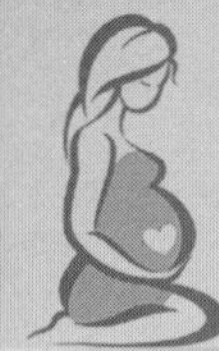

Postnatal Assessment for Mother and Baby

Mother

Postnatal day	1	2	3	4	5	6
Date						
Time						
Vital sign						
Temperature						
Pulse						
Respiration						
BP						
Fundal height						
Uterus						
Lochia						
Perineal care/episiotomy (REEDA)						
Breast						
Bowel/stool						
Bladder/urine						

Baby

Postnatal day	1	2	3	4	5	6
Date						
Time						
Vital sign						
Temperature						
Pulse						
Respiration						
Urine (time/day)						
Stool (time/day)						
Eye care						
Cord care						
Fontanels (Normal/Absent)						
Reflexes						
Activity						
Breastfeeding						
Anthropometric measurement						
Length (cm)						
Head circumference (cm)						
Chest (cm)						
Abdominal (cm)						
Weight (kg)						

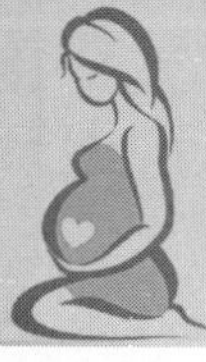

Chief Complaints

....

....

....

....

Condition of Mother at Discharge

....

....

....

....

Condition of Newborn at Discharge

....

....

....

....

Health Education (Diet, Family Planning/Follow-up)

....

....

....

....

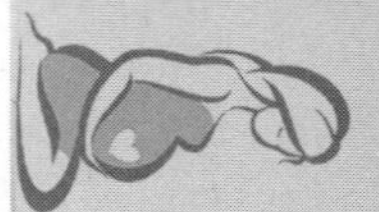

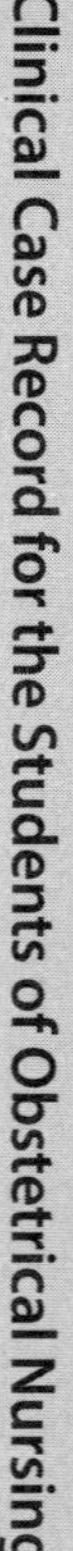

Nursing Care Plan

S.No.	Assessment	Nursing Diagnosis	Goal/Expected Out Come	Nursing Intervention	Rational	Implementation	Evaluation

Signature of Sister in Charge ________________

Signature of Supervisor ________________

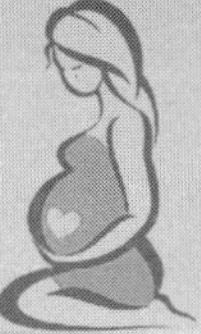

Postnatal Assessment (Case No. 16)

Client's Profile

Name : .... Occupation : ....

Age : .... Income per month : ....

Hospital name : .... W/o : ....

Date of booking : .... Period of gestation : ....

Reg. No : .... Religion : ....

Address : ....

Education : ....

Menstrual History

Age at menarche : ....year of age

Cycle of : .... days

Period duration of : .... days

Blood flow: Average/scanty/heavy ....

Dysmenorrhea: ....

Obstetric History

S.No.	Year	Term/ preterm	Abortion/ stillbirth	Nature of delivery	Child		Immunization	Growth and development	Nature of puerperium	Remark
					Alive	Sex/ weight				

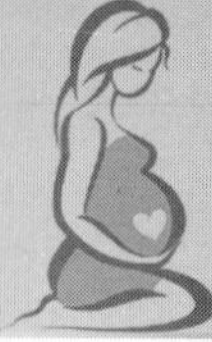

Personal History

Allergies to drug : .... Body built : ....

Habit : Smoking/alcohol/betel chewing/any drug addiction

Hobbies : ....

Dietary habits : Veg/nonvegetarian,....................... Diet per day : 2/3/4/5/6

Immunization status : TT: 1st dose .... 2nd dose ....

Present and Past Medical History

High BP/diabetes/breathlessness on exertion/palpitation/tuberculosis/asthma/renal disease/convulsion/jaundice/ malaria/RTI/STI/HIV/AIDS/no any/if any other specify ....

Family History

Family History of :

Systemic Illness : High BP/Diabetes/Tuberculosis/No Any

Blood Disorder : Thalassemia/Repeated blood transfusion

Delivery of : Twins/Congenital abnormalities

Notes on Admission for Labor

Present pregnancy : Full term/pre term .... Period of gestation : ....

Presentation of fetus : .... FHS : ....

Labor Notes

Membrane ruptured on : .... at: ....

Length of labor : ....

1st stage : .... 2nd stage : ....

3rd stage : .... **Total hours** : **...**

Maternal Condition on Shifting

Date and time of shifting (in postnatal ward) : ....

Newborn general condition on shifting : ....

Newborn date and time of shifting (in postnatal ward) : ....

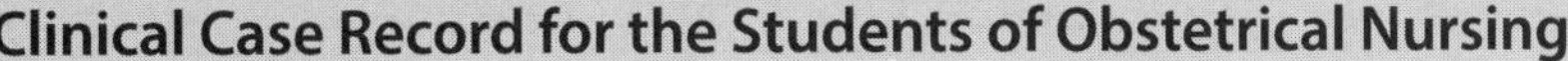
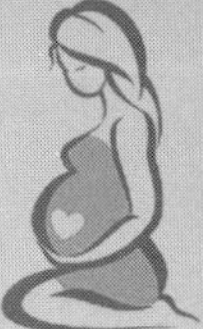

Postnatal Assessment for Mother and Baby

Mother

Postnatal day	1	2	3	4	5	6
Date						
Time						
Vital sign						
Temperature						
Pulse						
Respiration						
BP						
Fundal height						
Uterus						
Lochia						
Perineal care/episiotomy (REEDA)						
Breast						
Bowel/stool						
Bladder/urine						

Baby

Postnatal day	1	2	3	4	5	6
Date						
Time						
Vital sign						
Temperature						
Pulse						
Respiration						
Urine (time/day)						
Stool (time/day)						
Eye care						
Cord care						
Fontanels (Normal/Absent)						
Reflexes						
Activity						
Breastfeeding						
Anthropometric measurement						
Length (cm)						
Head circumference (cm)						
Chest (cm)						
Abdominal (cm)						
Weight (kg)						

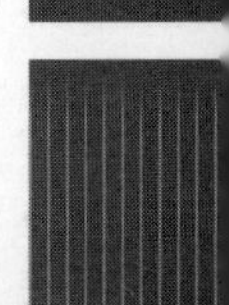

Chief Complaints

....

....

....

....

Condition of Mother at Discharge

....

....

....

....

Condition of Newborn at Discharge

....

....

....

....

Health Education (Diet, Family Planning/Follow-up)

....

....

....

....

Nursing Care Plan

S.No.	Assessment	Nursing Diagnosis	Goal/Expected Out Come	Nursing Intervention	Rational	Implementation	Evaluation

Signature of Sister in Charge

Signature of Supervisor

Postnatal Assessment (Case No. 17)

Client's Profile

Name : .... Occupation : ....

Age : .... Income per month : ....

Hospital name : .... W/o : ....

Date of booking : .... Period of gestation : ....

Reg. No : .... Religion : ....

Address : ....

Education : ....

Menstrual History

Age at menarche : ....year of age

Cycle of : .... days

Period duration of : .... days

Blood flow: Average/scanty/heavy ....

Dysmenorrhea: ....

Obstetric History

S.No.	Year	Term/ preterm	Abortion/ stillbirth	Nature of delivery	Child		Immunization	Growth and development	Nature of puerperium	Remark
					Alive	Sex/ weight				

Personal History

Allergies to drug : .... Body built : ....

Habit : Smoking/alcohol/betel chewing/any drug addiction

Hobbies : ....

Dietary habits : Veg/nonvegetarian,...................... Diet per day : 2/3/4/5/6

Immunization status : TT: 1st dose .... 2nd dose ....

Present and Past Medical History

High BP/diabetes/breathlessness on exertion/palpitation/tuberculosis/asthma/renal disease/convulsion/jaundice/malaria/RTI/STI/HIV/AIDS/no any/if any other specify ....

Family History

Family History of :

Systemic Illness : High BP/Diabetes/Tuberculosis/No Any

Blood Disorder : Thalassemia/Repeated blood transfusion

Delivery of : Twins/Congenital abnormalities

Notes on Admission for Labor

Present pregnancy : Full term/pre term .... Period of gestation : ....

Presentation of fetus : .... FHS : ....

Labor Notes

Membrane ruptured on : .... at: ....

Length of labor : ....

1st stage : .... 2nd stage : ....

3rd stage : .... **Total hours** : ....

Maternal Condition on Shifting

Date and time of shifting (in postnatal ward) : ....

Newborn general condition on shifting : ....

Newborn date and time of shifting (in postnatal ward) : ....

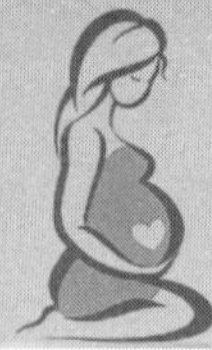

Postnatal Assessment for Mother and Baby

Mother

Postnatal day	1	2	3	4	5	6
Date						
Time						
Vital sign						
Temperature						
Pulse						
Respiration						
BP						
Fundal height						
Uterus						
Lochia						
Perineal care/episiotomy (REEDA)						
Breast						
Bowel/stool						
Bladder/urine						

Baby

Postnatal day	1	2	3	4	5	6
Date						
Time						
Vital sign						
Temperature						
Pulse						
Respiration						
Urine (time/day)						
Stool (time/day)						
Eye care						
Cord care						
Fontanels (Normal/Absent)						
Reflexes						
Activity						
Breastfeeding						
Anthropometric measurement						
Length (cm)						
Head circumference (cm)						
Chest (cm)						
Abdominal (cm)						
Weight (kg)						

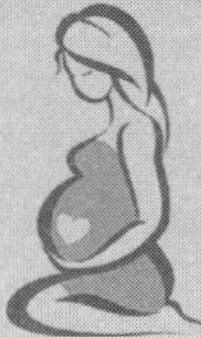

Chief Complaints

....

....

....

....

Condition of Mother at Discharge

....

....

....

....

Condition of Newborn at Discharge

....

....

....

....

Health Education (Diet, Family Planning/Follow-up)

....

....

....

....

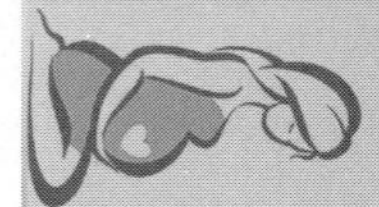

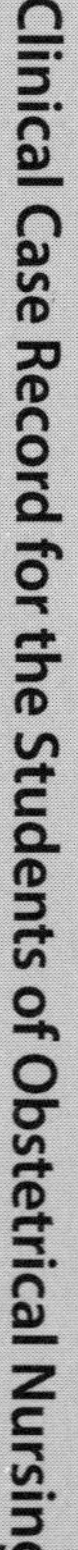

Nursing Care Plan

S.No.	Assessment	Nursing Diagnosis	Goal/Expected Out Come	Nursing Intervention	Rational	Implementation	Evaluation

Signature of Sister in Charge

Signature of Supervisor

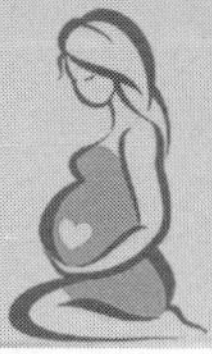

Postnatal Assessment (Case No. 18)

Client's Profile

Name : .... Occupation : ....

Age : .... Income per month : ....

Hospital name : .... W/o : ....

Date of booking : .... Period of gestation : ....

Reg. No : .... Religion : ....

Address : ....

Education : ....

Menstrual History

Age at menarche : ....year of age

Cycle of : .... days

Period duration of : .... days

Blood flow: Average/scanty/heavy ....

Dysmenorrhea: ....

Obstetric History

S.No.	Year	Term/ preterm	Abortion/ stillbirth	Nature of delivery	Child		Immunization	Growth and development	Nature of puerperium	Remark
					Alive	Sex/ weight				

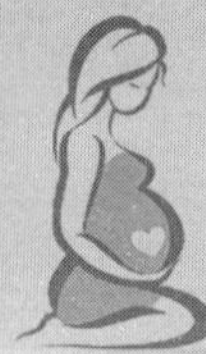

Personal History

Allergies to drug : .... Body built : ....

Habit : Smoking/alcohol/betel chewing/any drug addiction

Hobbies : ....

Dietary habits : Veg/nonvegetarian,...................... Diet per day : 2/3/4/5/6

Immunization status : TT: 1st dose .... 2nd dose ....

Present and Past Medical History

High BP/diabetes/breathlessness on exertion/palpitation/tuberculosis/asthma/renal disease/convulsion/jaundice/malaria/RTI/STI/HIV/AIDS/no any/if any other specify ....

Family History

Family History of :

Systemic Illness : High BP/Diabetes/Tuberculosis/No Any

Blood Disorder : Thalassemia/Repeated blood transfusion

Delivery of : Twins/Congenital abnormalities

Notes on Admission for Labor

Present pregnancy : Full term/pre term .... Period of gestation : ....

Presentation of fetus : .... FHS : ....

Labor Notes

Membrane ruptured on : .... at: ....

Length of labor : ....

1st stage : .... 2nd stage : ....

3rd stage : .... **Total hours** **: ....**

Maternal Condition on Shifting

Date and time of shifting (in postnatal ward) : ....

Newborn general condition on shifting : ....

Newborn date and time of shifting (in postnatal ward) : ....

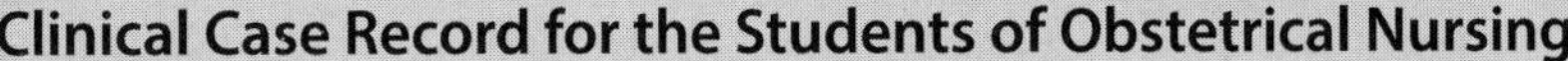

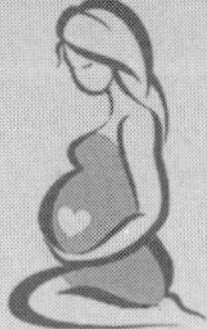

Postnatal Assessment for Mother and Baby

Mother

Postnatal day	1	2	3	4	5	6
Date						
Time						
Vital sign						
Temperature						
Pulse						
Respiration						
BP						
Fundal height						
Uterus						
Lochia						
Perineal care/episiotomy (REEDA)						
Breast						
Bowel/stool						
Bladder/urine						

Baby

Postnatal day	1	2	3	4	5	6
Date						
Time						
Vital sign						
Temperature						
Pulse						
Respiration						
Urine (time/day)						
Stool (time/day)						
Eye care						
Cord care						
Fontanels (Normal/Absent)						
Reflexes						
Activity						
Breastfeeding						
Anthropometric measurement						
Length (cm)						
Head circumference (cm)						
Chest (cm)						
Abdominal (cm)						
Weight (kg)						

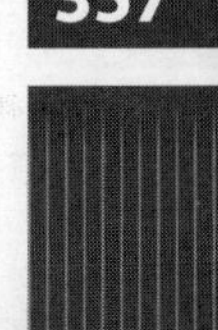

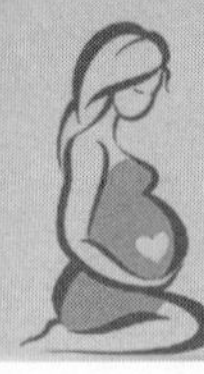

Chief Complaints

....

....

....

....

Condition of Mother at Discharge

....

....

....

....

Condition of Newborn at Discharge

....

....

....

....

Health Education (Diet, Family Planning/Follow-up)

....

....

....

....

Nursing Care Plan

S.No.	Assessment	Nursing Diagnosis	Goal/Expected Out Come	Nursing Intervention	Rational	Implementation	Evaluation

Signature of Sister in Charge

Signature of Supervisor

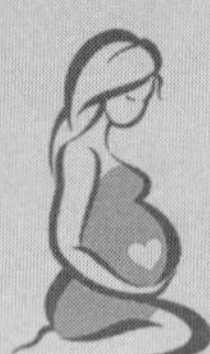

Postnatal Assessment (Case No. 19)

Client's Profile

Name : .... Occupation : ....

Age : .... Income per month : ....

Hospital name : .... W/o : ....

Date of booking : .... Period of gestation : ....

Reg. No : .... Religion : ....

Address : ....

Education : ....

Menstrual History

Age at menarche : ....year of age

Cycle of : .... days

Period duration of : .... days

Blood flow: Average/scanty/heavy ....

Dysmenorrhea: ....

Obstetric History

S.No.	Year	Term/ preterm	Abortion/ stillbirth	Nature of delivery	Child		Immunization	Growth and development	Nature of puerperium	Remark
					Alive	Sex/ weight				

Personal History

Allergies to drug : .... Body built : ....

Habit : Smoking/alcohol/betel chewing/any drug addiction

Hobbies : ....

Dietary habits : Veg/nonvegetarian,........................ Diet per day : 2/3/4/5/6

Immunization status : TT: 1st dose .... 2nd dose ....

Present and Past Medical History

High BP/diabetes/breathlessness on exertion/palpitation/tuberculosis/asthma/renal disease/convulsion/jaundice/malaria/RTI/STI/HIV/AIDS/no any/if any other specify ....

Family History

Family History of :

Systemic Illness : High BP/Diabetes/Tuberculosis/No Any

Blood Disorder : Thalassemia/Repeated blood transfusion

Delivery of : Twins/Congenital abnormalities

Notes on Admission for Labor

Present pregnancy : Full term/pre term .... Period of gestation : ....

Presentation of fetus : .... FHS : ....

Labor Notes

Membrane ruptured on : .... at: ....

Length of labor : ....

1st stage : .... 2nd stage : ....

3rd stage : .... **Total hours : ....**

Maternal Condition on Shifting

Date and time of shifting (in postnatal ward) : ....

Newborn general condition on shifting : ....

Newborn date and time of shifting (in postnatal ward) : ....

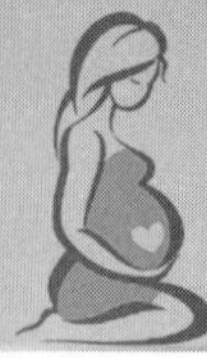

Postnatal Assessment for Mother and Baby

Mother

Postnatal day	1	2	3	4	5	6
Date						
Time						
Vital sign						
Temperature						
Pulse						
Respiration						
BP						
Fundal height						
Uterus						
Lochia						
Perineal care/episiotomy (REEDA)						
Breast						
Bowel/stool						
Bladder/urine						

Baby

Postnatal day	1	2	3	4	5	6
Date						
Time						
Vital sign						
Temperature						
Pulse						
Respiration						
Urine (time/day)						
Stool (time/day)						
Eye care						
Cord care						
Fontanels (Normal/Absent)						
Reflexes						
Activity						
Breastfeeding						
Anthropometric measurement						
Length (cm)						
Head circumference (cm)						
Chest (cm)						
Abdominal (cm)						
Weight (kg)						

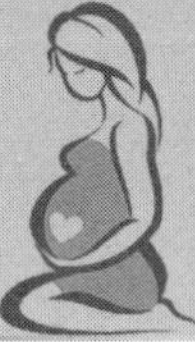

Chief Complaints

....

....

....

....

Condition of Mother at Discharge

....

....

....

....

Condition of Newborn at Discharge

....

....

....

....

Health Education (Diet, Family Planning/Follow-up)

....

....

....

....

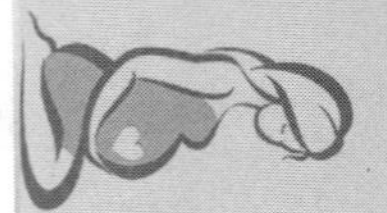

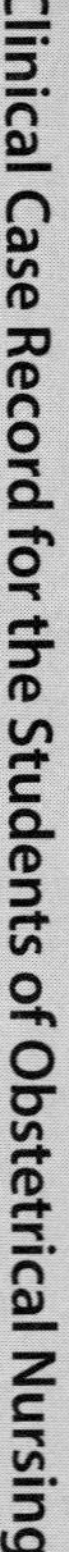

Nursing Care Plan

S.No.	Assessment	Nursing Diagnosis	Goal/Expected Out Come	Nursing Intervention	Rational	Implementation	Evaluation

Signature of Sister in Charge

Signature of Supervisor

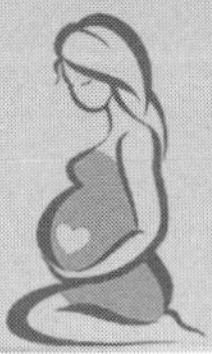

Postnatal Assessment (Case No. 20)

Client's Profile

Name : .... Occupation : ....

Age : .... Income per month : ....

Hospital name : .... W/o : ....

Date of booking : .... Period of gestation : ....

Reg. No : .... Religion : ....

Address : ....

Education : ....

Menstrual History

Age at menarche : ....year of age

Cycle of : .... days

Period duration of : .... days

Blood flow: Average/scanty/heavy ....

Dysmenorrhea: ....

Obstetric History

S.No.	Year	Term/ preterm	Abortion/ stillbirth	Nature of delivery	Child		Immunization	Growth and development	Nature of puerperium	Remark
					Alive	Sex/ weight				

Personal History

Allergies to drug : .... Body built : ....

Habit : Smoking/alcohol/betel chewing/any drug addiction

Hobbies : ....

Dietary habits : Veg/nonvegetarian, ... Diet per day : 2/3/4/5/6

Immunization status : TT: 1st dose .... 2nd dose ....

Present and Past Medical History

High BP/diabetes/breathlessness on exertion/palpitation/tuberculosis/asthma/renal disease/convulsion/jaundice/malaria/RTI/STI/HIV/AIDS/no any/if any other specify ....

Family History

Family History of :

Systemic Illness : High BP/Diabetes/Tuberculosis/No Any

Blood Disorder : Thalassemia/Repeated blood transfusion

Delivery of : Twins/Congenital abnormalities

Notes on Admission for Labor

Present pregnancy : Full term/pre term .... Period of gestation : ....

Presentation of fetus : .... FHS : ....

Labor Notes

Membrane ruptured on : .... at: ....

Length of labor : ....

1st stage : .... 2nd stage : ....

3rd stage : .... **Total hours** : ....

Maternal Condition on Shifting

Date and time of shifting (in postnatal ward) : ....

Newborn general condition on shifting : ....

Newborn date and time of shifting (in postnatal ward) : ....

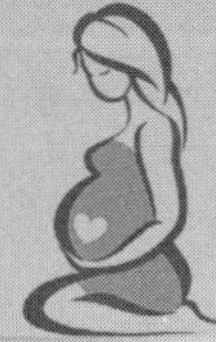

Postnatal Assessment for Mother and Baby

Mother

Postnatal day	1	2	3	4	5	6
Date						
Time						
Vital sign						
Temperature						
Pulse						
Respiration						
BP						
Fundal height						
Uterus						
Lochia						
Perineal care/episiotomy (REEDA)						
Breast						
Bowel/stool						
Bladder/urine						

Baby

Postnatal day	1	2	3	4	5	6
Date						
Time						
Vital sign						
Temperature						
Pulse						
Respiration						
Urine (time/day)						
Stool (time/day)						
Eye care						
Cord care						
Fontanels (Normal/Absent)						
Reflexes						
Activity						
Breastfeeding						
Anthropometric measurement						
Length (cm)						
Head circumference (cm)						
Chest (cm)						
Abdominal (cm)						
Weight (kg)						

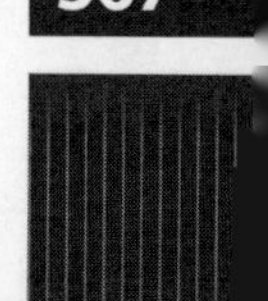

Chief Complaints

....

....

....

....

Condition of Mother at Discharge

....

....

....

....

Condition of Newborn at Discharge

....

....

....

....

Health Education (Diet, Family Planning/Follow-up)

....

....

....

....

Nursing Care Plan

S.No.	Assessment	Nursing Diagnosis	Goal/Expected Out Come	Nursing Intervention	Rational	Implementation	Evaluation

Signature of Sister in Charge

Signature of Supervisor

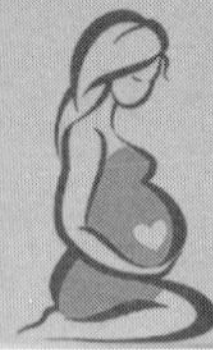

Vaginal Examination (Case No. 1)

Client's Profile

Name : ....
Age : ....
Hospital name : ....
Date of booking : ....
Reg. No : ....
Religion : ....
Education : ....
Occupation : ....
Income per month : ....
W/o : ....
Address : ....
GPLAS : ....
LMP : ....
EDD : ....
Date and time of admission : ....

Examination Finding

Vaginal Examination Findings

- Condition of vulva/perineum: ....
- Vaginal discharge—mucus/excessive watery/foul smelling: ....
- Degree of cervical dilation: ....
- Degree of effacement of cervix: ....
- Deciding stage of labor: ....
- Membrane—intact/rupture/umbilical cord/bag of membrane/any other specify: ....
- Color of amniotic fluid: ....
- Presenting part: ....
- Palpable (fontanels/suture): ....
- Position: ....
- Station of head: ....
- Degree of molding: ....

Pelvic Examination

- Sacral promontory: Felt or contracted/sacral hollow feel (favourable): ....
- Ischial spine: Felt or contracted/unfavorable: ....
- Finding: Adequate pelvis/inadequate pelvis: ....
- Remark for delivery mode: ....

Remark for Delivery Mode

....
....
....
....

Signature of Sister in Charge

Signature of Supervisor

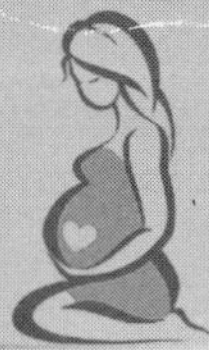

Vaginal Examination (Case No. 2)

Client's Profile

Name	:	Income per month	: ....
Age	:	W/o	: ....
Hospital name	:	Address	: ....
Date of booking	:	GPLAS	: ....
Reg. No	:	LMP	: ....
Religion	:	EDD	: ....
Education	:	Date and time of admission	: ....
Occupation	:		

Examination Finding

Vaginal Examination Findings

- Condition of vulva/perineum: ....
- Vaginal discharge—mucus/excessive watery/foul smelling: ....
- Degree of cervical dilation: ....
- Degree of effacement of cervix: ....
- Deciding stage of labor: ....
- Membrane—intact/rupture/umbilical cord/bag of membrane/any other specify: ....
- Color of amniotic fluid: ....
- Presenting part: ....
- Palpable (fontanels/suture): ....
- Position: ....
- Station of head: ....
- Degree of molding: ....

Pelvic Examination

- Sacral promontory: Felt or contracted/sacral hollow feel (favourable): ....
- Ischial spine: Felt or contracted/unfavorable: ....
- Finding: Adequate pelvis/inadequate pelvis: ....
- Remark for delivery mode: ....

Remark for Delivery Mode

....

....

....

....

Signature of Sister in Charge **Signature of Supervisor**

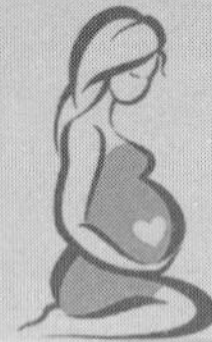

Vaginal Examination (Case No. 3)

Client's Profile

Name : ....
Age : ....
Hospital name : ....
Date of booking : ....
Reg. No : ....
Religion : ....
Education : ....
Occupation : ....

Income per month : ....
W/o : ....
Address : ....
GPLAS : ....
LMP : ....
EDD : ....
Date and time of admission : ....

Examination Finding

Vaginal Examination Findings

- Condition of vulva/perineum: ....
- Vaginal discharge—mucus/excessive watery/foul smelling: ....
- Degree of cervical dilation: ....
- Degree of effacement of cervix: ....
- Deciding stage of labor: ....
- Membrane—intact/rupture/umbilical cord/bag of membrane/any other specify: ....
- Color of amniotic fluid: ....
- Presenting part: ....
- Palpable (fontanels/suture): ....
- Position: ....
- Station of head: ....
- Degree of molding: ....

Pelvic Examination

- Sacral promontory: Felt or contracted/sacral hollow feel (favourable): ....
- Ischial spine: Felt or contracted/unfavorable: ....
- Finding: Adequate pelvis/inadequate pelvis: ....
- Remark for delivery mode: ....

Remark for Delivery Mode

....
....
....
....

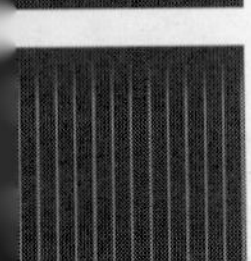

Signature of Sister in Charge

Signature of Supervisor

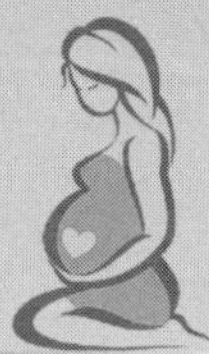

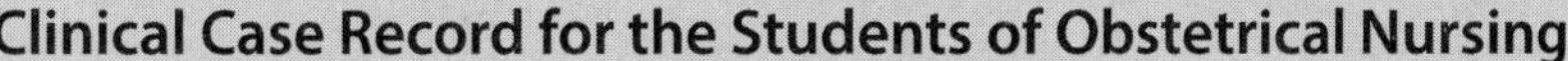

Vaginal Examination (Case No. 4)

Client's Profile

Name	:	Income per month	: ....
Age	:	W/o	: ....
Hospital name	:	Address	: ....
Date of booking	:	GPLAS	: ....
Reg. No	:	LMP	: ....
Religion	:	EDD	: ....
Education	:	Date and time of admission	: ....
Occupation	:		

Examination Finding

Vaginal Examination Findings

- Condition of vulva/perineum: ....
- Vaginal discharge—mucus/excessive watery/foul smelling: ....
- Degree of cervical dilation: ....
- Degree of effacement of cervix: ....
- Deciding stage of labor: ....
- Membrane—intact/rupture/umbilical cord/bag of membrane/any other specify: ....
- Color of amniotic fluid: ....
- Presenting part: ....
- Palpable (fontanels/suture): ....
- Position: ....
- Station of head: ....
- Degree of molding: ....

Pelvic Examination

- Sacral promontory: Felt or contracted/sacral hollow feel (favourable): ....
- Ischial spine: Felt or contracted/unfavorable: ....
- Finding: Adequate pelvis/inadequate pelvis: ....
- Remark for delivery mode: ....

Remark for Delivery Mode

....

....

....

....

Signature of Sister in Charge **Signature of Supervisor**

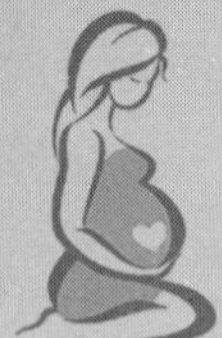

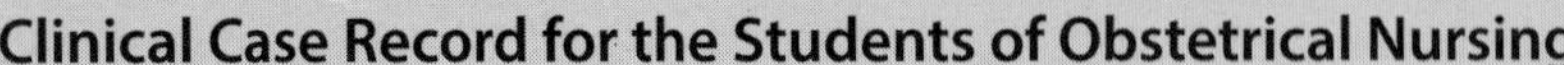

Vaginal Examination (Case No. 5)

Client's Profile

Name	:	Income per month	: ....
Age	:	W/o	: ....
Hospital name	:	Address	: ....
Date of booking	:	GPLAS	: ....
Reg. No	:	LMP	: ....
Religion	:	EDD	: ....
Education	:	Date and time of admission	: ....
Occupation	:		

Examination Finding

Vaginal Examination Findings

- Condition of vulva/perineum: ....
- Vaginal discharge—mucus/excessive watery/foul smelling: ....
- Degree of cervical dilation: ....
- Degree of effacement of cervix: ....
- Deciding stage of labor: ....
- Membrane—intact/rupture/umbilical cord/bag of membrane/any other specify: ....
- Color of amniotic fluid: ....
- Presenting part: ....
- Palpable (fontanels/suture): ....
- Position: ....
- Station of head: ....
- Degree of molding: ....

Pelvic Examination

- Sacral promontory: Felt or contracted/sacral hollow feel (favourable): ....
- Ischial spine: Felt or contracted/unfavorable: ....
- Finding: Adequate pelvis/inadequate pelvis: ....
- Remark for delivery mode: ....

Remark for Delivery Mode

....

....

....

....

Signature of Sister in Charge **Signature of Supervisor**

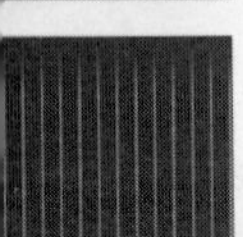

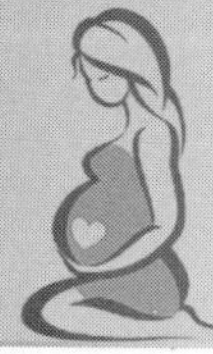

Assisted with Cesarean Section (Case No. 1)

Client's Profile

Name : ....
Age : ....
Hospital name : ....
Date of booking : ....
Reg. No : ....
Religion : ....
Education : ....
Occupation : ....
Income per month : ....
W/o : ....

Address : ....
GPLAS : ....
LMP : ....
EDD : ....
Type of cesarean section : ....
Position of baby : ....
Presentation of baby : ....
Date and time of admission : ....
Date and time of discharge or transfer: ....
Length of stay in hospital : ....

Cesarean Section Notes

Indication for Cesarean Section: 1. ....

2. ....

3. ....

4. ....

Date and time of admission : ....
Type of anesthesia given : ....
Total time of cesarean section operation : ....
Date and time of delivery/birth of baby : ....

Sex of baby : ....
Weight of baby : ....
Heath status of baby : ....

Umbilical blood vessels: ....a. Arteries: .... b. Veins : ....

Weight of placenta : ....
Amount of blood loss : ....
Condition of mother : ....

Number of suture : ....
Date of suture removable : ....

Health Education

Mother

....

....

Baby

....

....

Notes on Transfer

Condition of mother on transfer : ....

Healthy/unhealthy (if unhealthy specify : ....

Condition of baby on transfer or discharge : ....

....

....

Signature of Sister in Charge

Signature of Supervisor

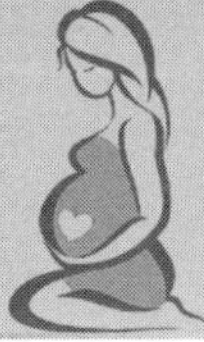

Assisted with Cesarean Section (Case No. 2)

Client's Profile

Name : ....
Age : ....
Hospital name : ....
Date of booking : ....
Reg. No : ....
Religion : ....
Education : ....
Occupation : ....
Income per month : ....
W/o : ....

Address : ....
GPLAS : ....
LMP : ....
EDD : ....
Type of cesarean section : ....
Position of baby : ....
Presentation of baby : ....
Date and time of admission : ....
Date and time of discharge or transfer: ....
Length of stay in hospital : ....

Cesarean Section Notes

Indication for Cesarean Section:
1. ....
2. ....
3. ....
4. ....

Date and time of admission : ....
Type of anesthesia given : ....
Total time of cesarean section operation : ....
Date and time of delivery/birth of baby : ....
Umbilical blood vessels: ....a. Arteries: ....
b. Veins : ....
Weight of placenta : ....
Amount of blood loss : ....
Condition of mother : ....

Sex of baby : ....
Weight of baby : ....
Heath status of baby : ....
Number of suture : ....
Date of suture removable : ....

Health Education

Mother

....

....

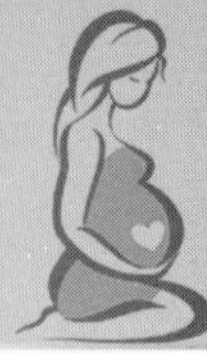

Baby

....

....

Notes on Transfer

Condition of mother on transfer : ....

Healthy/unhealthy (if unhealthy specify : ....

Condition of baby on transfer or discharge : ....

....

....

Signature of Sister in Charge **Signature of Supervisor**

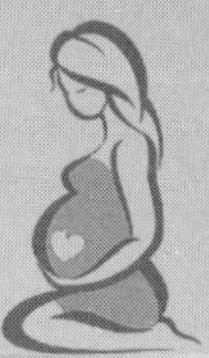

IUCD Insertion (Case No. 1)

Client's Profile

Hospital : ....
Registration no : ....
Name : ....
Age : ....
Address : ....
W/o : ....

Religion : ....
Date and type of last delivery : ....
Para : ....
Lactation- complete/incomplete : ....
Type of IUCD : ....
Date and time of IUCD insertion : ....

Specific Counseling

Counseling and Guidance (Yes/No) : ....
Consent for Contraceptive Method (Yes/No): ....
Type of IUCD : ....

History Taking

Medical/Surgical History : ....
Gynecological History : ....
Puerperium History : ....

Examination

Bladder : ....
Abdomen : ....
External Genitalia : ....

Bimanual Examination : ....
Rectovaginal Examination : ....
Speculum Examination : ....

Steps of IUCD Insertion

Preinsertion Steps

....

....

....

....

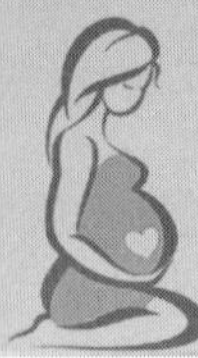

Post Insertion Steps

....

....

....

....

Health Education

....

....

....

....

Method for self examination of IUCD in place: ....
Time for IUCD removal : .... Date and day for follow-up : ....

Signature of Sister in Charge **Signature of Supervisor**

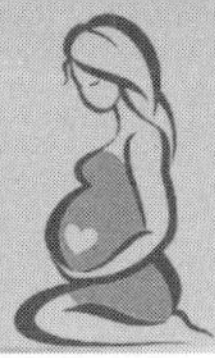

IUCD Insertion (Case No. 2)

Client's Profile

Hospital : ....
Registration no : ....
Name : ....
Age : ....
Address : ....
W/o : ....

Religion : ....
Date and type of last delivery : ....
Para : ....
Lactation- complete/incomplete : ....
Type of IUCD : ....
Date and time of IUCD insertion : ....

Specific Counseling

Counseling and Guidance (Yes/No) : ....
Consent for Contraceptive Method (Yes/No): ....
Type of IUCD : ....

History Taking

Medical/Surgical History : ....
Gynecological History : ....
Puerperium History : ....

Examination

Bladder : ....
Abdomen : ....
External Genitalia : ....

Bimanual Examination : ....
Rectovaginal Examination : ....
Speculum Examination : ....

Steps of IUCD Insertion

Preinsertion Steps

....

....

....

....

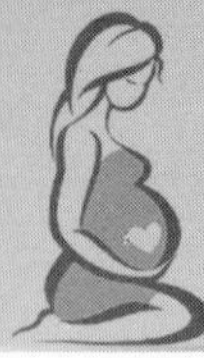

Post Insertion Steps

....

....

....

....

Health Education

....

....

....

....

Method for self examination of IUCD in place: ....

Time for IUCD removal : .... Date and day for follow-up : ....

Signature of Sister in Charge **Signature of Supervisor**

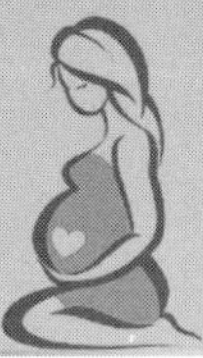

IUCD Insertion (Case No. 3)

Client's Profile

Hospital : ....
Registration no : ....
Name : ....
Age : ....
Address : ....
W/o : ....

Religion : ....
Date and type of last delivery : ....
Para : ....
Lactation- complete/incomplete : ....
Type of IUCD : ....
Date and time of IUCD insertion : ....

Specific Counseling

Counseling and Guidance (Yes/No) : ....
Consent for Contraceptive Method (Yes/No): ....
Type of IUCD : ....

History Taking

Medical/Surgical History : ....
Gynecological History : ....
Puerperium History : ....

Examination

Bladder : ....
Abdomen : ....
External Genitalia : ....

Bimanual Examination : ....
Rectovaginal Examination : ....
Speculum Examination : ....

Steps of IUCD Insertion

Preinsertion Steps

....

....

....

....

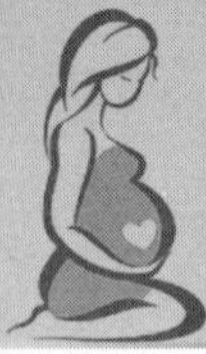

Post Insertion Steps

....

....

....

....

Health Education

....

....

....

....

Method for self examination of IUCD in place: ....

Time for IUCD removal : .... Date and day for follow-up : ....

Signature of Sister in Charge **Signature of Supervisor**

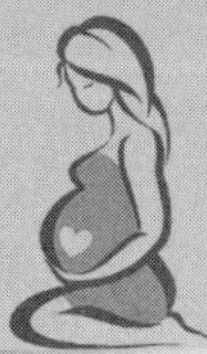

IUCD Insertion (Case No. 4)

Client's Profile

Hospital : ....

Registration no : ....

Name : ....

Age : ....

Address : ....

W/o : ....

Religion : ....

Date and type of last delivery : ....

Para : ....

Lactation- complete/incomplete : ....

Type of IUCD : ....

Date and time of IUCD insertion : ....

Specific Counseling

Counseling and Guidance (Yes/No) : ....

Consent for Contraceptive Method (Yes/No): ....

Type of IUCD : ....

History Taking

Medical/Surgical History : ....

Gynecological History : ....

Puerperium History : ....

Examination

Bladder : ....

Abdomen : ....

External Genitalia : ....

Bimanual Examination : ....

Rectovaginal Examination : ....

Speculum Examination : ....

Steps of IUCD Insertion

Preinsertion Steps

....

....

....

....

Post Insertion Steps

....

....

....

....

Health Education

....

....

....

....

Method for self examination of IUCD in place: ....
Time for IUCD removal : .... Date and day for follow-up : ....

Signature of Sister in Charge **Signature of Supervisor**

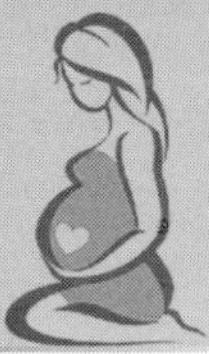

IUCD Insertion (Case No. 5)

Client's Profile

Hospital : ....

Registration no : ....

Name : ....

Age : ....

Address : ....

W/o : ....

Religion : ....

Date and type of last delivery : ....

Para : ....

Lactation- complete/incomplete : ....

Type of IUCD : ....

Date and time of IUCD insertion : ....

Specific Counseling

Counseling and Guidance (Yes/No) : ....

Consent for Contraceptive Method (Yes/No): ....

Type of IUCD : ....

History Taking

Medical/Surgical History : ....

Gynecological History : ....

Puerperium History : ....

Examination

Bladder : ....

Abdomen : ....

External Genitalia : ....

Bimanual Examination : ....

Rectovaginal Examination : ....

Speculum Examination : ....

Steps of IUCD Insertion

Preinsertion Steps

....

....

....

....

Post Insertion Steps

....

....

....

....

Health Education

....

....

....

....

Method for self examination of IUCD in place: ....
Time for IUCD removal : .... Date and day for follow-up : ....

Signature of Sister in Charge **Signature of Supervisor**

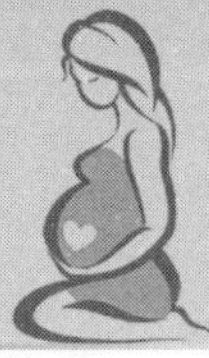

Episiotomy and Suturing (Case No. 1)

Client's Profile

Hospital name	:	W/o	: ....
Date of booking	:	Address	: ....
Reg. No	:	Date and time of admission	: ....
Name	:	Type of previous delivery (if any)	: ....
Age	:	Indication for episiotomy	: ....

Episiotomy and Suturing Notes

Necessary equipment : ....

Administration of local anesthetic : ....

Episiotomy type/time : ....

Repairing the episiotomy/number of skin suture : ....

Health Education (Episiotomy Care/Follow-up)

....

....

....

....

....

....

....

....

....

Signature of Sister in Charge

Signature of Supervisor

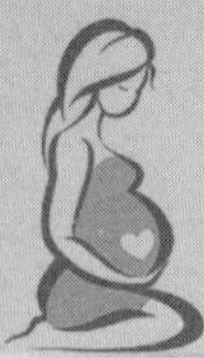

Episiotomy and Suturing (Case No. 2)

Client's Profile

Hospital name : ....

Date of booking : ....

Reg. No : ....

Name : ....

Age : ....

W/o : ....

Address : ....

Date and time of admission : ....

Type of previous delivery (if any) : ....

Indication for episiotomy : ....

Episiotomy and Suturing Notes

Necessary equipment : ....

Administration of local anesthetic : ....

Episiotomy type/time : ....

Repairing the episiotomy/number of skin suture : ....

Health Education (Episiotomy Care/Follow-up)

....

....

....

....

....

....

....

....

....

Signature of Sister in Charge ______________________

Signature of Supervisor ______________________

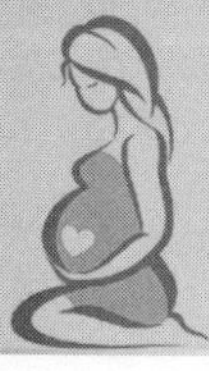

Episiotomy and Suturing (Case No. 3)

Client's Profile

Hospital name : ....

Date of booking : ....

Reg. No : ....

Name : ....

Age : ....

W/o : ....

Address : ....

Date and time of admission : ....

Type of previous delivery (if any) : ....

Indication for episiotomy : ....

Episiotomy and Suturing Notes

Necessary equipment : ....

Administration of local anesthetic : ....

Episiotomy type/time : ....

Repairing the episiotomy/number of skin suture : ....

Health Education (Episiotomy Care/Follow-up)

....

....

....

....

....

....

....

....

....

Signature of Sister in Charge

Signature of Supervisor

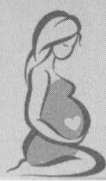

Episiotomy and Suturing (Case No. 4)

Client's Profile

Hospital name : .... W/o : ....

Date of booking : .... Address : ....

Reg. No : .... Date and time of admission : ....

Name : .... Type of previous delivery (if any) : ....

Age : .... Indication for episiotomy : ....

Episiotomy and Suturing Notes

Necessary equipment : ....

Administration of local anesthetic : ....

Episiotomy type/time : ....

Repairing the episiotomy/number of skin suture : ....

Health Education (Episiotomy Care/Follow-up)

....

....

....

....

....

....

....

....

....

Signature of Sister in Charge **Signature of Supervisor**

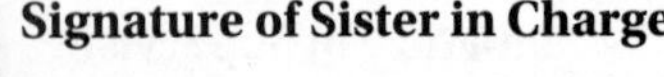

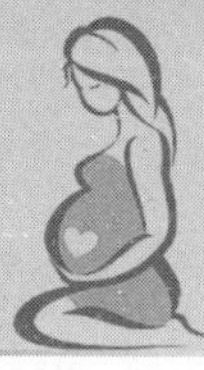

Episiotomy and Suturing (Case No. 5)

Client's Profile

Hospital name	:	W/o	: ....
Date of booking	:	Address	: ....
Reg. No	:	Date and time of admission	: ....
Name	:	Type of previous delivery (if any)	: ....
Age	:	Indication for episiotomy	: ....

Episiotomy and Suturing Notes

Necessary equipment : ....

Administration of local anesthetic : ....

Episiotomy type/time : ....

Repairing the episiotomy/number of skin suture : ....

Health Education (Episiotomy Care/Follow-up)

....

....

....

....

....

....

....

....

....

Signature of Sister in Charge **Signature of Supervisor**

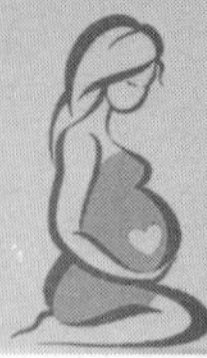

Witness/Assisted Abnormal Delivery (Case No. 1)

Client's Profile

Name : .... Religion : .... W/o : ....

Age : .... Education : .... Parity : ....

Hospital name : .... Occupation : .... LMP : ....

Date of booking : .... Income per month : .... EDD ....

Reg. No : .... Marriage duration : .... Period of gestation ....

Address : ....

....

Date and time of admission : ....

Date and time of discharge or transfer : ....

Admission Note

General Examinations

i. Temperature: .... iii. Respiration: ....

ii. Pulse: .... iv. BP: ....

Hydration: .... Anemia: (Present/absent) ....

Labor pain: (Present/absent).................................. Edema: (Generalized/ankle edema) ....

Abdominal Examination/Obstetrical Examination by Palpation

Height of uterus: .... cm Lie: .... Superficial grip: ....

Gestational weeks: .... Presentation: .... Deep pelvic grip: ....

Abdominal girth: ....cm Position of fetus:.. FHR: ....

Scar:.. Lateral grip: ....

Time/date of onset of contraction : ....

Uterine contraction: Present/absent/well contracted : ....

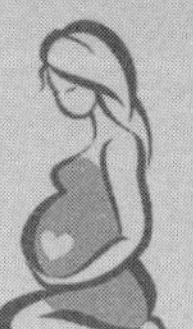

Investigation

Date	Hemoglobin	Blood Group/ Sugar	Urine		Bowel	Bladder	Any Other
			Albumin	Sugar			

Vaginal Examination

S.No	Date and time	Finding	Remark

Previous Obstetrical History

S.No	Year	Term/ preterm	Abortion/ stillbirth	Nature of delivery	Child		Immunization	Growth and development	Nature of puerperium	Remark
					Alive	Sex/ weight				

Admission History

Pregnancy complaints	
Menstrual history	
Medical history	
Surgical history	

Old Pattern Partograph

Parity: *Reg No:* *Date and Time of Admission:* *Date and Time of ROM:*

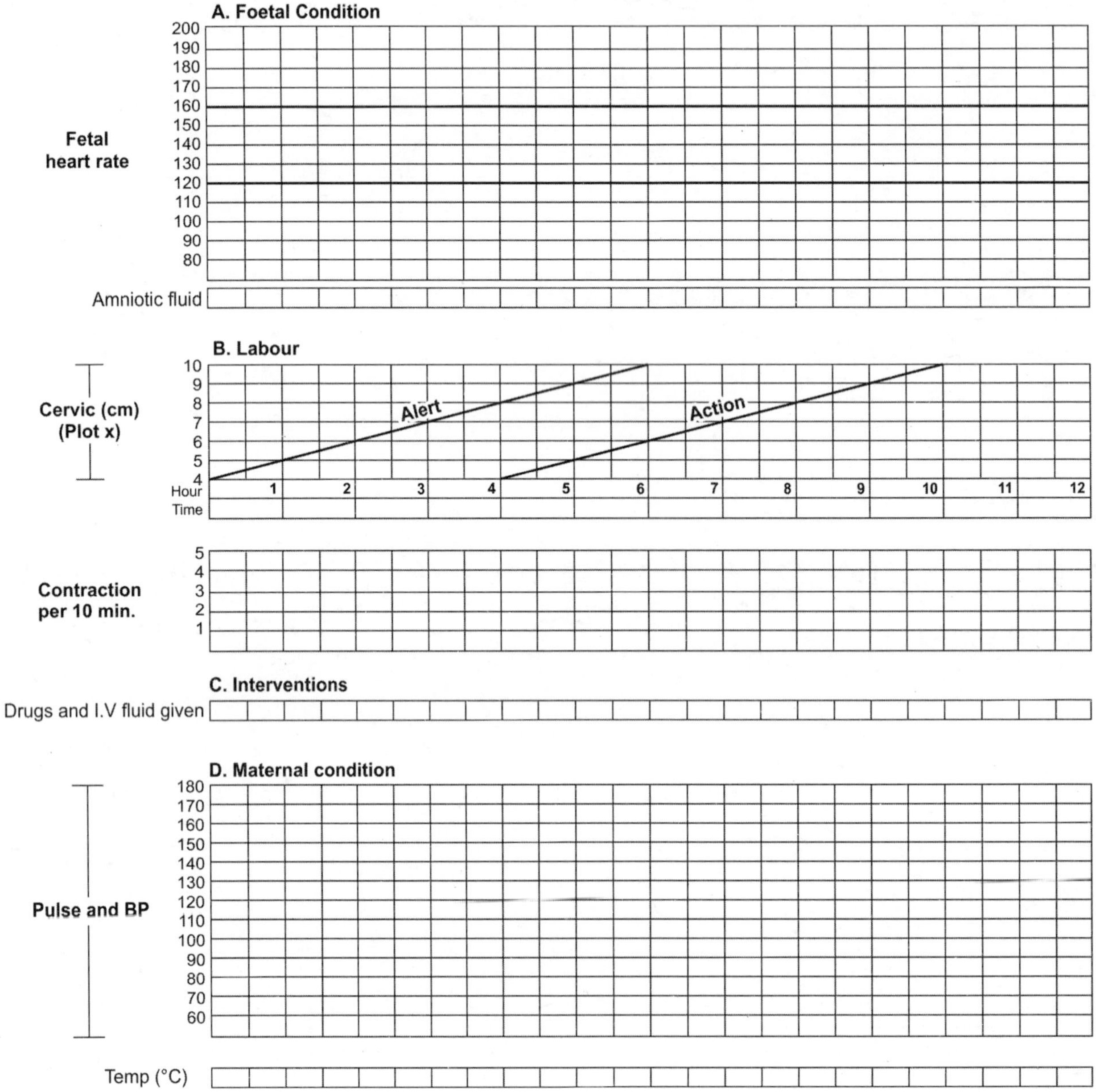

A. Foetal Condition

Fetal heart rate

200
190
180
170
160
150
140
130
120
110
100
90
80

Amniotic fluid

B. Labour

Cervic (cm)
(Plot x)

10
9
8
7
6
5
4

Alert

Action

Hour	1	2	3	4	5	6	7	8	9	10	11	12
Time												

Contraction per 10 min.

5
4
3
2
1

C. Interventions

Drugs and I.V fluid given

D. Maternal condition

Pulse and BP

180
170
160
150
140
130
120
110
100
90
80
70
60

Temp (°C)

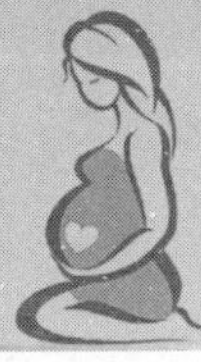

WHO Modified Partograph

Parity: *Reg No:* *Date and Time of Admission:* *Date and Time of ROM:*

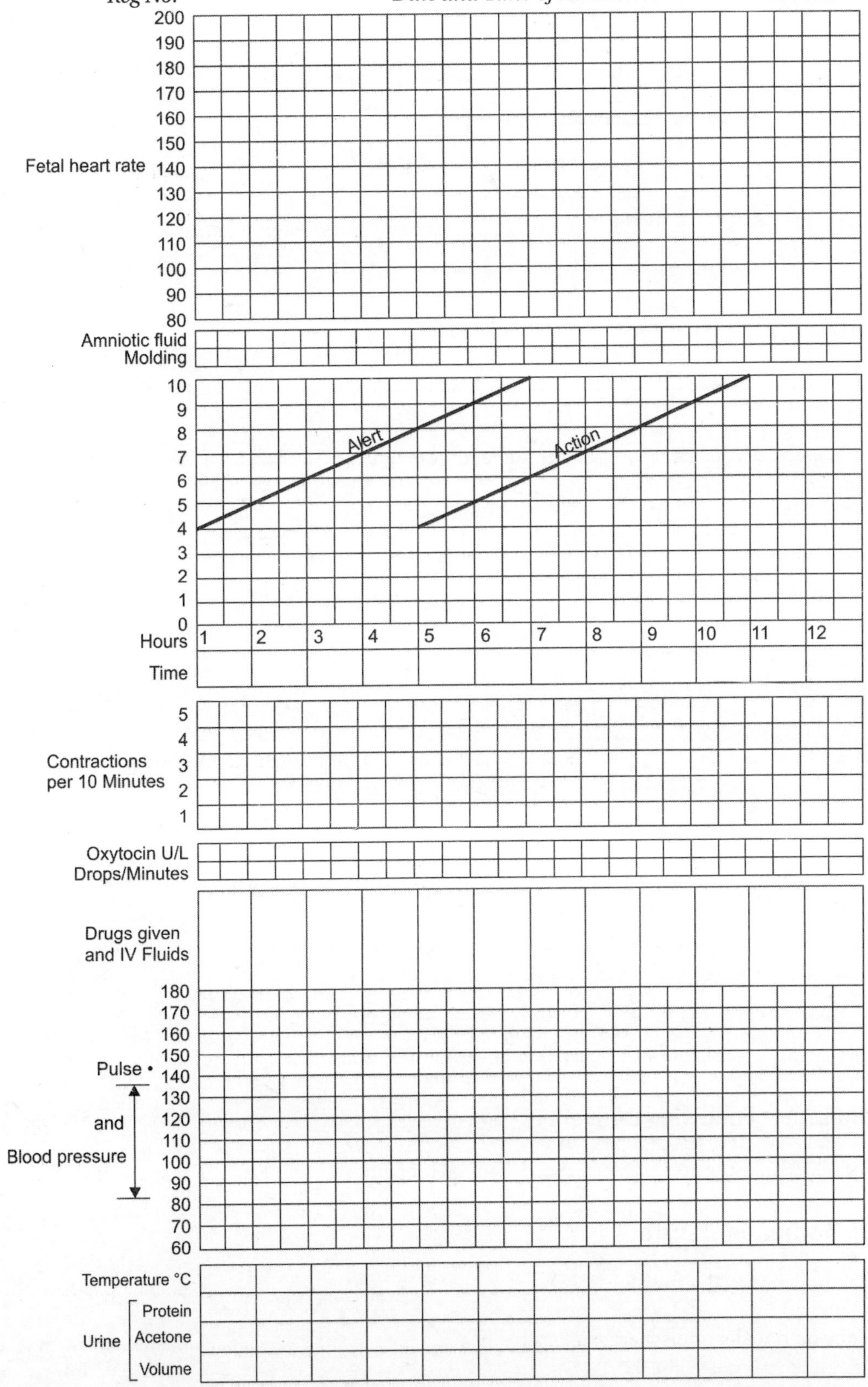

Delivery Note

Labor Progress Note Date and Time of Onset of Pain

Onset of true labor: On .... At: ....

Date and time of full cervix dilatation: .... Effacement: ....

Membrane ruptured (spontaneous/artificial/PROM) on .... At ....

Total duration of: 1st stage .... Hrs .... Min ....

2nd stage .... Hrs .... Min ....

3rd stage .... Hrs .... Min ....

Total hours = ... Hrs .... Min ....

Baby at Birth

Mode of delivery: .... Score at one minute ....

Baby born on:.. At: .... Sex: ....

Apgar scoring: .... Score at five minute................................ Anus patent: ....

Initiation of breastfeeding: ....

Drug administration: ....

Delivery of Placenta and Membrane

Delivery of placenta on: .... At:........................... Cord insertion: ....

Spontaneous/helped/manually removed .... Examination of placenta: Complete/Incomplete ....

Weight of placenta:..

Cord length: .... Examination of membrane: ....

Blood Loss

Before delivery of placenta : ....

During delivery of placenta : ....

After delivery of placenta : ....

Perineum

Intact : .... Episiotomy : .... Laceration : .... Repair : ....

Condition of Mother Following Delivery

Pulse: .... BP: .... Uterus: .... Vaginal bleeding: .... Breastfeeding initiated at: ....

Condition of Mother on Transfer

Healthy/unhealthy (if unhealthy specify): ....

Condition of baby on transfer or discharge: ....

Nursing Care Plan

S.No.	Assessment	Nursing Diagnosis	Goal/Expected Out Come	Nursing Intervention	Rational	Implementation	Evaluation

Signature of Sister in Charge

Signature of Supervisor

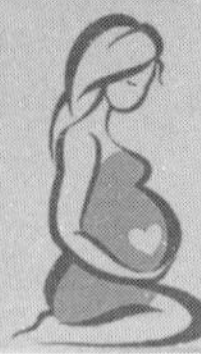

Witness/Assisted Abnormal Delivery (Case No. 2)

Client's Profile

Name : .... Religion : .... W/o : ....

Age : .... Education : .... Parity : ....

Hospital name : .... Occupation : .... LMP : ....

Date of booking : .... Income per month : .... EDD ....

Reg. No : .... Marriage duration : .... Period of gestation ....

Address : ....

....

Date and time of admission : ....

Date and time of discharge or transfer : ....

Admission Note

General Examinations

i. Temperature: .... iii. Respiration: ....

ii. Pulse: .... iv. BP: ....

Hydration: .... Anemia: (Present/absent) ....

Labor pain: (Present/absent).................................. Edema: (Generalized/ankle edema) ....

Abdominal Examination/Obstetrical Examination by Palpation

Height of uterus: .... cm Lie: .... Superficial grip: ....

Gestational weeks: .... Presentation: .... Deep pelvic grip: ....

Abdominal girth: ....cm Position of fetus: .... FHR: ....

Scar: .... Lateral grip: ....

Time/date of onset of contraction : ....

Uterine contraction: Present/absent/well contracted : ....

Investigation

Date	Hemoglobin	Blood Group/ Sugar	Urine		Bowel	Bladder	Any Other
			Albumin	Sugar			

Vaginal Examination

S.No	Date and time	Finding	Remark

Previous Obstetrical History

S.No	Year	Term/ preterm	Abortion/ stillbirth	Nature of delivery	Child		Immunization	Growth and development	Nature of puerperium	Remark
					Alive	Sex/ weight				

Admission History

Pregnancy complaints	
Menstrual history	
Medical history	
Surgical history	

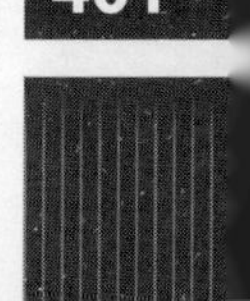

Old Pattern Partograph

Parity: *Reg No:* *Date and Time of Admission:* *Date and Time of ROM:*

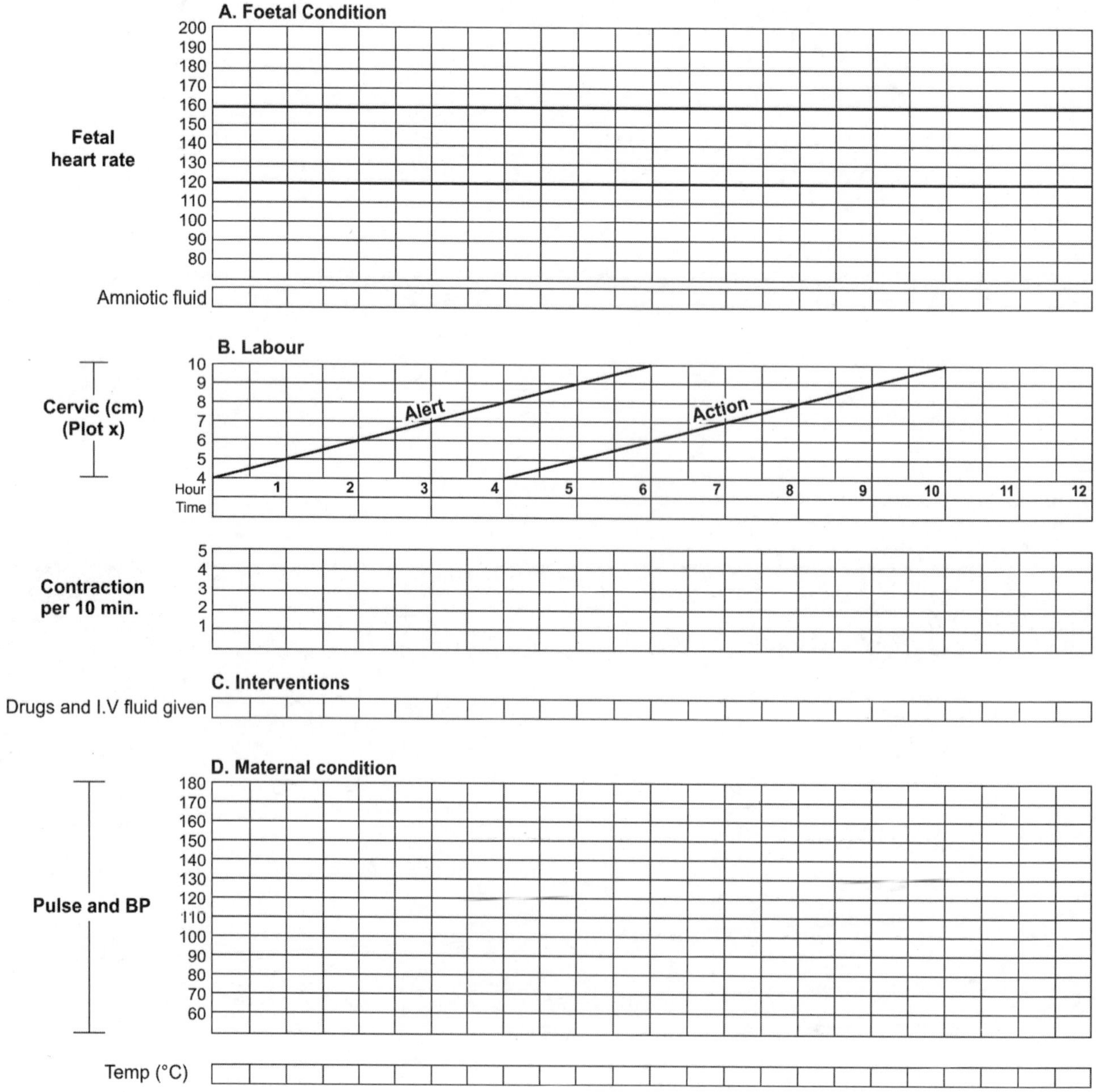

A. Foetal Condition

Fetal heart rate

200
190
180
170
160
150
140
130
120
110
100
90
80

Amniotic fluid

B. Labour

Cervic (cm) (Plot x)

10
9
8
7
6
5
4

Alert

Action

Hour 1 2 3 4 5 6 7 8 9 10 11 12

Time

Contraction per 10 min.

5
4
3
2
1

C. Interventions

Drugs and I.V fluid given

D. Maternal condition

Pulse and BP

180
170
160
150
140
130
120
110
100
90
80
70
60

Temp (°C)

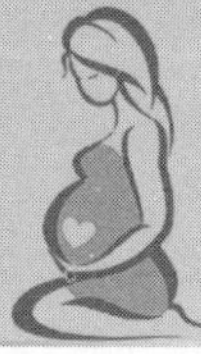

WHO Modified Partograph

Parity: *Reg No:* *Date and Time of Admission:* *Date and Time of ROM:*

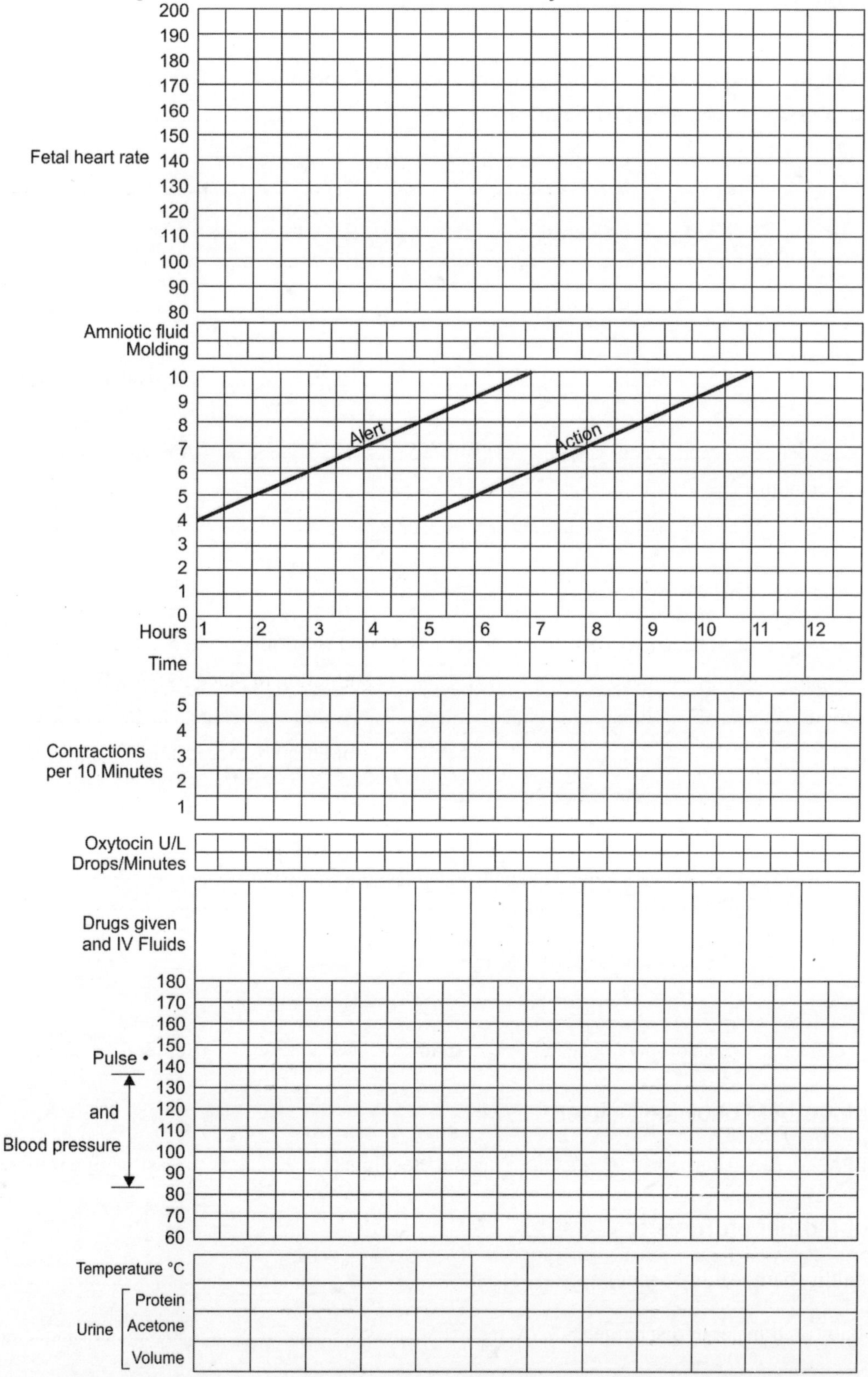

Fetal heart rate: 200, 190, 180, 170, 160, 150, 140, 130, 120, 110, 100, 90, 80

Amniotic fluid
Molding

10, 9, 8, 7, 6, 5, 4, 3, 2, 1, 0

Hours	1	2	3	4	5	6	7	8	9	10	11	12
Time												

Contractions per 10 Minutes: 5, 4, 3, 2, 1

Oxytocin U/L
Drops/Minutes

Drugs given and IV Fluids

Pulse •
and
Blood pressure ↕
180, 170, 160, 150, 140, 130, 120, 110, 100, 90, 80, 70, 60

Temperature °C	
Urine – Protein	
Urine – Acetone	
Urine – Volume	

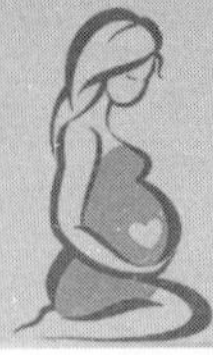

Delivery Note

Labor Progress Note Date and Time of Onset of Pain

Onset of true labor: On .... At: ....

Date and time of full cervix dilatation: .... Effacement: ....

Membrane ruptured (spontaneous/artificial/PROM) on .... At ....

Total duration of: 1st stage .... Hrs .... Min ....

2nd stage .... Hrs .... Min ....

3rd stage .... Hrs .... Min ....

Total hours = ... Hrs .... Min ....

Baby at Birth

Mode of delivery: .... Score at one minute ....

Baby born on:.......................... At: .... Sex: ....

Apgar scoring: .... Score at five minute.......................... Anus patent: ....

Initiation of breastfeeding: ....

Drug administration: ....

Delivery of Placenta and Membrane

Delivery of placenta on: .... At:.......................... Cord insertion: ....

Spontaneous/helped/manually removed .... Examination of placenta: Complete/Incomplete ....

Weight of placenta:..

Cord length: .... Examination of membrane: ....

Blood Loss

Before delivery of placenta : ....

During delivery of placenta : ....

After delivery of placenta : ....

Perineum

Intact : .... Episiotomy :............. Laceration :.............................. Repair : ....

Condition of Mother Following Delivery

Pulse: .... BP: .... Uterus: .... Vaginal bleeding: .... Breastfeeding initiated at: ....

Condition of Mother on Transfer

Healthy/unhealthy (if unhealthy specify): ....

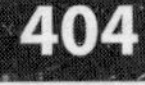

Condition of baby on transfer or discharge: ....

Nursing Care Plan

S.No.	Assessment	Nursing Diagnosis	Goal/Expected Out Come	Nursing Intervention	Rational	Implementation	Evaluation

Signature of Sister in Charge

Signature of Supervisor

Witness/Assisted Abnormal Delivery (Case No. 3)

Client's Profile

Name : .... Religion : .... W/o : ....

Age : .... Education : .... Parity : ....

Hospital name : .... Occupation : .... LMP : ....

Date of booking : .... Income per month : .... EDD ....

Reg. No : .... Marriage duration : .... Period of gestation ....

Address : ....

....

Date and time of admission : ....

Date and time of discharge or transfer : ....

Admission Note

General Examinations

i. Temperature: .... iii. Respiration: ....

ii. Pulse: .... iv. BP: ....

Hydration: .... Anemia: (Present/absent) ....

Labor pain: (Present/absent).................................. Edema: (Generalized/ankle edema) ....

Abdominal Examination/Obstetrical Examination by Palpation

Height of uterus: .... cm Lie: .... Superficial grip: ....

Gestational weeks: .... Presentation: .... Deep pelvic grip: ....

Abdominal girth: ....cm Position of fetus: .... FHR: ....

Scar: .... Lateral grip: ....

Time/date of onset of contraction : ....

Uterine contraction: Present/absent/well contracted : ....

Investigation

Date	Hemoglobin	Blood Group/ Sugar	Urine		Bowel	Bladder	Any Other
			Albumin	Sugar			

Vaginal Examination

S.No	Date and time	Finding	Remark

Previous Obstetrical History

S.No	Year	Term/ preterm	Abortion/ stillbirth	Nature of delivery	Child		Immunization	Growth and development	Nature of puerperium	Remark
					Alive	Sex/ weight				

Admission History

Pregnancy complaints	
Menstrual history	
Medical history	
Surgical history	

Old Pattern Partograph

Parity: *Reg No:* *Date and Time of Admission:* *Date and Time of ROM:*

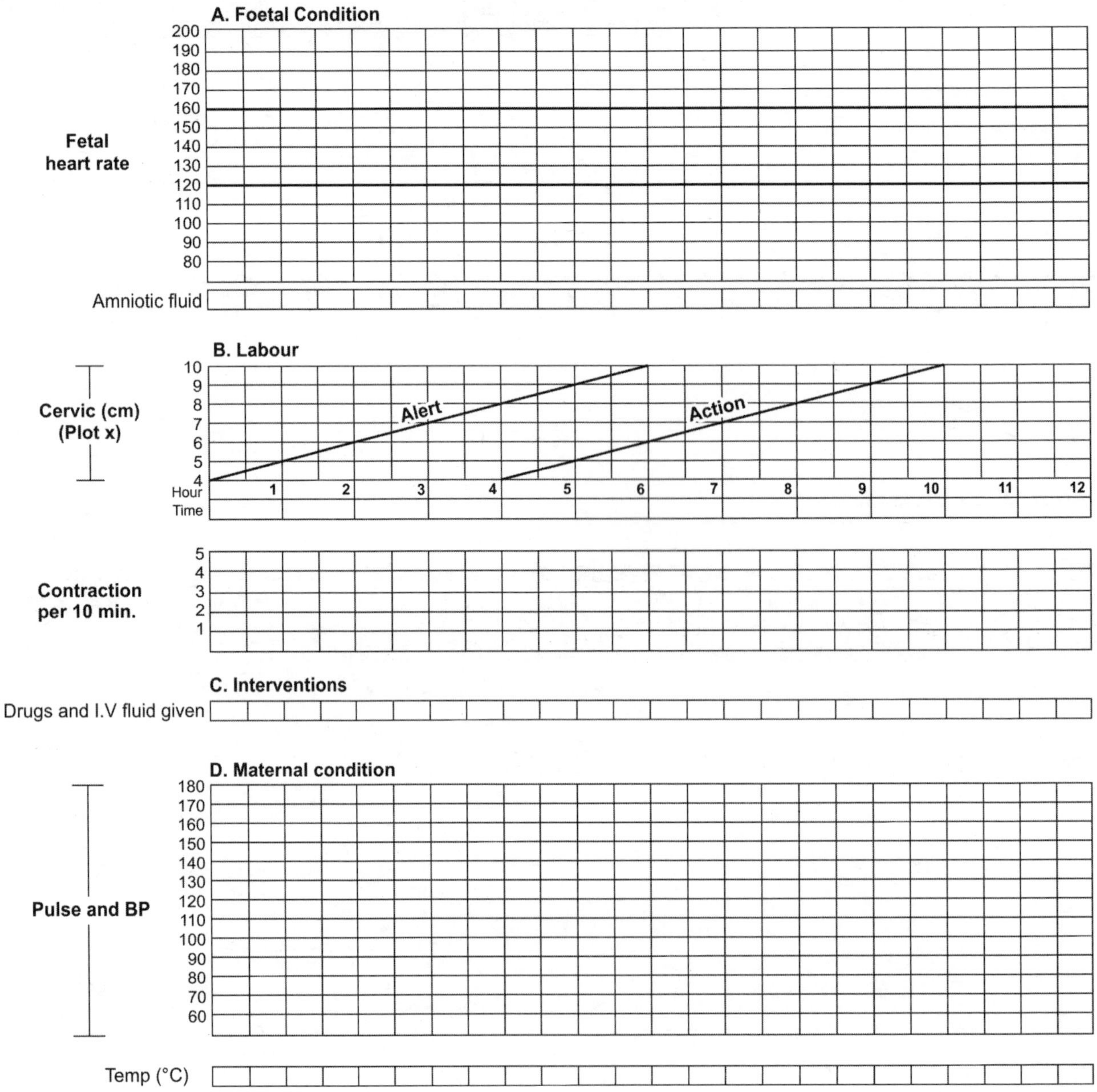

A. Foetal Condition

Fetal heart rate: 200, 190, 180, 170, 160, 150, 140, 130, 120, 110, 100, 90, 80

Amniotic fluid

B. Labour

Cervic (cm) (Plot x): 10, 9, 8, 7, 6, 5, 4

Alert

Action

Hour: 1, 2, 3, 4, 5, 6, 7, 8, 9, 10, 11, 12

Time

Contraction per 10 min.: 5, 4, 3, 2, 1

C. Interventions

Drugs and I.V fluid given

D. Maternal condition

Pulse and BP: 180, 170, 160, 150, 140, 130, 120, 110, 100, 90, 80, 70, 60

Temp (°C)

WHO Modified Partograph

Parity: *Reg No:* *Date and Time of Admission:* *Date and Time of ROM:*

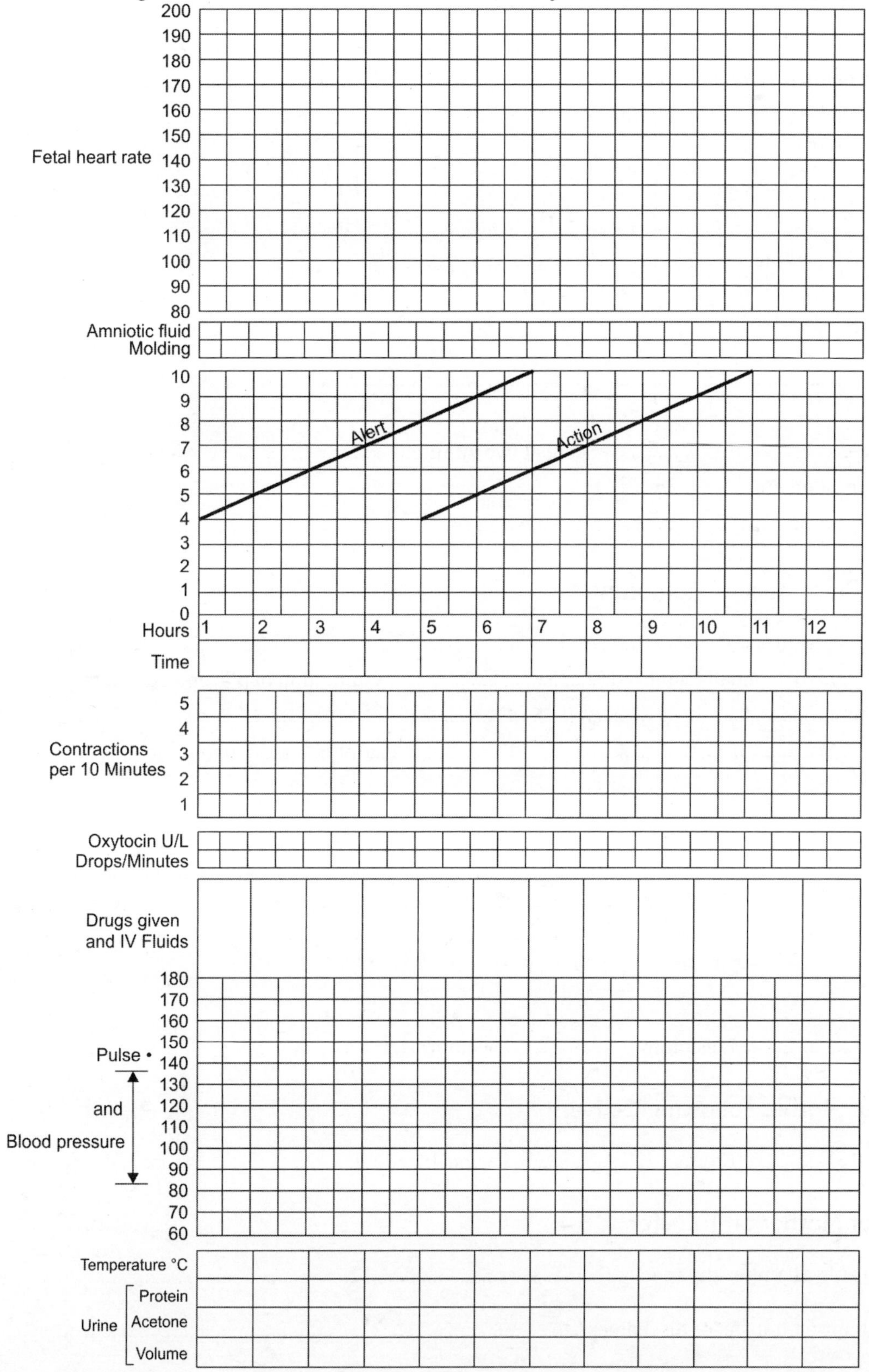

Fetal heart rate: 200, 190, 180, 170, 160, 150, 140, 130, 120, 110, 100, 90, 80

Amniotic fluid

Molding

Cervical dilatation: 10, 9, 8, 7, 6, 5, 4, 3, 2, 1, 0

Alert

Action

Hours	1	2	3	4	5	6	7	8	9	10	11	12
Time												

Contractions per 10 Minutes: 5, 4, 3, 2, 1

Oxytocin U/L

Drops/Minutes

Drugs given and IV Fluids

Pulse • and Blood pressure ↕: 180, 170, 160, 150, 140, 130, 120, 110, 100, 90, 80, 70, 60

Temperature °C

Urine: Protein, Acetone, Volume

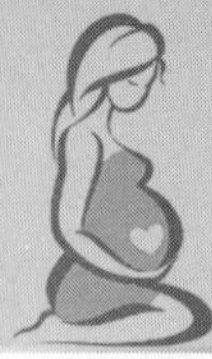

Delivery Note

Labor Progress Note Date and Time of Onset of Pain

Onset of true labor: On .... At: ....

Date and time of full cervix dilatation: .... Effacement: ....

Membrane ruptured (spontaneous/artificial/PROM) on .... At ....

Total duration of: 1st stage .... Hrs .... Min ....

2nd stage .... Hrs .... Min ....

3rd stage .... Hrs .... Min ....

Total hours = ... Hrs .... Min ....

Baby at Birth

Mode of delivery: .... Score at one minute ....

Baby born on:.. At: .... Sex: ....

Apgar scoring: .... Score at five minute.. Anus patent: ....

Initiation of breastfeeding: ....

Drug administration: ....

Delivery of Placenta and Membrane

Delivery of placenta on:.......................... At:.......................... Cord insertion: ....

Spontaneous/helped/manually removed .... Examination of placenta: Complete/Incomplete ....

Weight of placenta:..

Cord length: .... Examination of membrane: ....

Blood Loss

Before delivery of placenta : ....

During delivery of placenta : ....

After delivery of placenta : ....

Perineum

Intact : .... Episiotomy :............. Laceration :.............................. Repair : ....

Condition of Mother Following Delivery

Pulse: .... BP: .... Uterus: .... Vaginal bleeding: .... Breastfeeding initiated at: ....

Condition of Mother on Transfer

Healthy/unhealthy (if unhealthy specify): ....

Condition of baby on transfer or discharge: ....

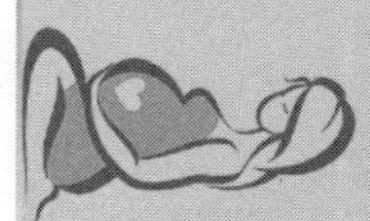

Nursing Care Plan

S.No.	Assessment	Nursing Diagnosis	Goal/Expected Out Come	Nursing Intervention	Rational	Implementation	Evaluation

Signature of Sister in Charge

Signature of Supervisor

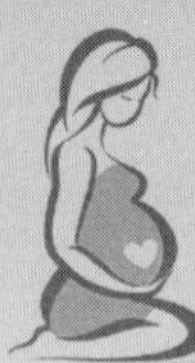

Witness/Assisted Abnormal Delivery (Case No. 4)

Client's Profile

Name : .... Religion : .... W/o : ....

Age : .... Education : .... Parity : ....

Hospital name : .... Occupation : .... LMP : ....

Date of booking : .... Income per month : .... EDD.................................

Reg. No : .... Marriage duration : .... Period of gestation ....

Address : ....

....

Date and time of admission : ....

Date and time of discharge or transfer : ....

Admission Note

General Examinations

i. Temperature: ....

ii. Pulse: ....

iii. Respiration: ....

iv. BP: ....

Hydration: ....

Anemia: (Present/absent) ....

Labor pain: (Present/absent)..................................

Edema: (Generalized/ankle edema) ....

Abdominal Examination/Obstetrical Examination by Palpation

Height of uterus: .... cm Lie: .... Superficial grip: ....

Gestational weeks: .... Presentation: .... Deep pelvic grip: ....

Abdominal girth: ....cm Position of fetus: .... FHR: ....

Scar: .... Lateral grip: ....

Time/date of onset of contraction : ....

Uterine contraction: Present/absent/well contracted : ....

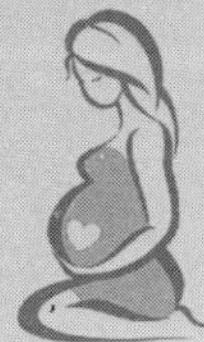

Investigation

Date	Hemoglobin	Blood Group/ Sugar	Urine		Bowel	Bladder	Any Other
			Albumin	Sugar			

Vaginal Examination

S.No	Date and time	Finding	Remark

Previous Obstetrical History

S.No	Year	Term/ preterm	Abortion/ stillbirth	Nature of delivery	Child		Immunization	Growth and development	Nature of puerperium	Remark
					Alive	Sex/ weight				

Admission History

Pregnancy complaints	
Menstrual history	
Medical history	
Surgical history	

Old Pattern Partograph

Parity: *Reg No:* *Date and Time of Admission:* *Date and Time of ROM:*

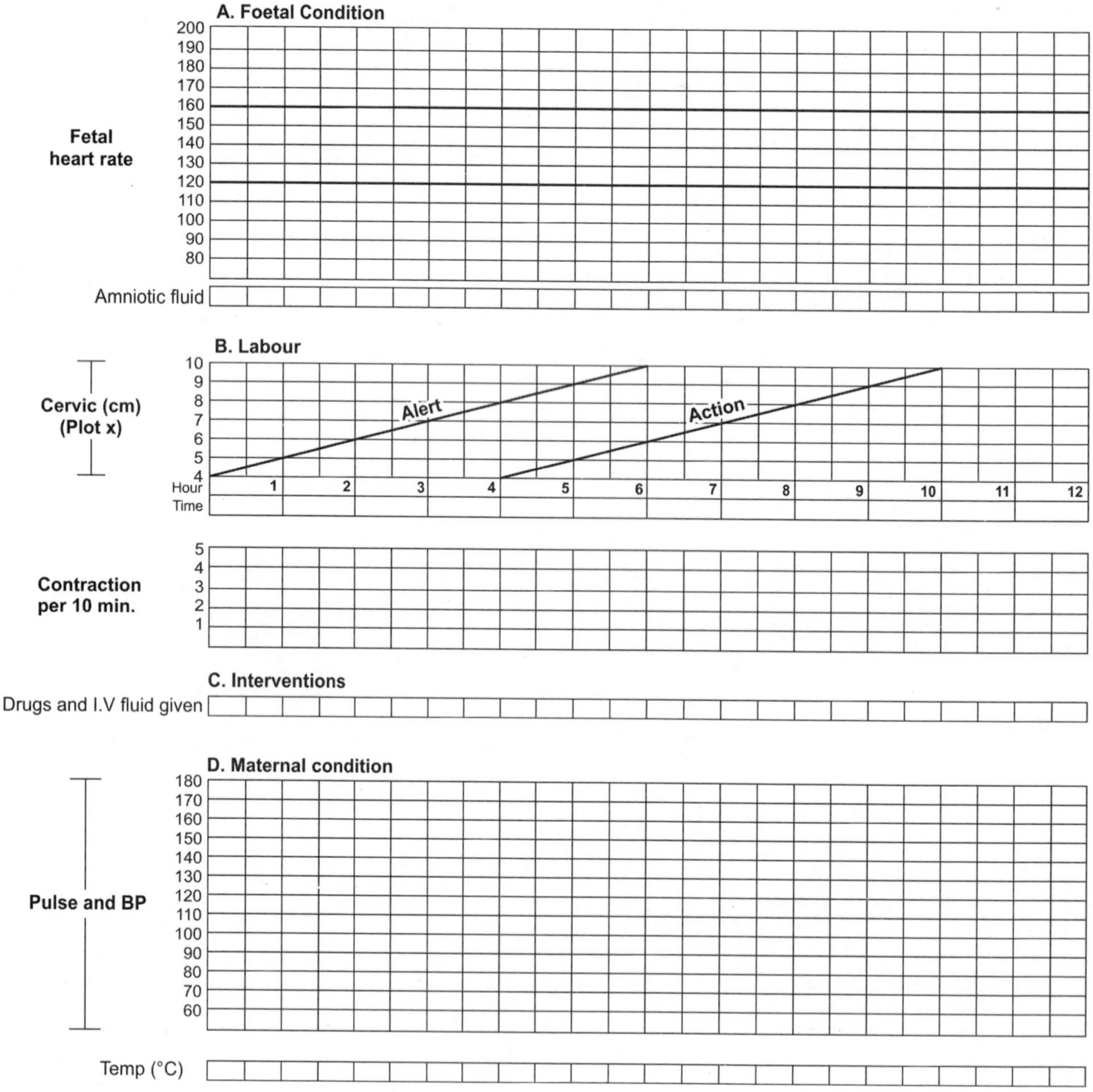

A. Foetal Condition

Fetal heart rate: 200, 190, 180, 170, 160, 150, 140, 130, 120, 110, 100, 90, 80

Amniotic fluid

B. Labour

Cervic (cm) (Plot x): 10, 9, 8, 7, 6, 5, 4

Alert

Action

Hour	1	2	3	4	5	6	7	8	9	10	11	12
Time												

Contraction per 10 min.: 5, 4, 3, 2, 1

C. Interventions

Drugs and I.V fluid given

D. Maternal condition

Pulse and BP: 180, 170, 160, 150, 140, 130, 120, 110, 100, 90, 80, 70, 60

Temp (°C)

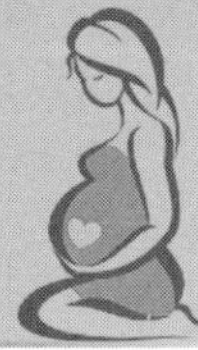

WHO Modified Partograph

Parity: *Reg No:* *Date and Time of Admission:* *Date and Time of ROM:*

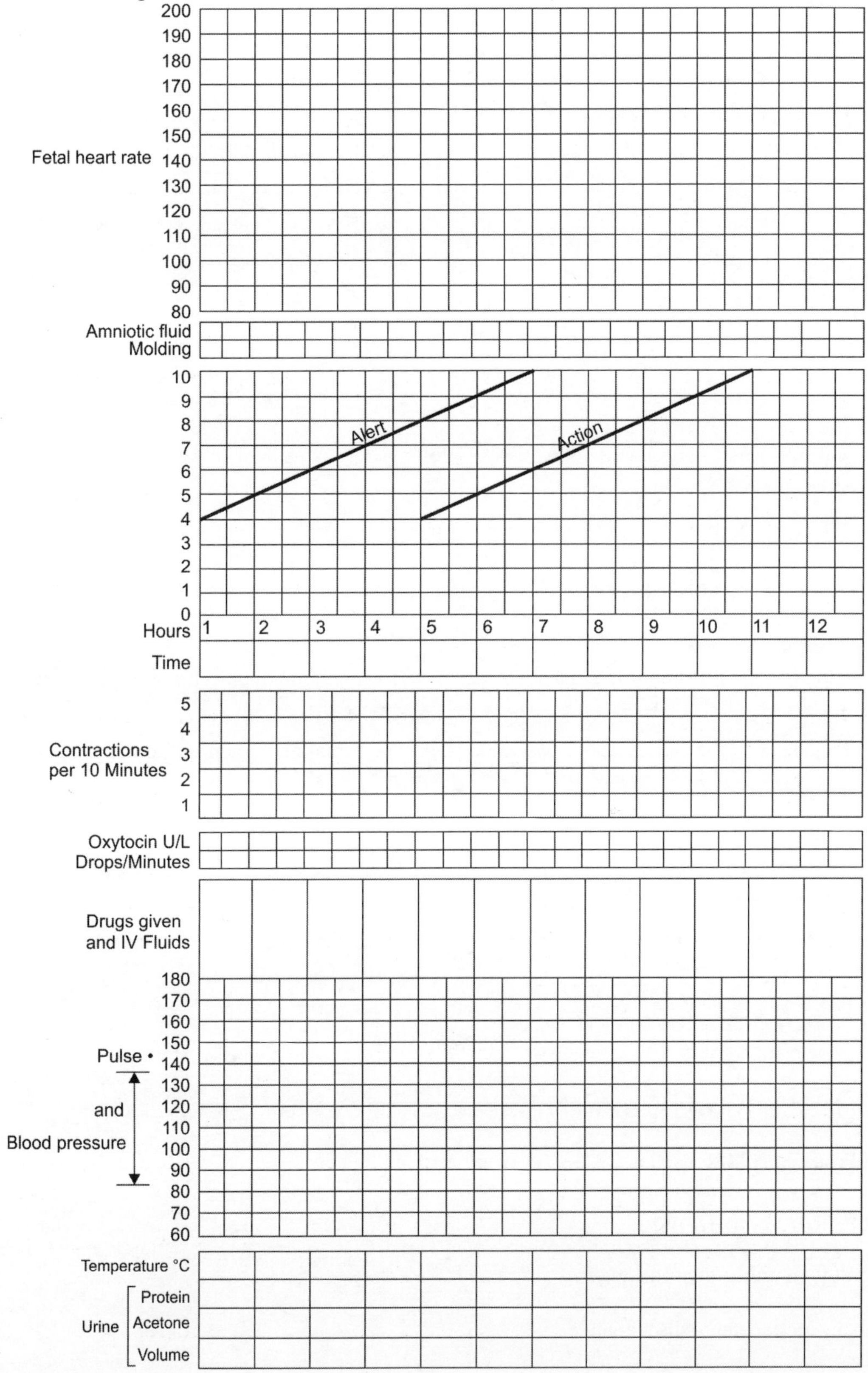

Fetal heart rate: 200, 190, 180, 170, 160, 150, 140, 130, 120, 110, 100, 90, 80

Amniotic fluid

Molding

Cervical dilatation: 10, 9, 8, 7, 6, 5, 4, 3, 2, 1, 0

Alert

Action

Hours	1	2	3	4	5	6	7	8	9	10	11	12
Time												

Contractions per 10 Minutes: 5, 4, 3, 2, 1

Oxytocin U/L

Drops/Minutes

Drugs given and IV Fluids

Pulse • and Blood pressure: 180, 170, 160, 150, 140, 130, 120, 110, 100, 90, 80, 70, 60

Temperature °C

Urine: Protein, Acetone, Volume

Delivery Note

Labor Progress Note Date and Time of Onset of Pain

Onset of true labor: On .... At: ....
Date and time of full cervix dilatation: .... Effacement: ....
Membrane ruptured (spontaneous/artificial/PROM) on .... At ....

Total duration of: 1st stage .... Hrs .... Min ....
2nd stage .... Hrs .... Min ....
3rd stage .... Hrs .... Min ....
Total hours = ... Hrs .... Min ....

Baby at Birth

Mode of delivery: .... Score at one minute ....
Baby born on:................................ At: .... Sex: ....
Apgar scoring: .... Score at five minute................................ Anus patent: ....
Initiation of breastfeeding: ....
Drug administration: ....

Delivery of Placenta and Membrane

Delivery of placenta on: .... At:........................ Cord insertion: ....
Spontaneous/helped/manually removed .... Examination of placenta: Complete/Incomplete ....
Weight of placenta:...
Cord length: .... Examination of membrane: ....

Blood Loss

Before delivery of placenta : ....
During delivery of placenta : ....
After delivery of placenta : ....

Perineum

Intact : .... Episiotomy :............. Laceration :.............................. Repair : ....

Condition of Mother Following Delivery

Pulse: .... BP: .... Uterus: .... Vaginal bleeding: .... Breastfeeding initiated at: ....

Condition of Mother on Transfer

Healthy/unhealthy (if unhealthy specify): ....

Condition of baby on transfer or discharge: ....

Nursing Care Plan

S.No.	Assessment	Nursing Diagnosis	Goal/Expected Out Come	Nursing Intervention	Rational	Implementation	Evaluation

Signature of Sister in Charge

Signature of Supervisor

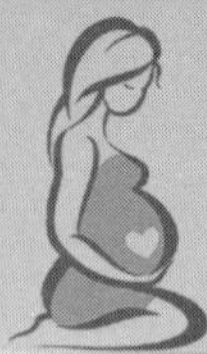

Witness/Assisted Abnormal Delivery (Case No. 5)

Client's Profile

Name : .... Religion : .... W/o : ....

Age : .... Education : .... Parity : ....

Hospital name : .... Occupation : .... LMP : ....

Date of booking : .... Income per month : .... EDD ....

Reg. No : .... Marriage duration : .... Period of gestation ....

Address : ....

....

Date and time of admission : ....

Date and time of discharge or transfer : ....

Admission Note

General Examinations

i. Temperature: ....

ii. Pulse: ....

iii. Respiration: ....

iv. BP: ....

Hydration: ....

Anemia: (Present/absent) ....

Labor pain: (Present/absent).................................

Edema: (Generalized/ankle edema) ....

Abdominal Examination/Obstetrical Examination by Palpation

Height of uterus: .... cm

Lie: ....

Superficial grip: ....

Gestational weeks: ....

Presentation: ....

Deep pelvic grip: ....

Abdominal girth: ....cm

Position of fetus: ....

FHR: ....

Scar: ....

Lateral grip: ....

Time/date of onset of contraction : ....

Uterine contraction: Present/absent/well contracted : ....

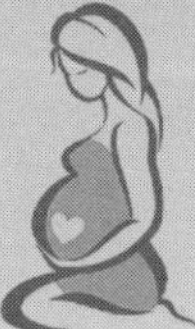

Investigation

Date	Hemoglobin	Blood Group/ Sugar	Urine		Bowel	Bladder	Any Other
			Albumin	Sugar			

Vaginal Examination

S.No	Date and time	Finding	Remark

Previous Obstetrical History

S.No	Year	Term/ preterm	Abortion/ stillbirth	Nature of delivery	Child		Immunization	Growth and development	Nature of puerperium	Remark
					Alive	Sex/ weight				

Admission History

Pregnancy complaints	
Menstrual history	
Medical history	
Surgical history	

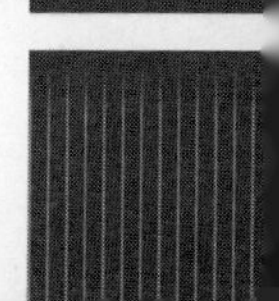

Old Pattern Partograph

Parity: *Reg No:* *Date and Time of Admission:* *Date and Time of ROM:*

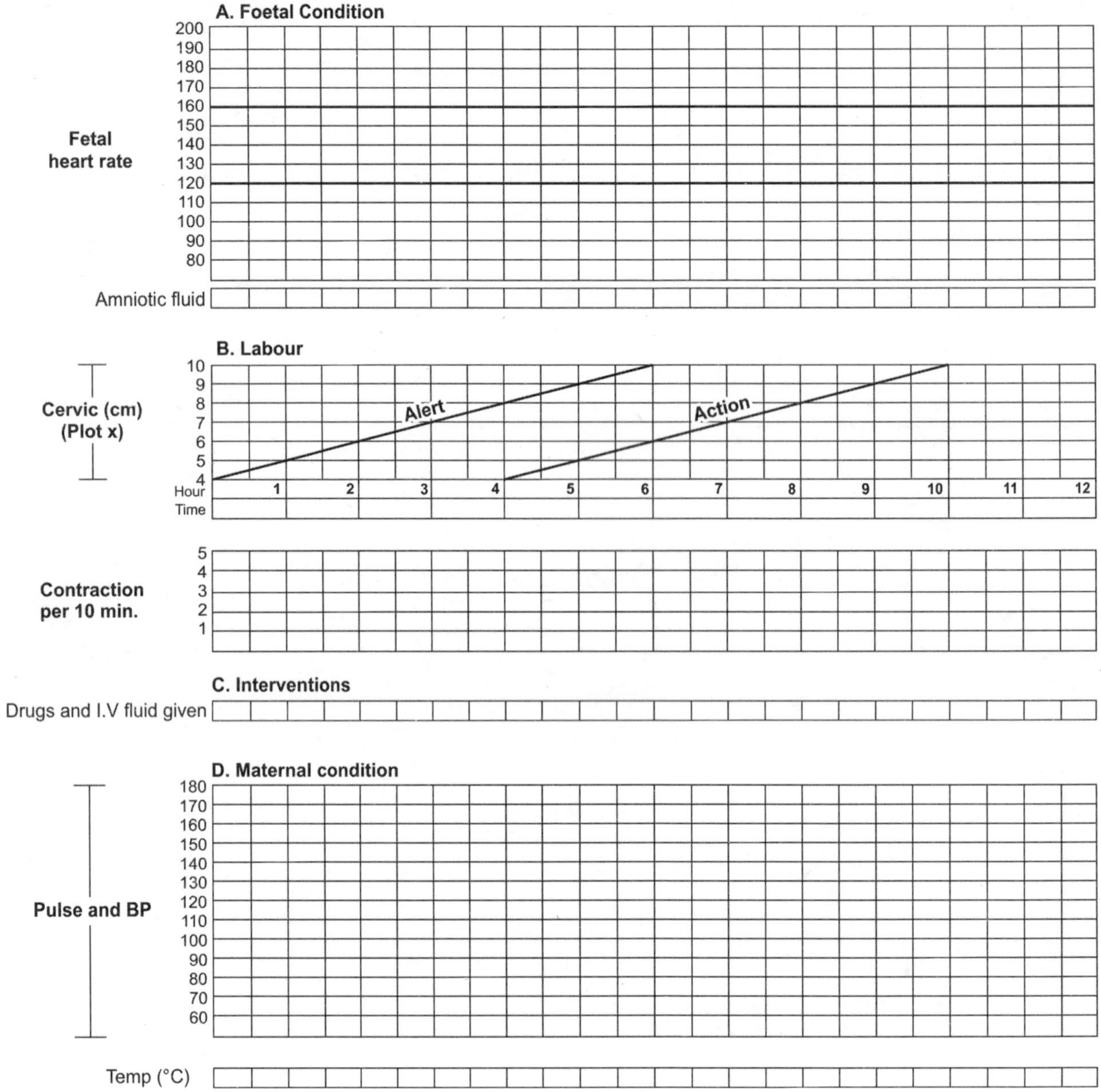

A. Foetal Condition

Fetal heart rate

200
190
180
170
160
150
140
130
120
110
100
90
80

Amniotic fluid

B. Labour

Cervic (cm) (Plot x)

10
9
8
7
6
5
4

Alert

Action

Hour	1	2	3	4	5	6	7	8	9	10	11	12
Time												

Contraction per 10 min.

5
4
3
2
1

C. Interventions

Drugs and I.V fluid given

D. Maternal condition

Pulse and BP

180
170
160
150
140
130
120
110
100
90
80
70
60

Temp (°C)

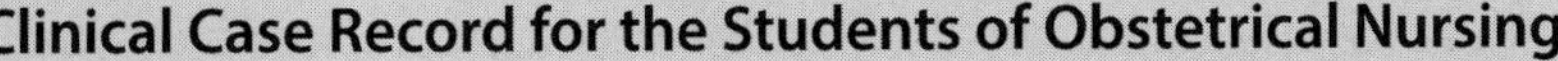
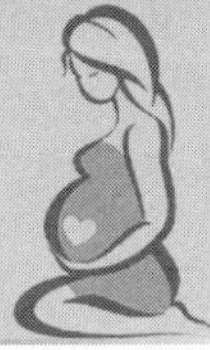

WHO Modified Partograph

Parity: *Reg No:* *Date and Time of Admission:* *Date and Time of ROM:*

Fetal heart rate
200
190
180
170
160
150
140
130
120
110
100
90
80

Amniotic fluid
Molding

10
9
8
7
6
5
4
3
2
1
0

Alert

Action

Hours	1	2	3	4	5	6	7	8	9	10	11	12
Time												

Contractions per 10 Minutes
5
4
3
2
1

Oxytocin U/L
Drops/Minutes

Drugs given and IV Fluids

Pulse •
and
Blood pressure
180
170
160
150
140
130
120
110
100
90
80
70
60

Temperature °C

Urine
Protein
Acetone
Volume

Delivery Note

Labor Progress Note Date and Time of Onset of Pain

Onset of true labor: On .... At: ....
Date and time of full cervix dilatation: .... Effacement: ....
Membrane ruptured (spontaneous/artificial/PROM) on .... At ....

Total duration of:			
	1st stage	Hrs	Min ....
	2nd stage	Hrs	Min ....
	3rd stage	Hrs	Min ....
	Total hours = ...	Hrs	Min ....

Baby at Birth

Mode of delivery: .... Score at one minute ....
Baby born on: .... At: .... Sex: ....
Apgar scoring: .... Score at five minute .... Anus patent: ....
Initiation of breastfeeding: ....
Drug administration: ....

Delivery of Placenta and Membrane

Delivery of placenta on: .... At: .... Cord insertion: ....
Spontaneous/helped/manually removed .... Examination of placenta: Complete/Incomplete ....
Weight of placenta: ....
Cord length: .... Examination of membrane: ....

Blood Loss

Before delivery of placenta : ....
During delivery of placenta : ....
After delivery of placenta : ....

Perineum

Intact : .... Episiotomy : .... Laceration : .... Repair : ....

Condition of Mother Following Delivery

Pulse: ...... BP: .... Uterus: .... Vaginal bleeding: .... Breastfeeding initiated at: ....

Condition of Mother on Transfer

Healthy/unhealthy (if unhealthy specify): ....

Condition of baby on transfer or discharge: ....

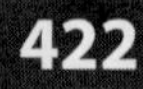

Nursing Care Plan

S.No.	Assessment	Nursing Diagnosis	Goal/Expected Out Come	Nursing Intervention	Rational	Implementation	Evaluation

Signature of Sister in Charge ____________________

Signature of Supervisor ____________________

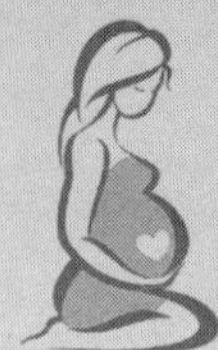

Newborn Resuscitation (Case No. 1)

Client's Profile

Hospital name	:	Mode of delivery	: ....
Date of booking	:	Gestational age of birth	: ....
Reg. No.	:	Newborn birthweight	: ....
B/O	:	Placenta weight	: ....
Date and time of birth	:	Total hours of delivery	: ....

Indication for Resuscitation

....

....

Delivery History Notes

Delivery Note

Labor progress note date and time of onset of pain

Date and time of full dilation: ....

Mode of delivery: ....

Total duration of : 1st stage .... 3rd stage ....

2nd stage .... Total hours ....

Baby at birth .... Delivery of placenta on at.....................................

Baby born on .... at .... Weight of placenta.......................................

Sex .... Cord length..

Anus patent.. Examination of placenta: (Complete/incomplete)...........

Initiation of breastfeeding ....

Drug administration .... Examination of membrane ....

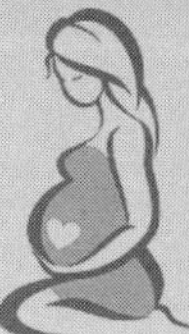

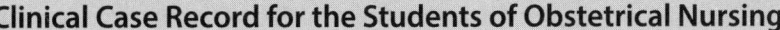

Newborn Assessment

Baby

Postnatal days	1	2	3	4	5	6
Date						
Time						
Vital sign						
Temperature						
Pulse						
Respiration						
Urine (time/day)						
Stool (time/day)						
Eye care						
Cord care						
Fontanels (Normal/Absent)						
Reflexes						
Activity						
Bresastfeeding						
Anthropometric measurement						
Length (cm)						
Head circumference (cm)						
Chest (cm)						
Abdominal (cm)						
Weight (kg)						

Resuscitation Notes

....

....

....

....

....

....

....

....

Drug Administered During Resuscitation

....

....

....

....

After Resuscitation Newborn Health Status

....

....

....

....

Health Education to Mother/Family Member

....

....

....

....

Signature of Sister in Charge ____________________

Signature of Supervisor ____________________

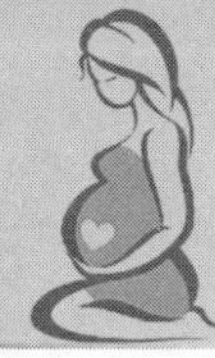

Newborn Resuscitation (Case No. 2)

Client's Profile

Hospital name : .... Mode of delivery : ....

Date of booking : .... Gestational age of birth : ....

Reg. No. : .... Newborn birthweight : ....

B/O : .... Placenta weight : ....

Date and time of birth : .... Total hours of delivery : ....

Indication for Resuscitation

....

....

Delivery History Notes

Delivery Note

Labor progress note date and time of onset of pain

Date and time of full dilation: ....

Mode of delivery: ....

Total duration of : 1st stage .... 3rd stage ....

2nd stage .... Total hours ....

Baby at birth .... Delivery of placenta on at...

Baby born on .... at .... Weight of placenta...

Sex .... Cord length...

Anus patent.. Examination of placenta: (Complete/incomplete)...........

Initiation of breastfeeding ....

Drug administration .... Examination of membrane ....

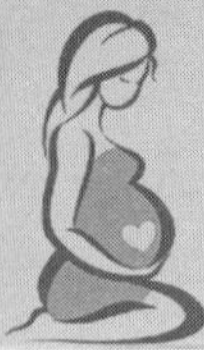

Newborn Assessment

Baby

Postnatal days	1	2	3	4	5	6
Date						
Time						
Vital sign						
Temperature						
Pulse						
Respiration						
Urine (time/day)						
Stool (time/day)						
Eye care						
Cord care						
Fontanels (Normal/Absent)						
Reflexes						
Activity						
Bresastfeeding						
Anthropometric measurement						
Length (cm)						
Head circumference (cm)						
Chest (cm)						
Abdominal (cm)						
Weight (kg)						

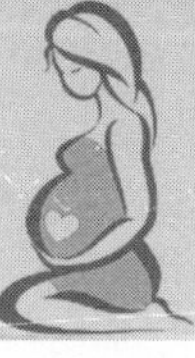

Resuscitation Notes

....

....

....

....

....

....

....

....

Drug Administered During Resuscitation

....

....

....

....

After Resuscitation Newborn Health Status

....

....

....

....

Health Education to Mother/Family Member

....

....

....

....

Signature of Sister in Charge **Signature of Supervisor**

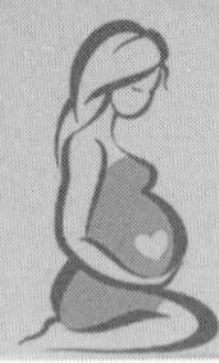

Newborn Resuscitation (Case No. 3)

Client's Profile

Hospital name : ....
Date of booking : ....
Reg. No. : ....
B/O : ....
Date and time of birth : ....

Mode of delivery : ....
Gestational age of birth : ....
Newborn birthweight : ....
Placenta weight : ....
Total hours of delivery : ....

Indication for Resuscitation

....

....

Delivery History Notes

Delivery Note

Labor progress note date and time of onset of pain

Date and time of full dilation: ....

Mode of delivery: ....

Total duration of : 1st stage ....

2nd stage ....

3rd stage ....

Total hours ....

Baby at birth ....

Baby born on .... at ....

Sex ....

Anus patent..

Delivery of placenta on at..

Weight of placenta..

Cord length..

Examination of placenta: (Complete/incomplete)...........

Initiation of breastfeeding ....

Drug administration ....

Examination of membrane ....

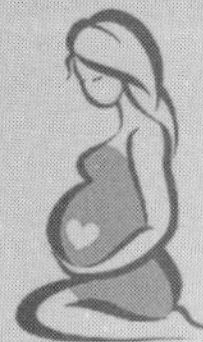

Newborn Assessment

Baby

Postnatal days	1	2	3	4	5	6
Date						
Time						
Vital sign						
Temperature						
Pulse						
Respiration						
Urine (time/day)						
Stool (time/day)						
Eye care						
Cord care						
Fontanels (Normal/Absent)						
Reflexes						
Activity						
Bresastfeeding						
Anthropometric measurement						
Length (cm)						
Head circumference (cm)						
Chest (cm)						
Abdominal (cm)						
Weight (kg)						

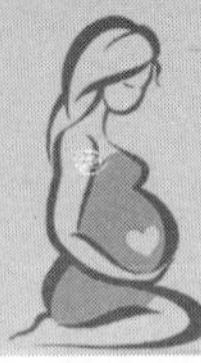

Resuscitation Notes

....

....

....

....

....

....

....

....

Drug Administered During Resuscitation

....

....

....

....

After Resuscitation Newborn Health Status

....

....

....

....

Health Education to Mother/Family Member

....

....

....

....

Signature of Sister in Charge **Signature of Supervisor**

________________________ ________________________

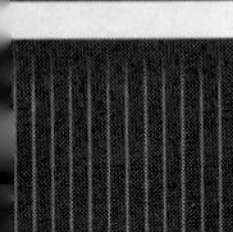

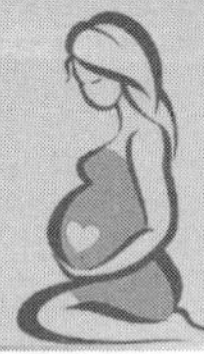

Newborn Resuscitation (Case No. 4)

Client's Profile

Hospital name : .... Mode of delivery : ....

Date of booking : .... Gestational age of birth : ....

Reg. No. : .... Newborn birthweight : ....

B/O : .... Placenta weight : ....

Date and time of birth : .... Total hours of delivery : ....

Indication for Resuscitation

....

....

Delivery History Notes

Delivery Note

Labor progress note date and time of onset of pain

Date and time of full dilation: ....

Mode of delivery: ....

Total duration of : 1st stage .... 3rd stage ....

2nd stage .... Total hours ....

Baby at birth .... Delivery of placenta on at..

Baby born on .... at .... Weight of placenta..

Sex .... Cord length..

Anus patent.. Examination of placenta: (Complete/incomplete)............

Initiation of breastfeeding ....

Drug administration .... Examination of membrane ....

Newborn Assessment

Baby

Postnatal days	1	2	3	4	5	6
Date						
Time						
Vital sign						
Temperature						
Pulse						
Respiration						
Urine (time/day)						
Stool (time/day)						
Eye care						
Cord care						
Fontanels (Normal/Absent)						
Reflexes						
Activity						
Bresastfeeding						
Anthropometric measurement						
Length (cm)						
Head circumference (cm)						
Chest (cm)						
Abdominal (cm)						
Weight (kg)						

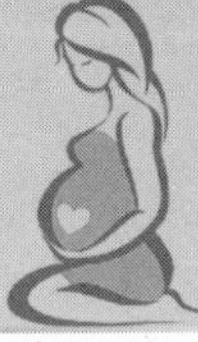

Resuscitation Notes

....

....

....

....

....

....

....

....

Drug Administered During Resuscitation

....

....

....

....

After Resuscitation Newborn Health Status

....

....

....

....

Health Education to Mother/Family Member

....

....

....

....

Signature of Sister in Charge ______________________

Signature of Supervisor ______________________

Newborn Resuscitation (Case No. 5)

Client's Profile

Hospital name	:	Mode of delivery	: ....
Date of booking	:	Gestational age of birth	: ....
Reg. No.	:	Newborn birthweight	: ....
B/O	:	Placenta weight	: ....
Date and time of birth	:	Total hours of delivery	: ....

Indication for Resuscitation

....

....

Delivery History Notes

Delivery Note

Labor progress note date and time of onset of pain

Date and time of full dilation: ....

Mode of delivery: ....

Total duration of	: 1st stage	3rd stage ....
	2nd stage	Total hours ....

Baby at birth .... Delivery of placenta on at.......................................

Baby born on .... at .... Weight of placenta...

Sex .... Cord length...

Anus patent... Examination of placenta: (Complete/incomplete)...........

Initiation of breastfeeding ....

Drug administration .... Examination of membrane ....

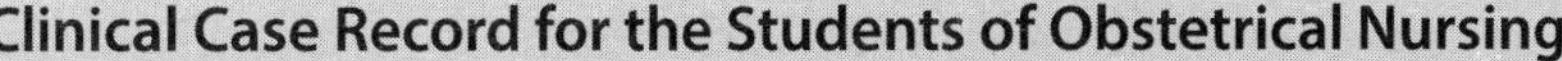

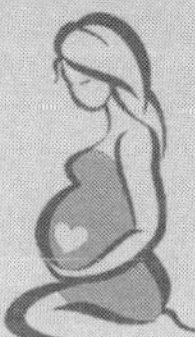

Newborn Assessment

Baby

Postnatal days	1	2	3	4	5	6
Date						
Time						
Vital sign						
Temperature						
Pulse						
Respiration						
Urine (time/day)						
Stool (time/day)						
Eye care						
Cord care						
Fontanels (Normal/Absent)						
Reflexes						
Activity						
Bresastfeeding						
Anthropometric measurement						
Length (cm)						
Head circumference (cm)						
Chest (cm)						
Abdominal (cm)						
Weight (kg)						

Resuscitation Notes

....
....
....
....
....
....
....
....

Drug Administered During Resuscitation

....
....
....
....

After Resuscitation Newborn Health Status

....
....
....
....

Health Education to Mother/Family Member

....
....
....
....

Signature of Sister in Charge **Signature of Supervisor**

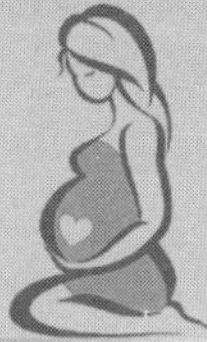

Medical Abbreviations

Abbreviations	Meanings
'a	Before
AAT	Auscultated acceleration test
aa	of each
ac	Before meals
abd	Abdomen
ABC	Alternative birth center
accel	Acceleration of fetal heart rate (FHR)
ad lib	As desired
aq	Water
AFP	Alpha fetoprotein (test)
AMA	Against medical advice
AROM	Artificial rupture of (fetal) membranes
ACOG	American College of Obstetricians And Gynecologists
ACS	American Cancer Society
ACTH	Adrenocorticotropic hormone
AFE	Amniotic fluid embolism
AFP	Alpha-fetoprotein
ALT	Alanine transaminase
APGO	Association of professors of Gynecology and Obstetrics
AROM	Artificial rupture of membranes
ART	Assisted reproductive technology
ASC	Atypical squamous cells
ASCCP	American society for colposcopy and cervical pathology
ASC-H	Atypical squamous cells, cannot exclude HSIL
ASC-US	Atypical squamous cells of uncertain significance
BBT	Basal body temperature
BCA	Bichloroacetic acid
BMI	Body mass index
BP	Blood pressure
BPD	Biparietal diameter
BPM	Beats per minute
BRCA-1, BRCA-2	Breast cancer genes
BUN	Blood urea nitrogen
BV	Bacterial vaginosis

Abbreviations	Meanings
bid	Two times per day
bl	Baseline
bm	Bowel movement
bmr	Basal metabolic rate
bow	Bag of waters
bbow	Bulging bag of waters
bbv	Beat to beat variability (FHR)
bp	Blood pressure
bid	Two times per day
bl	Baseline
bpm	Beats per minute
br	Breech
BV	Bacterial vaginosis
'c	With
C	Celsius
CBC	Complete blood count
cc	Chief complaint
cc	Cubic centimeter
CMV	Cytomegalovirus
CM	Certified midwife
CNS	Central nervous system
C0 2	Carbon dioxide
c/o	Complains of
CPD	Cephalopelvic disproportion
CPR	Cardiopulmonary resuscitation
C/S	Cesarean section
CST	Contraction stress test
CVA	Cerebrovascular anomaly
CVA	Costovertebral angle
CX	Cervix
CBC	Complete blood count
CC	Chief complaint
CDC [U.S.]	Centers for Disease Control and Prevention
CEE	Conjugated equine estrogens
CF	Cystic fibrosis
CIN	Cervical intraepithelial neoplasia
CLE	Continuous lumbar epidural
CMV	Cytomegalovirus

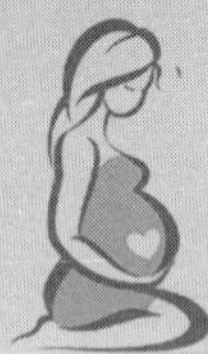

Abbreviations	Meanings
CNS	Central nervous system
CPD	Cephalopelvic disproportion
CPP	Chronic pelvic pain
CSF	Cerebrospinal fluid
CT	Computed tomography
CVS	Chorionic villus sampling
CXR	Chest x-ray
DCIS	Ductal carcinoma in situ
DES	Diethylstilbestrol
DHEA	Dehydroepiandrosterone
DHEAS	Dehydroepiandrosterone sulfate
DIC	Disseminated intravascular coagulation
DMSO	Dimethyl sulfoxide
DNA	Deoxyribonucleic acid
DSM-IV-TR	Diagnostic and statistical manual of mental
DTR	Deep tendon reflex
DUB	Dysfunctional uterine bleeding
DVT	Deep vein thrombosis
DandC	Dilation and curettage
dc	Discontinue
decels	Deceleration of FHT
DEM	Direct entry midwife
DIC	Disseminated intravascular coagulation
dil	Dilation
DM	Diabetes mellitus
DNKA	Did not keep appointment
DPT	Diphtheria-pertussis-tetanus
dr	Dram
DTR	Deep tendon reflex
DX	Diagnosis
EASI	Extra-amniotic saline infusion
ECC	Endocervical curettage
EDC	Estimated date of confinement
EE	Ethinylestradiol
ELISA	Enzyme-linked immunosorbent assay
EMB	Endometrial biopsy
EMG	Electromyography
EMTALA [U.S.]	Emergency Medical Treatment and Active Labor Act
EPDS	Edinburgh Postnatal Depression Scale
ET	Estrogen therapy; embryo transfer
EASI	Extra-amniotic saline infusion

Abbreviations	Meanings
ECC	Endocervical curettage
EDC	Estimated date of confinement
ELISA	Enzyme-linked immunosorbent assay
EMB	Endometrial biopsy
EMG	Electromyography
EMTALA [US]	Emergency Medical Treatment and Active Labor Act
EPDS	Edinburgh postnatal depression scale
ET	Estrogen therapy; embryo transfer
FAS	Fetal alcohol syndrome
FDA [U.S.]	Food and drug administration
FEV1	Forced expiratory volume in 1 second
FHR	Fetal heart rate
FHT	Fetal heart tone
FIGO	International Federation of Gynecology and Obstetrics
FISH	Fluorescent in situ hybridization
FSH	Follicle-stimulating hormone
FTA-ABS	Fluorescent treponemal antibody absorbed
F	Fahrenheit
FB	Finger breadths
FHT	Fetal heart tones
FHR	Fetal heart rate
FM	Fetal movement
FMC	Fetal movement count
FUO	Fever of unknown origins
G	Gravida
GC	Gonorrhea culture
GFT or GTT?	Drops
GI	Gastrointestinal
GTT	Glucose tolerance test
GU	Genitourinary
GYN	Gynecology
GAG	Glycosaminoglycan
GBS	Group B streptococcus
GI	Gastrointestinal
GIFT	Gamete intrafallopian transfer
GnRH	Gonadotropin-releasing hormone
GTN	Gestational trophoblastic neoplasm
GU	Genitourinary
H	Hour

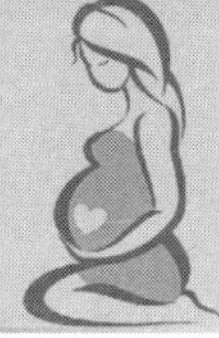

Abbreviations	Meanings
Hb or HGB	Hemoglobin
HCT	Hematocrit
Hx	History
h.s.	At bedtime (hora somni)
HBIG	Hepatitis B immune globulin
HCG, hCG	Human chorionic gonadotropin
HDL	High-density lipoprotein
HELLP	Hemolysis, Elevated Liver Enzymes, Low Platelets (Syndrome)
HIPAA [U.S.]	Health insurance Portability and Accountability Act
HIV	Human immunodeficiency virus
HMG, hMG	Human menopausal gonadotropin
HNPCC	Hereditary nonpolyposis colorectal cancer
HPI	History of present illness
HPV	Human papillomavirus
HRT	Hormone replacement therapy
HSG	Hysterosalpingogram
HSIL	High-grade squamous intraepithelial lesion
HSV	Herpes simplex virus
HT	Hormone therapy
HUMI	Harris-Kronner uterine manipulator injector
IBS	Irritable bowel syndrome
IC	Interstitial cystitis
ICSI	Intracytoplasmic sperm injection
ICU	Intensive care unit
IFE	Internal fetal electrode
IGF	Insulin-like growth factor
IM	Intramuscular
ITP	Idiopathic thrombocytopenic purpura
IUD	Intrauterine device
IUFD	Intrauterine fetal demise
IUGR	Intrauterine growth restriction
IUI	Intrauterine insemination
IUPC	Intrauterine pressure catheter
IV	Intravenous
IVF	In vitro fertilization
IVPB	Intravenous piggyback
IM	Intramuscular
IUP	Intrauterine pregnancy
I and O	In and out
inf.	Infusion
IUD	Intrauterine device

Abbreviations	Meanings
IUFD	Intrauterine fetal death
IUGR	Intrauterine growth retardation
L	Left
LB lb	Pound
LBW	Low birthweight
LDEM	Licensed direct entry midwife
LGA	Large for gestational age
LM	Licensed midwife
LMA	Left mentum anterior
LMP	Last menstrual period
LMP	Left mentum posterior
LMT	Left mentum transverse
LNMP	Last normal menstrual period
LOA	Left occipital anterior
LOP	Left occipital posterior
LOT	Left occipital transverse
L/S	Lecithin/sphingomyelin ratio
LSA	Left sacrum anterior
LSP	Left sacrum posterior
LST	Left sacrum transverse
LAM	Lactational amenorrhea method
LCIS	Lobular carcinoma in situ
LDH	Lactate dehydrogenase
LDL	Low-density lipoprotein
LEEP	Loop electrosurgical excision procedure
LH	Luteinizing hormone
LLETZ	Large-loop excision of the transformation zone
LMP	Last menstrual period
LOA	Left occiput anterior
LOP	Left occiput posterior
LSIL	Low-grade squamous intraepithelial lesion
LTV	Long-term variability
LUNA	Laparoscopic uterine nerve ablation
MAO	Monoamine oxidase
MCV	Mean corpuscular volume
MP	Micronized progesterone
MPA	Medroxyprogesterone acetate
MRI	Magnetic resonance imaging
MTHFR	Methylenetetrahydrofolate reductase
mec	Meconium
mecst	Meconium staining
Meth	Methergine

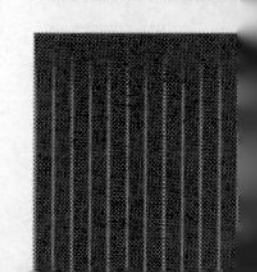

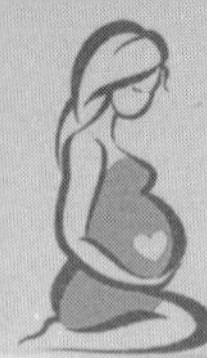

Abbreviations	Meanings
MTLP	Metabolic toxemia of late pregnancy
multip	Multipara
MW	Midwife
mcg	Microgram
mg	Milligram
ml	Milliliter
neg	Negative
NGU	Nongonococcal urethritis
NKA	None known about
NKA	No known allergies
NKDA	No known drug allergy
NPO	Nothing by mouth
N/R	Nonreactive
NST	Nonstress test
NSVB	Normal spontaneous vaginal birth
N/V	Nausea/vomiting
NAAT	Nucleic acid amplification test
NICHD [US]	National institute of child health and human development
NIH [US]	National institutes of health
NSAID	Nonsteroidal anti-inflammatory drug
NST	Nonstress test
NTD	Neural tube defect
02	Oxygen
OA	Occiput anterior
OB	Obstetrics/obstetrician
OCT	Oxytocin challenge test
OOP	Out of the pelvis
OP	Occiput posterior
Oz	Ounce
os	Opening
OTC	Over the counter
OAB	Overactive bladder
OCP	Oral contraceptive pill
OHSS	Ovarian hyperstimulation syndrome
OR	Operating room
OTC	Over-the-counter
PAPP	-A pregnancy-associated plasma protein a
PCOS	Polycystic ovarian syndrome
PCR	Polymerase chain reaction
PDE	Phosphodiesterase
PDS	Polydioxanone suture
PE	Pulmonary embolism

Abbreviations	Meanings
PEEP	Positive end-expiratory pressure
PEPI	Postmenopausal estrogen/progestin interventions trial
PGE	Prostaglandin E
PGY	Postgraduate year (PGY-1, PGY-2, etc.)
PI	Protease inhibitor
PID	Pelvic inflammatory disease
PIH	Pregnancy-induced hypertension
PMDD	Premenstrual dysphoric disorder
PMH	Past medical history
PMS	Premenstrual syndrome
POP-Q	Pelvic organ prolapse quantification system
PRBC	Packed red blood cell
PROM	Premature rupture of membrane
PT	Prothrombin time
PTT	Partial thromboplastin time
PUBS	Percutaneous umbilical cord blood sampling
'p	After
PERLA	Pupils equal and reactive to light, asymmetrical
PERRLA	Pupils equal, round, react to light, accommodation
PPhem	Postpartum hemorrhage
P	Para
P	Pulse
PAP	Papanicolaou smear
'pc	After meal
Ped	Pediatrician/pediatrics
PID	Pelvic inflammatory disease
PIH	Pregnancy induced hypertension
Pit	Pitocin
PKU	Phenylketonuria
pos	Positive
p.r.n.	As needed
po	By mouth
premie	Premature infant
primip	Primipara
PROM	Premature rupture of the (fetal) membranes
PROM	Prolonged rupture of the (fetal) membranes
PTT	Partial thromboplastin test
RBC	Red blood cell
RNA	Ribonucleic acid
ROA	Right occiput anterior

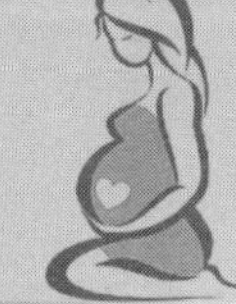

Abbreviations	Meanings
ROP	Right occiput posterior
ROS	Review of systems
RPR	Rapid plasma reagin
RR	Relative risk; respiratory rate
RTI	Reverse transcriptase inhibitor
R	Right
RBC	Red blood cell (count)
RDA	Recommended daily allowance
RDS	Respiratory distress syndrome
RMA	Right mentum anterior
RMP	Right mentum posterior
RMT	Right mentum transverse
RSA	Right sacrum anterior
R/O	Rule out
ROM	Rupture of (fetal) membranes
ROP	Right occiput posterior
ROT	Right occiput transverse
ROS	Review of symptoms
RPR	Rapid plasma reagin (syphilis test)
Rx	Treatment
SAB	Spontaneous abortion (miscarriage)
's	Without
Sig	Write
SGA	Small for gestational age
SIDS	Sudden infant death syndrome
SOAP	Subjective, objective, analysis, plan
S.O.S	Single dose only
SROM	Spontaneous rupture of (the fetal) membranes
St	Stage
sta	Station
STD	Sexually transmitted disease
Sp gr	Specific gravity
s.s.	One half
stat	Immediately
Sx	Symptom
S>D	Size is greater than dates
S<D	Size is small for dates
SD	Standard deviation
SERM	Selective estrogen receptor modulator
SLE	Systemic lupus erythematosus
SNRI	Serotonin-norepinephrine reuptake inhibitor
SROM	Spontaneous rupture of membrane

Abbreviations	Meanings
SSRI	Selective serotonin reuptake inhibitor
STD	Sexually transmitted disease
STI	Sexually transmitted infection
STV	Short-term variability
SUI	Stress urinary incontinence
TCA	Trichloroacetic acid
TENS	Transcutaneous electrical nerve stimulation
TNM	Tumor, node, metastasis
TPN	Total parenteral nutrition
TP-PA T	Pallidum particle agglutination
TRALI	Transfusion-related acute lung injury
TSH	Thyroid-stimulating hormone
TVT	Tension-free vaginal tape
TAB	Therapeutic abortion
TC	Telephone conversation
t.i.d.	Three time a day
TOP	Termination of pregnancy
TORCH	Toxoplasmosis, other, rubella, cytomegalovirus, herpes
TPR	Temperature, pulse, respirations
TSS	Toxic shock syndrome
u/a	Urinalysis
U	Unit
UC	Uterine contractions
U/S	Ultrasound
UTI	Urinary tract infection
VBAC	Vaginal birth after cesarean section
V.S.	Vital signs
VDRL	Venereal disease research lab
VE	Vacuum extractor
VTX	Vertex
WBC	White blood cells
WIC	Woman, infants and children
WNL	Within normal limits
Wt	Weight

Abbreviations Related to Time

Abbreviation s	Definitions
A.M	Before noon
ac, AC	Before meals
bid	Twice a day

Abbreviation s	Definitions
h,H	Hour
MN	Mid night
pc, PC	After meals
P.M	Afternoon, evening
q1h	Every hours
q2h	Every 2 hours
q3h	Every 3 hours
q4h	Every 4 hours
q6h	Every 6 hours
q8h	Every 8 hours
qid	Four times a day
tid	Three times a day

Abbreviations Related to Form

Abbreviations	Definitions
ac, AC	Before meals
amp	ampule
cap	capsule
comp	Compound
dil	Dilute
elix	Elixir
ext	Extract
H	Hypodermic

Abbreviation Related to Measurement

Abbreviations	Definitions
cm	Centimeter
g, gm	Gram
gr	Grain
kg	Kilogram
L	Liter
mcg	Microgram
mEq	Milliequivalent
mg	Milligram
mL	Milliliter
tsp	Teaspoon
tbsp	Tablespoon

BIBLIOGRAPHY

1. Dutta D.C "*Textbook of Obstetrics*", 5th Edition, New Central Book Agencies
2. Fraser Diane, M. Cooper, Margaret Amyls, "*Textbook of Midwives*" 4th Edition, Churchill Living Stone Publication.
3. Helen Varney Janm Kriesbs and Carbonyl Gegor, *Varney's Midwifery*, 4th Edition, Jones and Bartlett Learning
4. Jacob Annamma "*A Comprehensive Textbook of Midwifery* 4th Edition, Jaypee Publication
5. Jacob Annamma, *A Practical Record of Maternal and Newborn Nursing*, 4th Edition, Jaypee Brothers.
6. Nettina, Sandra M.; Mills, Elizabeth Jacqueline, "*Lippincott Manual of Nursing Practice*", 8th Edition, Lippincott Williams and Wilkins
7. National Rural Health Mission, "*Guidelines for Antenatal Care and Skilled Attendance at Birth*" April 2010, Maternal Health Division, Ministry of Health and Family Welfare, Government of India
8. Susan C. Dewit, *Fundamental Concepts and Skills for Nursing*, 3rd Edition, Sunders Elsevier

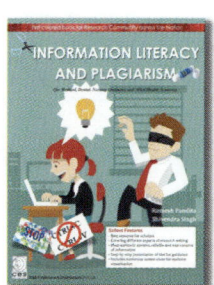

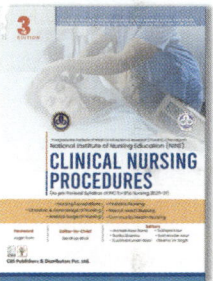

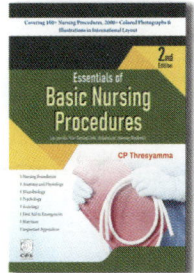

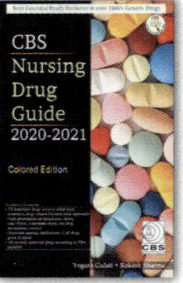

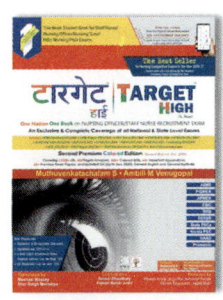

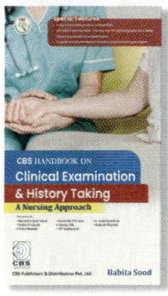

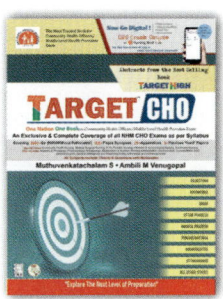

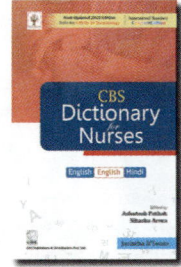

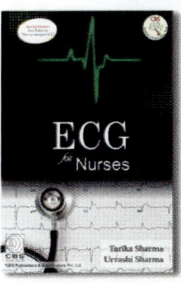

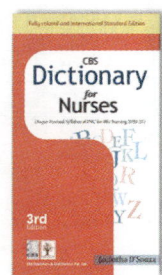

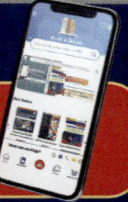

Community Health Nursing

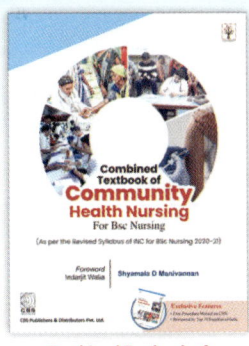

Combined Textbook of Community Health Nursing For BSc Nursing
Shyamala D Manivannan
978-93-90619-37-5
1/e, 2022
TBA

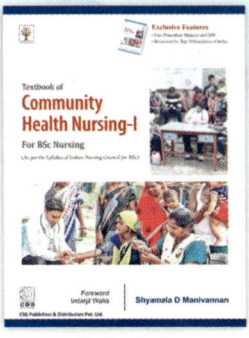

Textbook of Community Health Nursing-I For BSc Nursing
Shyamala D Manivannan
978-81-23927-01-5
1/e, 2018
MRP: ₹750/-

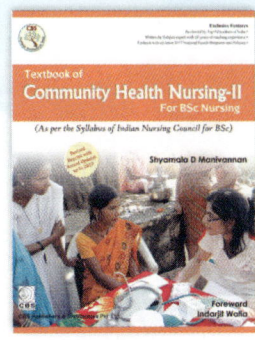

Textbook of Community Health Nursing-II For BSc Nursing
Shyamala D Manivannan
978-93-86827-22-7
1/e, 2018
MRP: ₹450/-

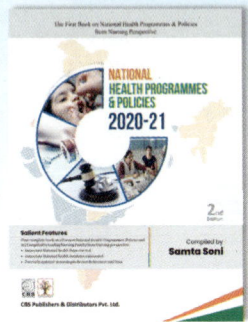

National Health Programmes & Policies 2020-21
Samta Soni
978-93-90619-13-9
2/e, 2022
MRP: ₹695/-

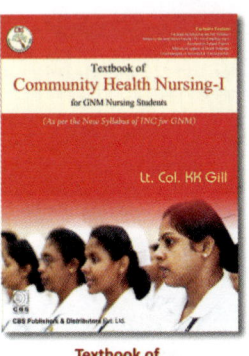

Textbook of Community Health Nursing-I For GNM Nursing Students
Lt. Col. KK Gill
978-93-86827-17-3
1/e, 2018
MRP: ₹550/-

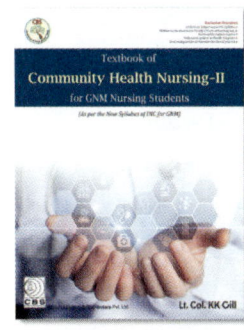

Textbook of Community Health Nursing-II for GNM Nursing Students
Lt. Col. KK Gill
978-93-88178-57-0
1/e, 2019
MRP: ₹525/-

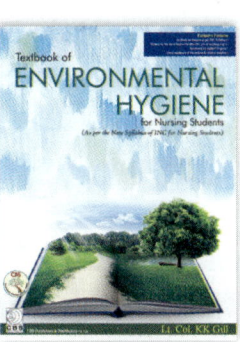

Textbook of Environmental Hygiene for Nursing Students
Lt. Col. KK Gill
978-93-88178-56-3
1/e, 2018-19
MRP: ₹225/-

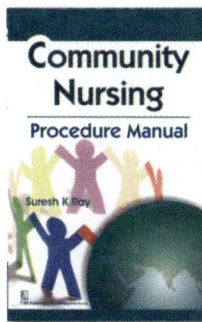

Community Nursing Procedure Manual
Suresh K Ray
978-81-23929-35-4
1/e, 2017
MRP: ₹265/-

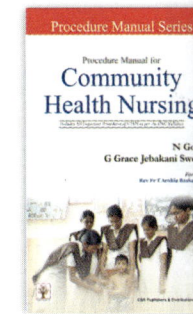

Procedure Manual fo Community Health Nur
N Gowri et al.
978-81-948693-6-
1/e, 2021
MRP: ₹195/-

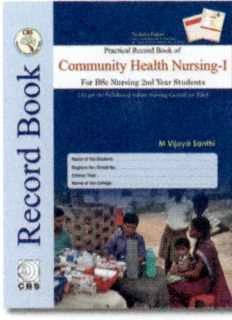

Practical Record Book of Community Health Nursing-I for BSc Nursing 2nd Year Students
M Vijaya Santhi
978-81-23926-84-1
1/e, 2016
MRP: ₹450/-

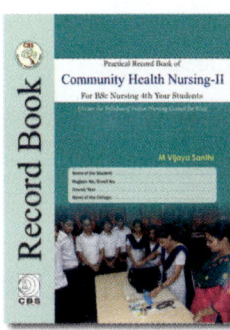

Practical Record Book of Community Health Nursing-II for BSc Nursing 4th Year Students
M Vijaya Santhi
978-93-88108-77-5
1/e, 2018-19
MRP: ₹575/-

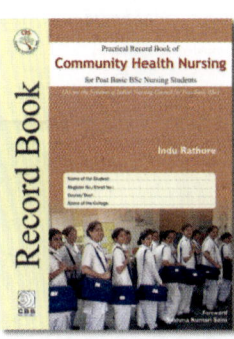

Practical Record Book of Community Health Nursing for Post Basic BSc Nursing Students
Indu Rathore
978-93-86827-06-7
1/e, 2017
MRP: ₹475/-

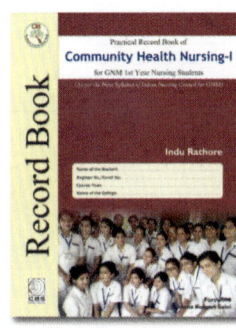

Practical Record Book of Community Health Nursing-I for GNM 1st Year Nursing Students
Indu Rathore
978-93-86827-07-4
1/e, 2018-19
MRP: ₹350/-

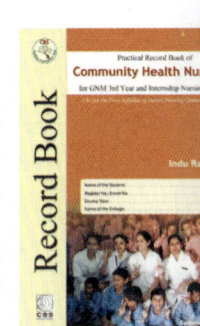

Practical Record Book Community Health Nur for GNM 3rd Year and Internship Nursing Stude
Indu Rathore
978-93-86827-30-
1/e, 2018-19
MRP: ₹395/-

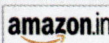

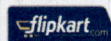

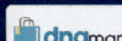

Nursing Foundation

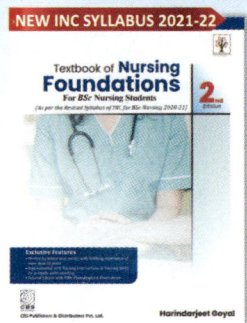

Textbook of
Nursing Foundations
for BSc Nursing Students
Harindarjeet Goyal
978-93-90619-12-2
2/e, 2022
MRP: ₹950/-

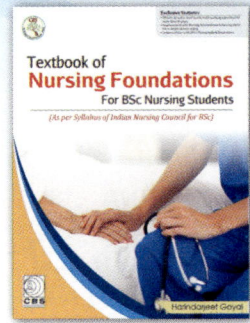

Textbook of
Nursing Foundations
for BSc Nursing Students
Harindarjeet Goyal
978-93-88108-94-2
1/e, 2020
MRP: ₹950/-

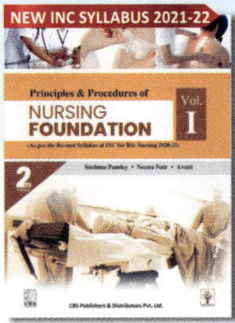

Principles & Procedures of
Nursing Foundation Vol-I
for BSc Nursing
Sushma Pandey et al.
978-93-90619-57-3
2/e, 2022
TBA

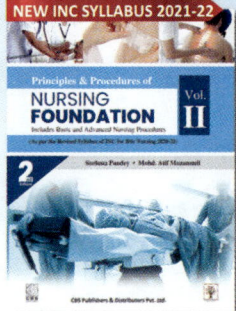

Principles & Procedures of
Nursing Foundation Vol-II
for BSc Nursing
Sushma Pandey et al.
978-93-90619-19-1
2/e, 2022
TBA

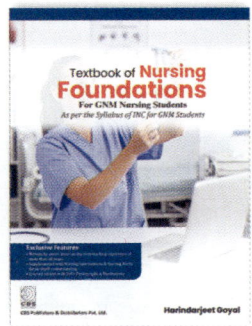

Textbook of
Nursing Foundations
for GNM Nursing Students
Harindarjeet Goyal
978-93-90619-70-2
1/e, 2022
MRP: ₹850/-

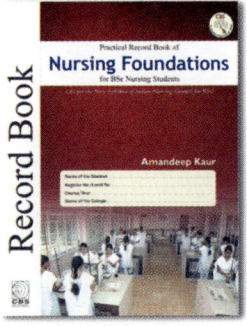

Practical Record Book of
Nursing Foundations
for BSc Nursing Students
Amandeep Kaur
978-93-88108-96-6
1/e, 2018-19
MRP: ₹425/-

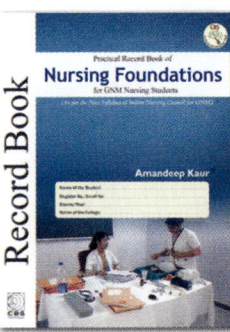

Practical Record Book of
Nursing Foundations
for GNM Nursing Students
Amandeep Kaur
978-93-88178-50-1
1/e, 2018-19
MRP: ₹350/-

Medical Surgical Nursing

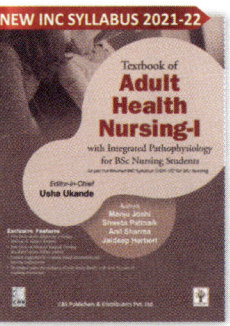

Textbook of
Adult Health Nursing-I
with Integrated Pathophysiology
for BSc Nursing Students
Usha Ukande
978-93-90619-20-7
1/e, 2022
TBA

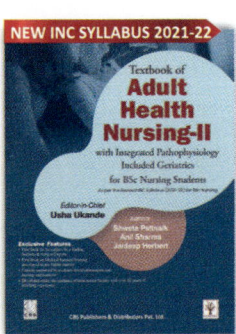

Textbook of
Adult Health Nursing-II
with Integrated Pathophysiology
Included Geriatrics for BSc Nursing Students
Usha Ukande
978-93-90619-86-3
1/e, 2022
TBA

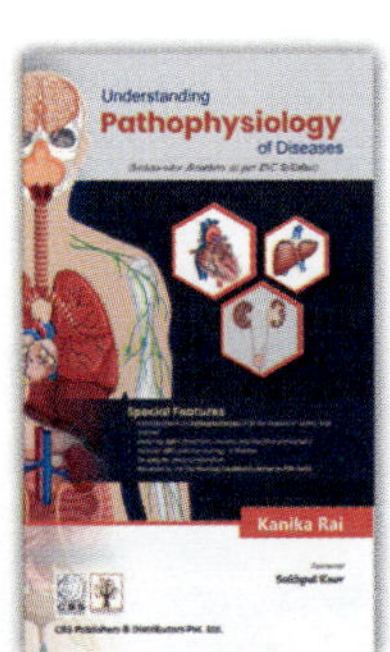

Understanding
Pathophysiology of Diseases
Kanika Rai
978-93-90619-11-5
1/e, 2022
MRP: ₹395/-

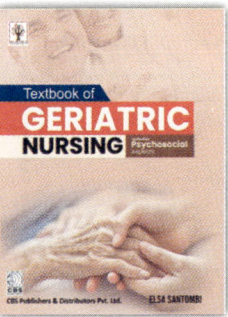

Textbook of
Geriatric Nursing
Including Psychosocial Aspects
Elsa Santombi
978-93-90619-79-5
1/e, 2022
TBA

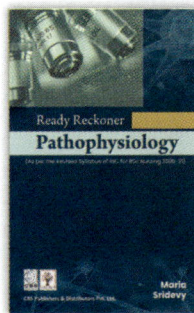

Ready Reckoner
Pathophysiology
for Nurses
Maria et al.
978-93-90619-05-4
1/e, 2022
TBA

MSN/Pharmacology/Pathology

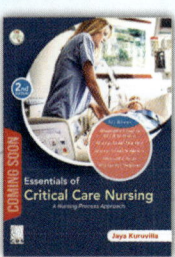

Essentials of
Critical Care Nursing
A Nursing Process Approach
Jaya Kuruvilla
978-93-90619-61-0
2/e, 2022
TBA

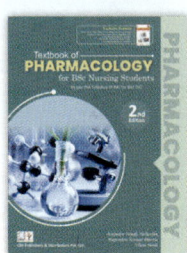

Textbook of
Pharmacology
For BSc Nursing Students
Joginder Singh Pathania et al.
978-93-90619-27-6
2/e, 2022
MRP: ₹650/-

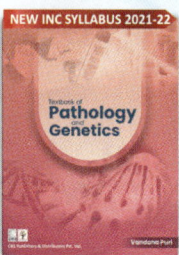

Textbook of
Pathology and Genetics
Vandana Puri
978-93-90619-87-0
1/e, 2022
TBA

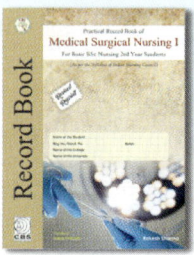

Practical Record Book of
Medical Surgical Nursing I
for Basic BSc Nursing 2nd Year Students
Rakesh Sharma
978-81-23928-00-5
1/e, 2018-19
MRP: ₹550/-

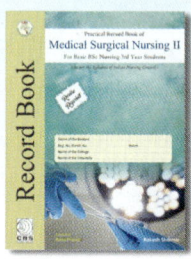

Practical Record Book of
Medical Surgical Nursing II
for Basic BSc Nursing 3nd Year Students
Rakesh Sharma
978-81-23928-01-2
1/e, 2018-19
MRP: ₹475/-

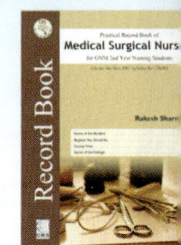

Practical Record Book
Medical Surgical Nurs
for GNM 2nd Year Nursing S
Rakesh Sharma
978-93-86827-04-3
1/e, 2017
MRP: ₹475/-

Child Health Nursing & Pediatric Nursing

Exclusive Marketing & Distribution Rights

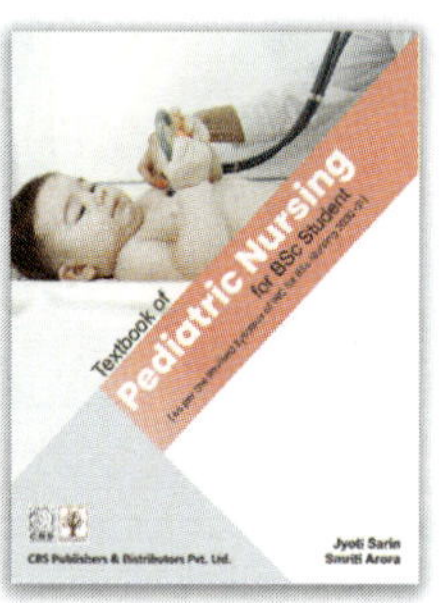

Textbook of
Pediatric Nursing
for BSc Nursing Students
Panchali Pal
978-81-948693-2-0
2/e, 2021
MRP: ₹795/-

Textbook of
Pediatric Nursing
for BSc Nursing Students
Jyoti Sarin et al.
978-93-90619-78-8
1/e, 2022
TBA

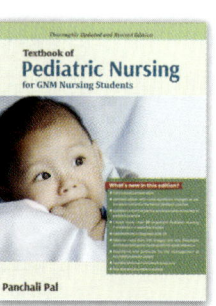

Textbook of
Pediatric Nursing
for GNM Nursing Students
Panchali Pal
978-93-90619-71-9
1/e, 2022
TBA

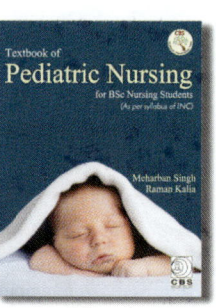

Textbook of
Pediatric Nursing
for BSc Nursing Students
Meharban Singh et al.
978-93-88108-72-0
1/e, 2018
MRP: ₹725/-

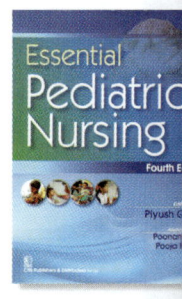

Essential
Pediatric Nursing
Piyush Gupta
978-93-86217-87-5
4/e, 2017
MRP: ₹750/-

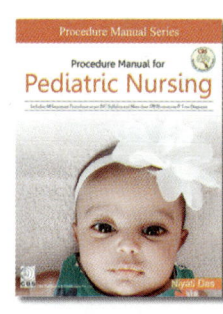

Procedure Manual for
Pediatric Nursing
Niyati Das
978-93-88108-86-7
1/e, 2018
MRP: ₹325/-

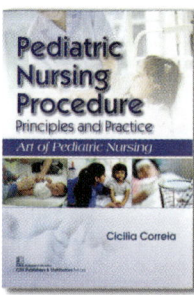

Pediatric Nursing Procedure
Principles and Practice
Cicilia Correia
978-93-86310-74-3
1/e, 2017
MRP: ₹450/-

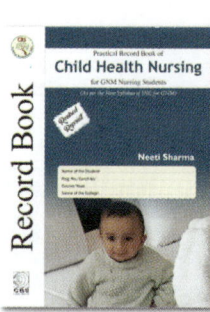

Practial Record Book of
Child Health Nursing
for GNM Nursing Students
Neeti Sharma
978-93-86827-53-1
1/e, 2017
MRP: ₹325/-

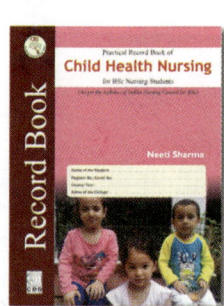

Practial Record Book of
Child Health Nursing
for BSc Nursing Students
Neeti Sharma
978-93-86827-05-0
1/e, 2017
MRP: ₹310/-

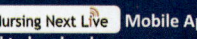

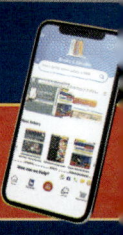

Mental Health Nursing & Psychiatric Nursing

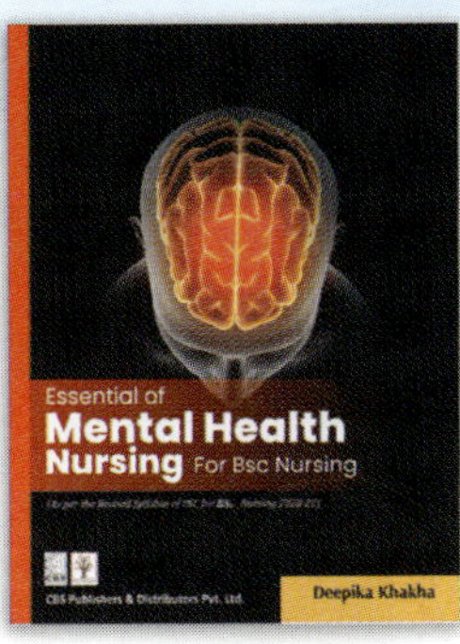
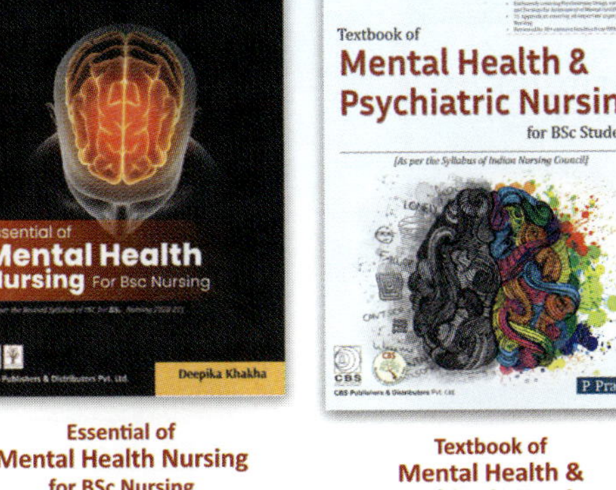

Essential of Mental Health Nursing for BSc Nursing
Deepika Khakha
978-93-90619-73-3
1/e, 2022
TBA

Textbook of Mental Health & Psychiatric Nursing
P Prakash
978-93-89261-91-2
1/e, 2019
MRP: ₹625/-

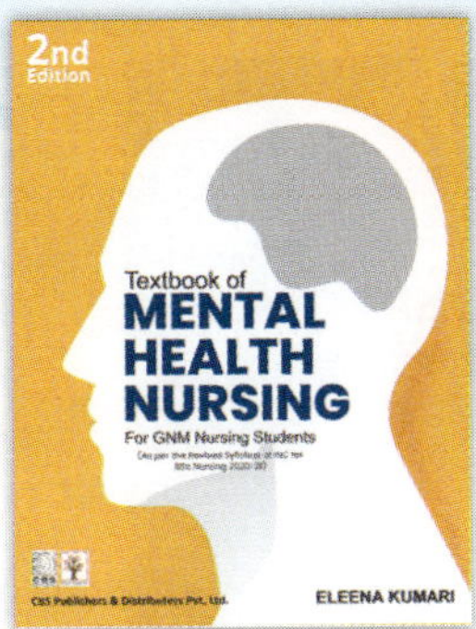

Textbook of Mental Health Nursing for GNM Nursing Students
Eleena Kumari
978-93-90619-72-6
2/e, 2022
MRP: ₹395/-

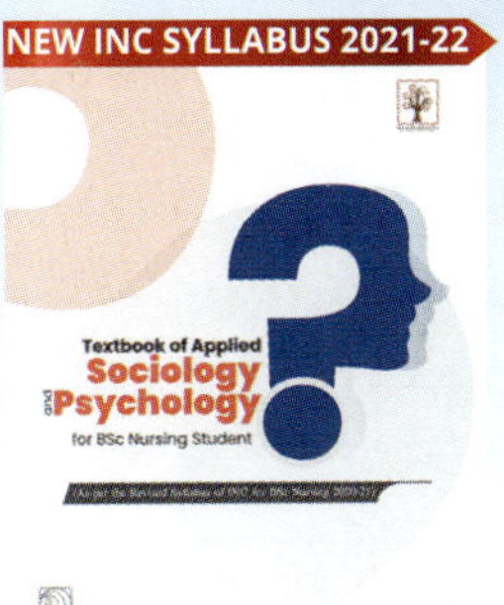

Textbook of Applied Sociology and Psychology for BSc Nursing Students
P Prakash
978-93-90619-54-2
1/e, 2022
MRP: ₹395/-

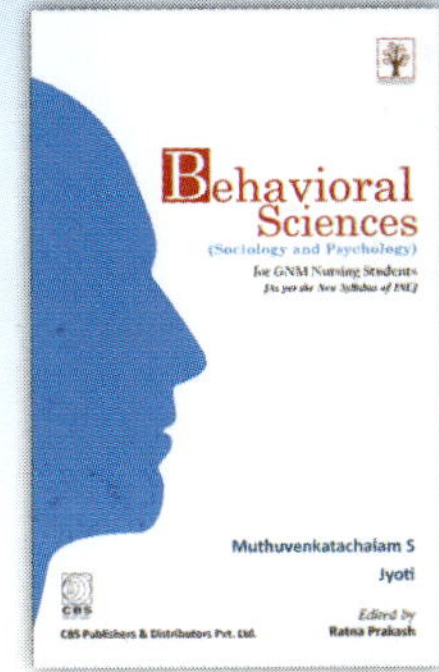

Behavioral Sciences (Sociology and Psychology)
Muthuvenkatachalam S et al.
978-93-90619-04-7
1/e , 2021
MRP: ₹350/-

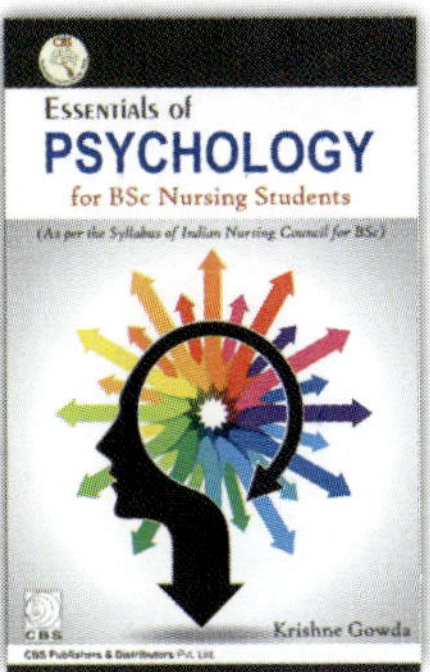

Essentials of Psychology for BSc Nursing Students
Krishne Gowda
978-81-23927-11-4
1/e, 2017
MRP: ₹340/-

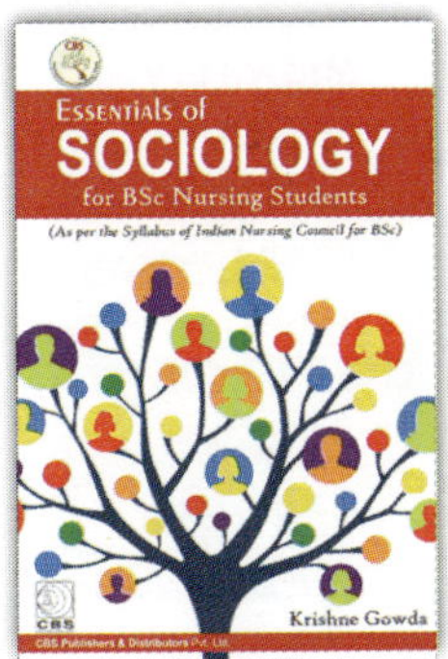

Essentials of Sociology for BSc Nursing Students
Krishne Gowda
978-93-86217-51-6
1/e, 2017
MRP: ₹395/-

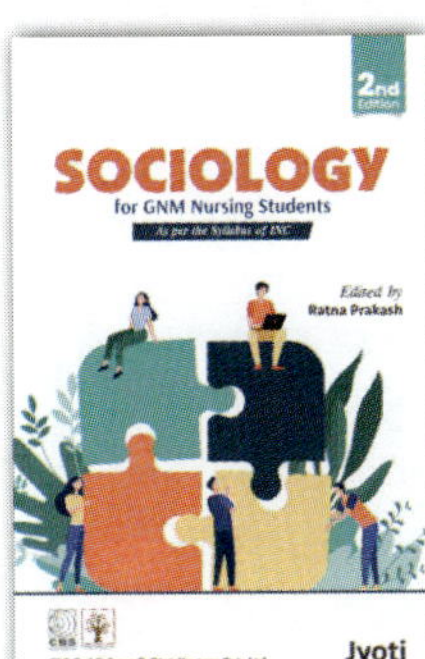

Sociology for GNM Nursing Students
Jyoti
978-81-948693-1-3
2/e, 2022
MRP: ₹210/-

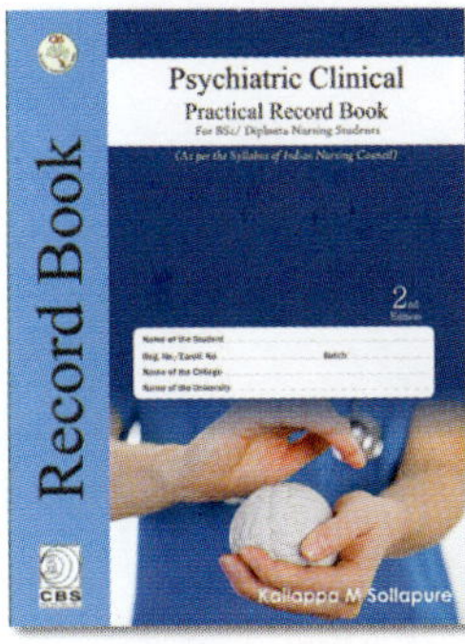

Psychiatric Clinical Practical Record Book for BSc/Diploma Nursing Students
Kallappa M Sollapure
978-93-88108-81-2
2/e, 2018-19
MRP: ₹395/-

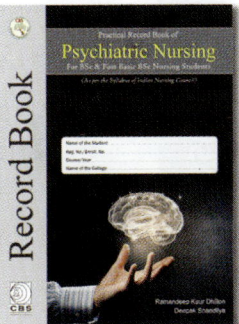

Practial Record Book of Psychiatric Nursing for BSc & Post Basic BSc Nursing Students
Ramandeep Kaur Dhillon
978-93-88108-80-5
1/e, 2019
MRP: ₹415/-

Midwifery, Obstetrical & Gynecological Nursing

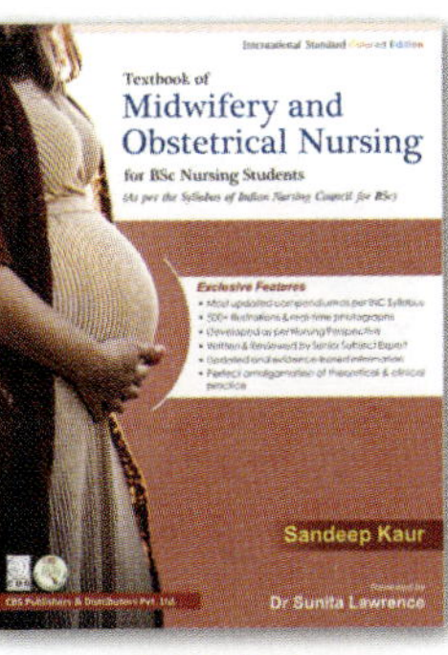

Textbook of Midwifery & Obstetrical Nursing for BSc Nursing Students
Sandeep Kaur
978-93-89261-90-5
1/e, 2020
MRP: ₹995/-

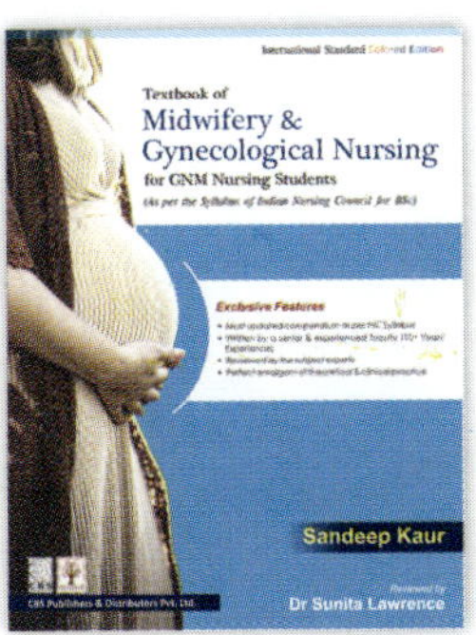

Textbook of Midwifery & Gynecological Nursing for GNM Nursing Students
Sandeep Kaur
978-93-90619-18-4
2/e, 2022
MRP: ₹895/-

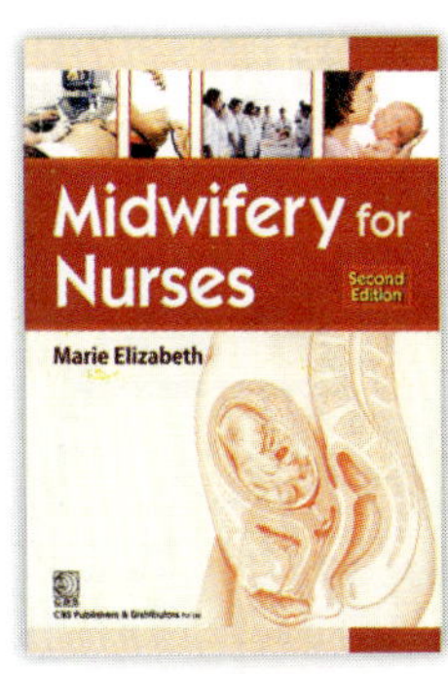

Textbook of Midwifery for Nurses
Marie Elizabeth
978-81-23922-14-0
2/e, 2018
MRP: ₹650/-

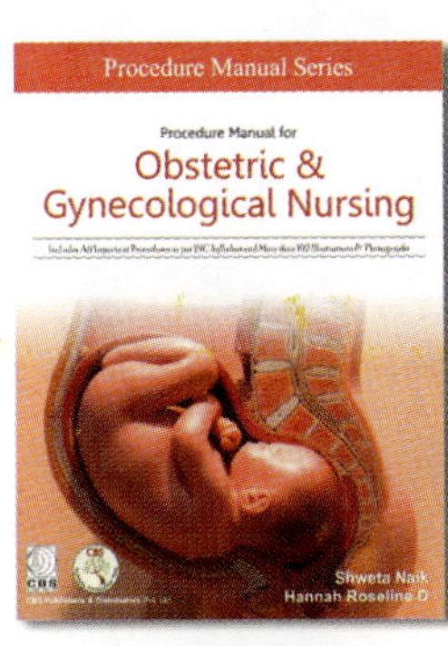

Procedure Manual for Obstetric & Gynecological Nursing
Sheweta Naik et al.
978-93-88178-60-0
1/e, 2018-19
MRP: ₹235/-

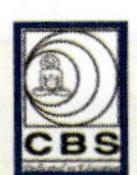
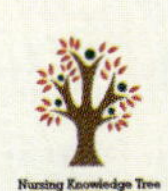

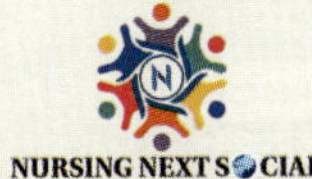

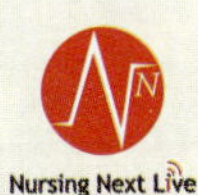

Midwifery, Obstetrical & Gynecological Nursing

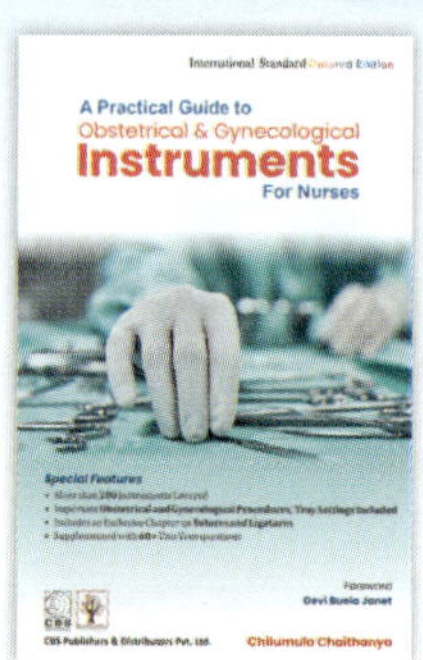

A Practical Guide to Obstetric & Gynecological Instruments for Nurses
Chilumula Chaithanya
978-93-90619-03-0
1/e, 2022
MRP: ₹250/-

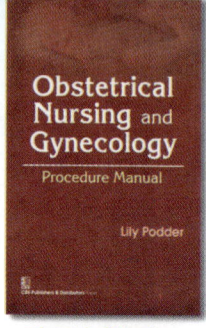

Obstetrical Nursing and Gynecology Procedure Manual
Lily Podder
978-81-23925-81-3
1/e, 2017
MRP: ₹265/-

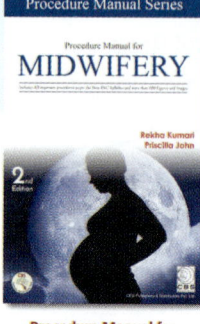

Procedure Manual for Midwifery
Rekha Kumari et al.
978-93-89261-94-3
2/e, 2019
MRP: ₹225/-

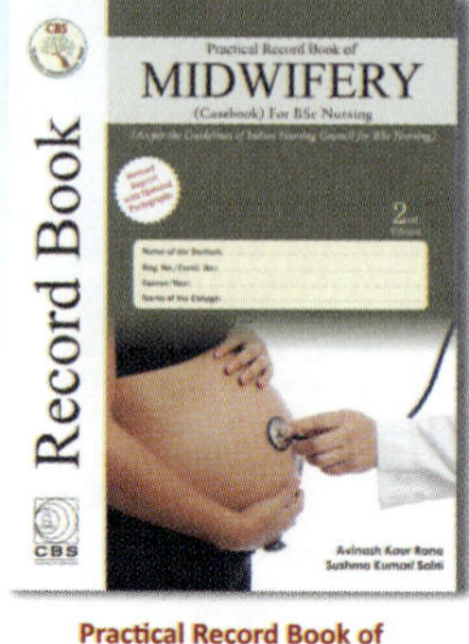

Practical Record Book of Midwifery (Casebook) for BSc Nursing
Avinash Kaur Rana et al.
978-93-88178-65-5
2/e (R/R), 2018-19
MRP: ₹675/-

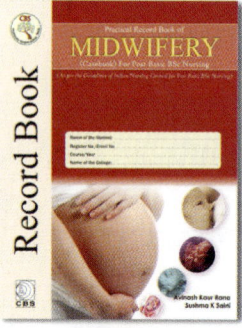

Practical Record Book of Midwifery (Casebook) for Post Basic BSc Nursing
Avinash Kaur Rana et al.
978-81-23927-07-7
1/e, 2016
MRP: ₹375/-

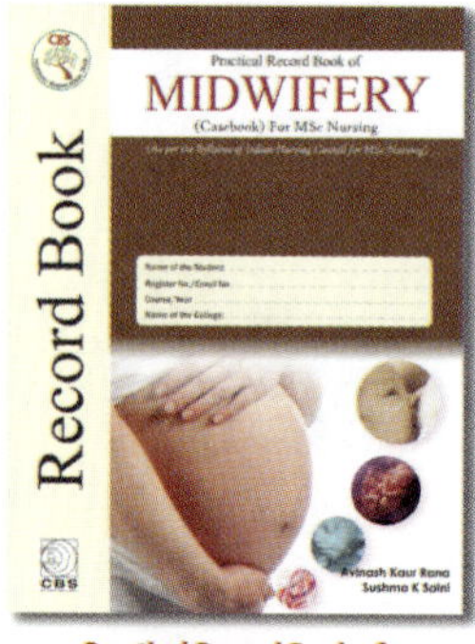

Practical Record Book of Midwifery (Casebook) for MSc Nursing
Avinash Kaur Rana et al.
978-93-86217-97-4
1/e, 2017
MRP: ₹625/-

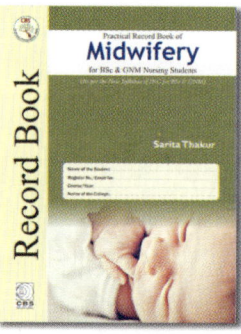

Practical Record Book of Midwifery for BSc & GNM Nursing Students
Sarita Thakur
978-93-86827-33-3
1/e, 2017
MRP: ₹415/-

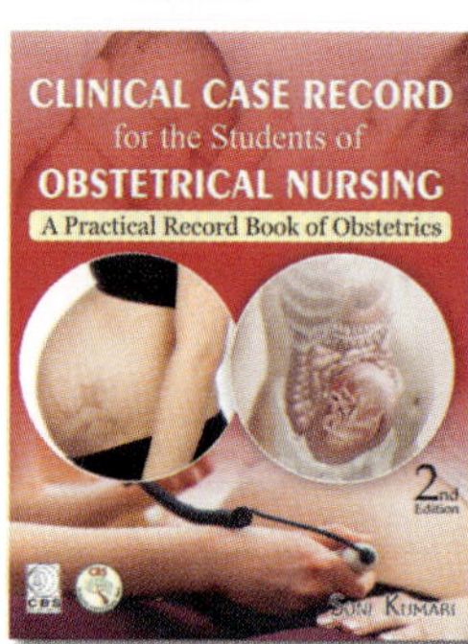

Clinical Case Record for the Students of Obstetrical Nursing A Practical Record Book of Obstetrics
Soni Kumari
978-93-88178-51-8
2/e, 2018
MRP: ₹475/-

Nursing Research/Biostatistics

Nursing Research in 21st Century
Sukhpal Kaur et al.
978-93-89261-89-9
1/e, 2020
MRP: ₹725/-

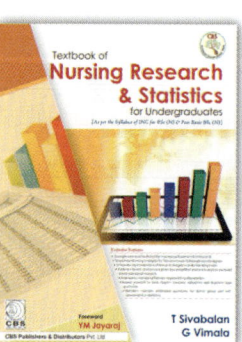

Textbook of Nursing Research & Statistics for Undergraduates
T Sivabalan et al.
978-93-88178-61-7
1/e, 2018
MRP: ₹525/-

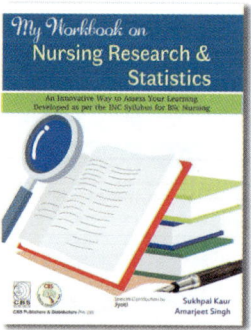

My Workbook on Nursing Research & Statistics
Sukhpal Kaur et al.
978-93-88108-75-1
1/e, 2019
MRP: ₹150/-

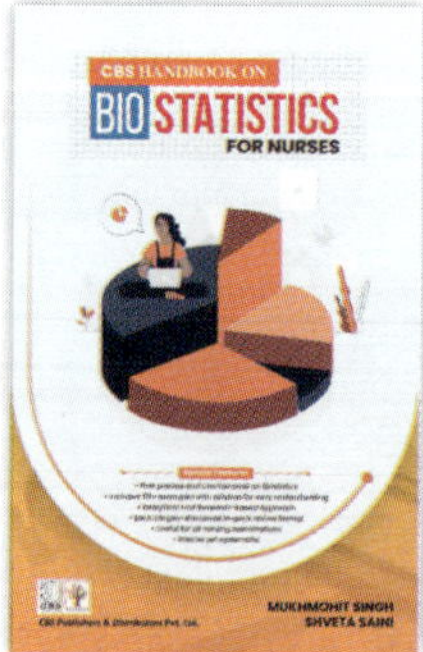

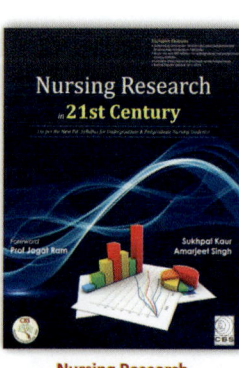

CBS Handbook on Biostatistics for Nurses
Mukhmohit Singh et al.
978-93-90619-10-8
1/e, 2022
MRP: ₹195/-

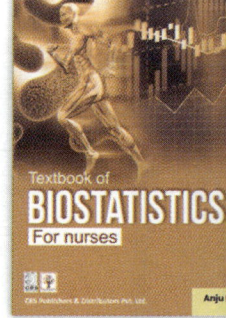

Textbook of Biostatistics for Nurses
Anju Dhir
978-93-90619-47-4
1/e, 2022
TBA

CET/Nursing Education

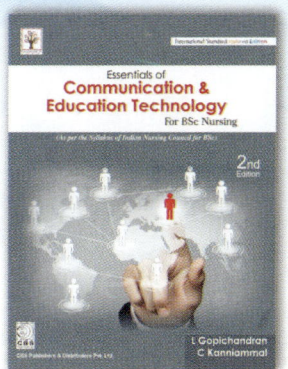

Essentials of
Communication & Education Technology
for BSc Nursing
L Gopichandran et al.
978-93-88178-58-7
2/e, 2019
MRP: ₹495/-

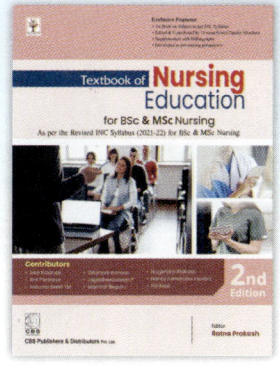

Textbook of
Nursing Education
for BSc & MSc Nursing
Ratna Prakash
978-93-90619-53-5
2/e, 2022
TBA

Nursing Management & Services

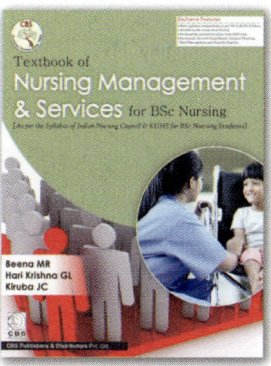

Textbook of
Nursing Management & Services
for BSc Nursing
Beena MR et al.
978-93-88178-62-4
1/e, 2019
MRP: ₹625/-

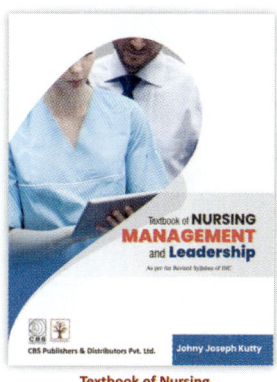

Textbook of Nursing
Management & Leadership
Johny Joseph Kutty
978-93-90619-40-5
1/e, 2022
MRP: ₹695/-

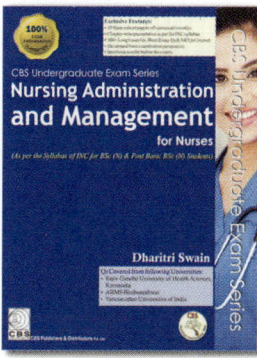

CBS Undergraduate Exam Series
Nursing Administration
and Management for Nurses
Dharitri Swain
978-93-86827-42-5
1/e, 2018
MRP: ₹350/-

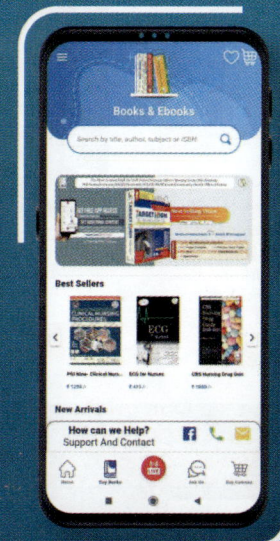

Microbiology

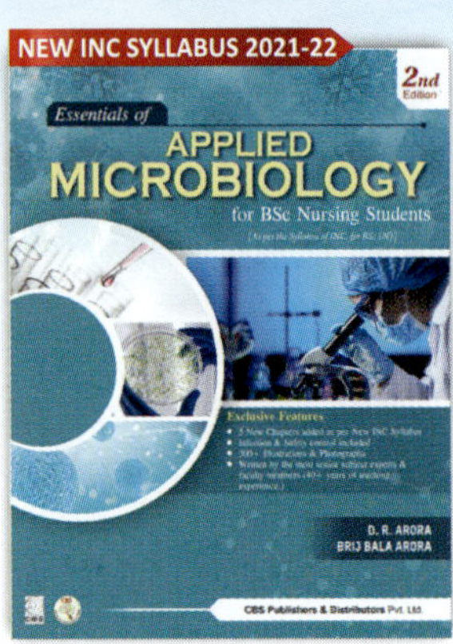

Essentials of Applied Microbiology for BSc Nursing Students
D.R. Arora et al.
978-81-945234-4-4
2/e, 2020

MRP: ₹575/-

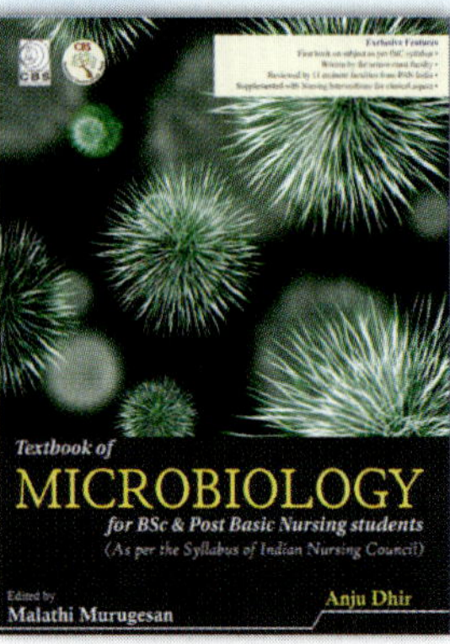

Textbook of Microbiology for BSc & Post Basic Nursing Students
Anju Dhir
978-93-88108-82-9
1/e, 2018

MRP: ₹725/-

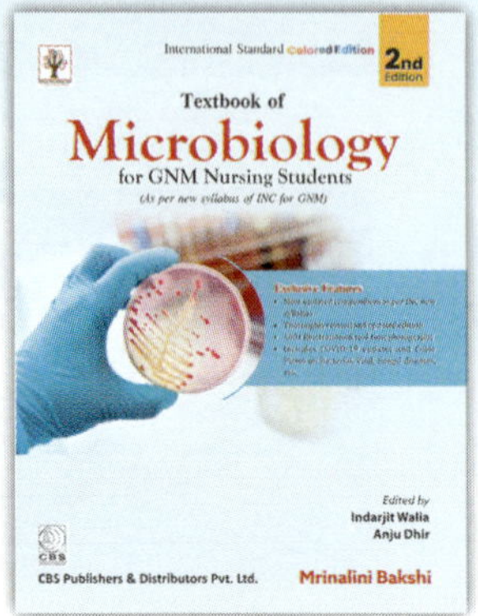

Textbook of Microbiology for GNM Nursing Students
Mrinalini Bakshi
978-93-90619-12-2
2/e, 2021

MRP: ₹225/-

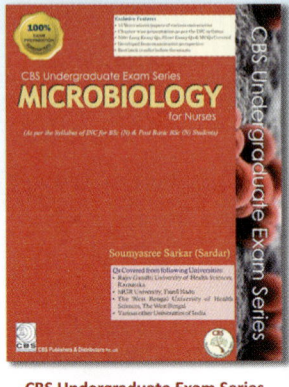

CBS Undergraduate Exam Series Microbiology for Nurses
Soumyasree Sarkar
978-93-86310-49-1
1/e, 2017

MRP: ₹275/-

English/First Aid/Computer

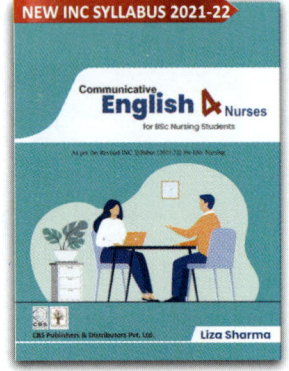

Communicative English 4 Nurses for BSc Nursing Students
Liza Sharma
978-93-90619-26-9
1/e, 2022

TBA

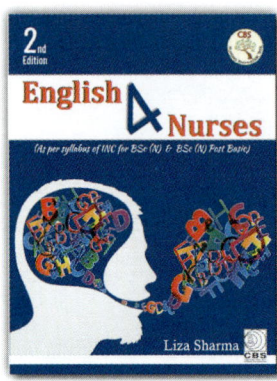

English 4 Nurses (BSc)
Liza Sharma
978-93-89261-95-0
2/e, 2019

MRP: ₹415/-

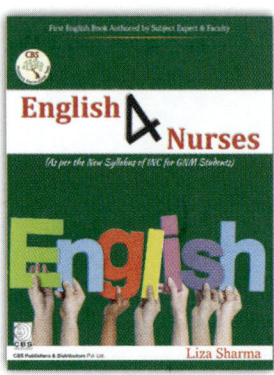

English 4 Nurses (GNM)
Liza Sharma
978-93-86827-09-8
1/e, 2017

MRP: ₹350/-

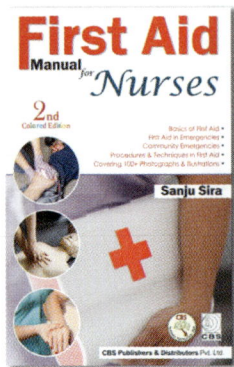

First Aid Manual for Nurses
Sanju Sira
978-93-88178-55-6
2/e, 2019

MRP: ₹310/-

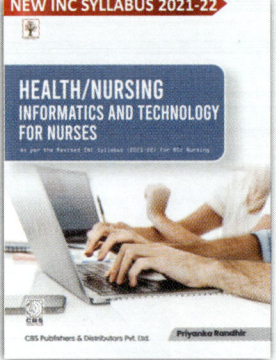

Health/Nursing Informatics and Technology for Nurses
Priyanka Randhir
978-93-90619-21-4
1/e, 2022

TBA

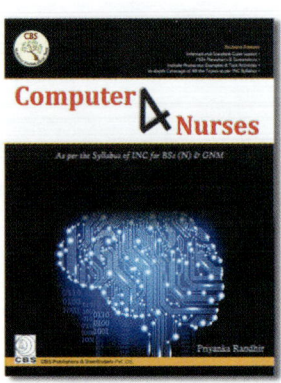

Computer 4 Nurses
Priyanka Randhir
978-93-86310-48-4
1/e, 2017

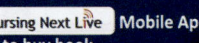

MRP: ₹370/-

Anatomy & Physiology/Biochemistry & Nutrition

Exclusive Marketing & Distribution Rights

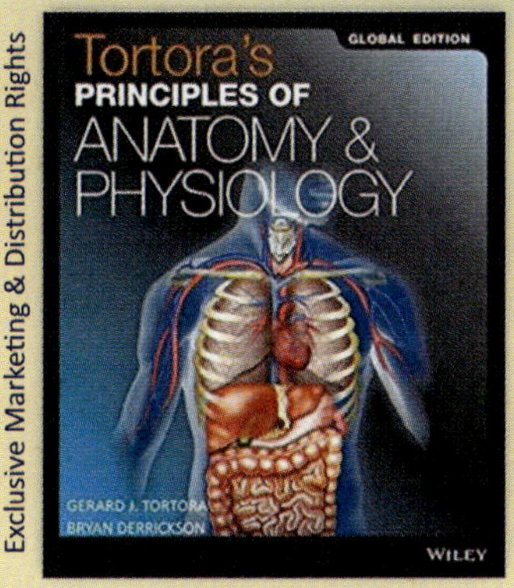

Tortora's Principles of
Anatomy & Physiology
Gerard J. Tortora
978-81-26567-61-4
GLOBAL Edition, 2017
MRP: ₹3495/-

BD Chaurasia's
Applied Anatomy and Physiology
for BSc Nursing Students
Krishna Garg
978-93-90619-65-8
1/e, 2022
TBA

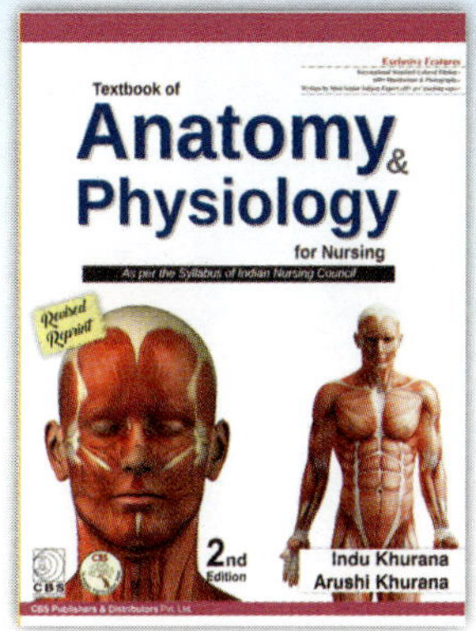

Textbook of
Anatomy & Physiology for Nursing
Indu Khurana et al.
978-93-86827-12-8
2/e, 2018
MRP: ₹995/-

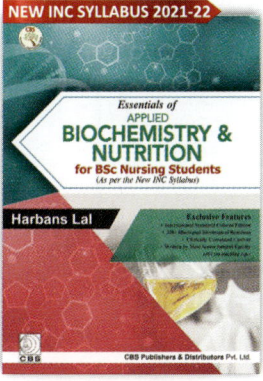

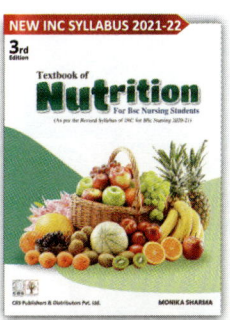

Essentials of APPLIED
Biochemistry & Nutrition
for BSc Nursing Students
Harbans Lal
978-93-90619-41-2
1/e, 2022
MRP: ₹450/-

Essentials of
Biochemistry
for BSc Nursing Students
Harbans Lal
978-81-948693-3-7
2/e, 2022
MRP: ₹450/-

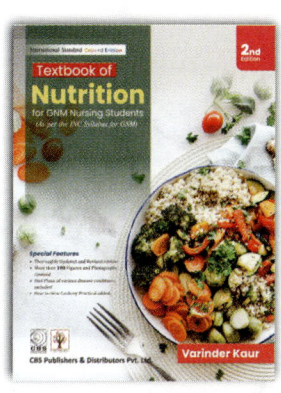

Textbook of
Nutrition
for GNM Nursing Students
Varinder Kaur
978-93-90619-02-3
2/e, 2022
MRP: ₹295/-

Essentials of
Anatomy & Physiology for GNM
with Clinical Importance
Krishna Garg et al.
978-93-86827-11-1
1/e, 2018
MRP: ₹475/-

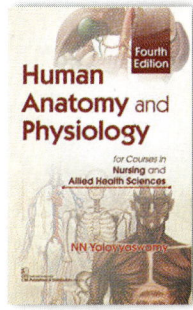

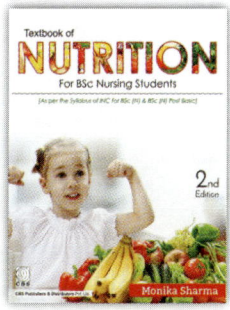

Human Anatomy and Physiology
for Nurses
N.N. Yalayyaswamy
978-93-87085-16-9
4/e, 2018
MRP: ₹395/-

Textbook of
Nutrition
for BSc Nursing Students
Monika Sharma
978-93-90619-02-3
3/e, 2022
MRP: ₹370/-

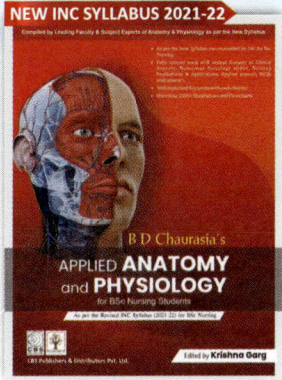

Textbook of Nutrition
for BSc Nursing Students
Monika Sharma
978-93-89261-92-9
2/e, 2019
MRP: ₹370/-

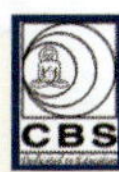

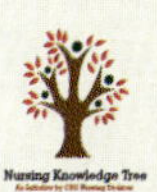

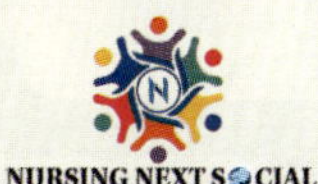

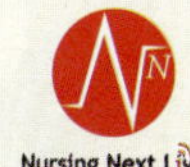

Others

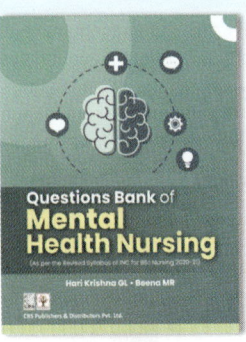

Questions Bank of Mental Health Nursing
Hari Krishna GL et al.
978-93-90619-46-7
1/e, 2022
TBA

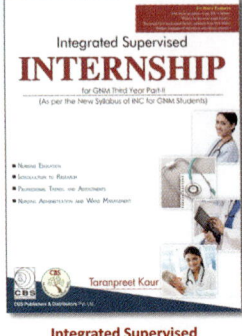

Integrated Supervised Internship for GNM Third Year Part-II
Taranpreet Kaur
978-93-88108-89-8
1/e, 2018
MRP: ₹415/-

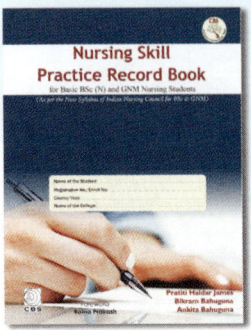

Nursing Skill Practice Record Book for Basic BSc (N) and GNM Nursing Students
Pratiti Haldar James et al.
978-93-86827-38-8
1/e, 2018-19
MRP: ₹310/-

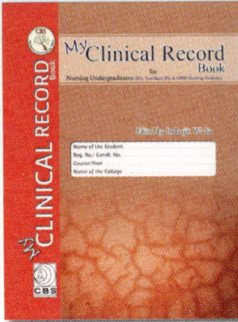

***My* Clinical Record Book for Nursing Undergraduates (BSc, Post Basic BSc & GNM Nursing Stude**
Indarjit Walia
978-81-23927-04-6
1/e, 2017-18
MRP: ₹325/-

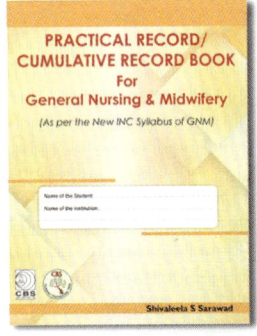

Practical Record/Cumulative Record Book for General Nursing & Midwifery
Shivaleela S Sarawad
978-93-86827-03-6
1/e, 2018
MRP: ₹225/-

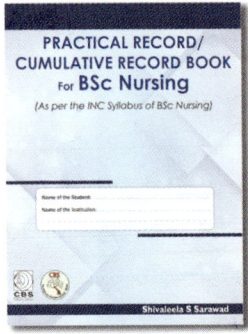

Practical Record/Cumulative Record Book for BSc Nursing
Shivaleela S Sarawad
978-93-86827-01-2
1/e, 2017
MRP: ₹210/-

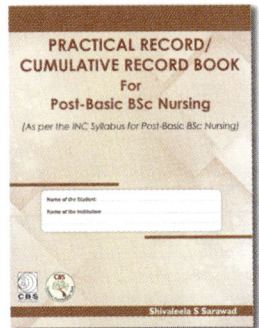

Practical Record/Cumulative Record Book for Post-Basic BSc Nursing
Shivaleela S Sarawad
978-93-86827-02-9
1/e, 2018
MRP: ₹225/-

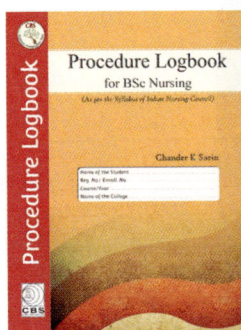

Procedure Logbook for BSc Nursing
Chander K Sarin
978-93-86310-46-0
1/e, 2017
MRP: ₹210/-

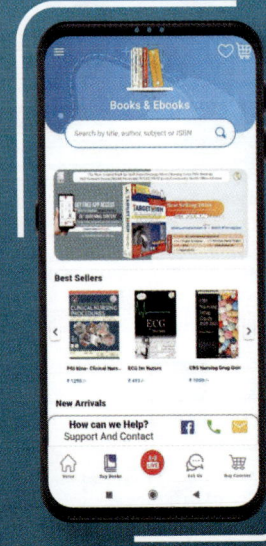

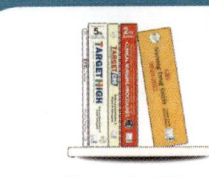

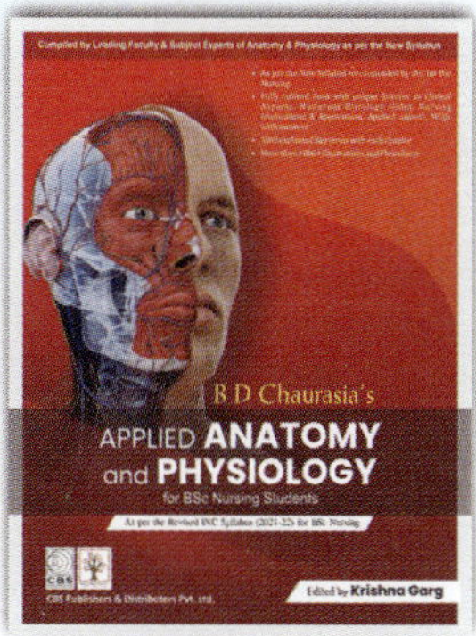

BD Chaurasia's
Applied Anatomy and Physiology
for BSc Nursing Students
Krishna Garg
978-93-90619-65-8
1/e, 2022
TBA

Essentials of Biochemistry
for BSc Nursing Students (As per KUHS)
Harbans Lal
978-81-948693-3-7
2/e, 2022
MRP: ₹450/-

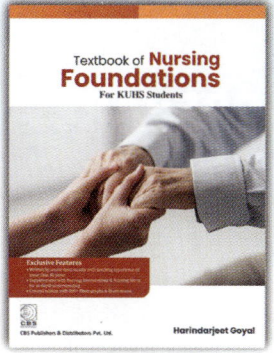

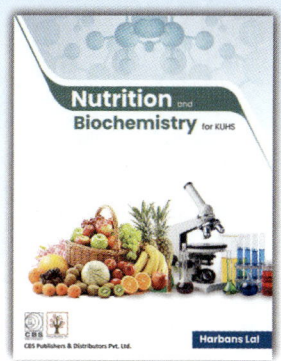

Textbook of
Nursing Foundations
for BSc Nursing (As per KUHS)
Harindarjeet Goyal
978-93-90619-38-2
1/e, 2022
MRP: ₹950/-

Textbook of
Nutrition & Biochemistry
for BSc Nursing (As per KUHS)
Harbans Lal
978-93-90619-32-0
1/e, 2022
MRP: ₹450/-

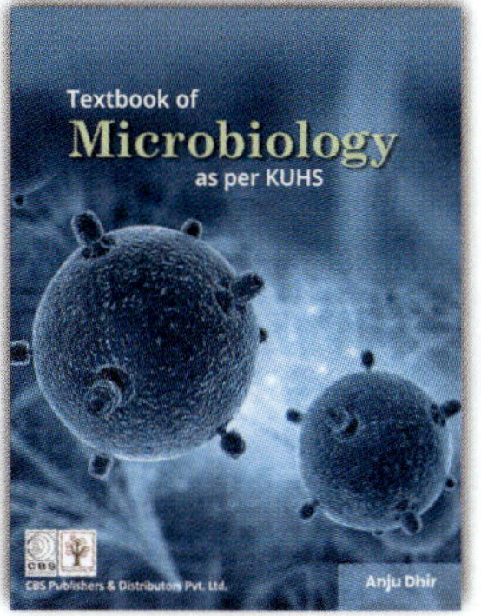

Textbook of
Microbiology
for BSc Nursing (As per KUHS)
Anju Dhir
978-93-90619-49-8
1/e, 2022
MRP: ₹725/-

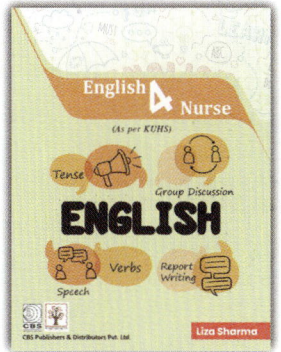

English 4 Nurses
for BSc Nursing (As per KUHS)
Liza Sharma
978-93-90619-33-7
1/e, 2022
MRP: ₹495/-

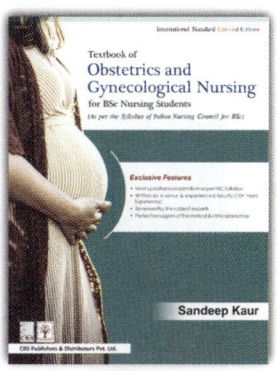

Textbook of
Obstetrics & Gynecological Nursing
for BSc Nursing (As per KUHS)
Sandeep Kaur
978-93-90619-48-1
1/e, 2022
MRP: ₹895/-

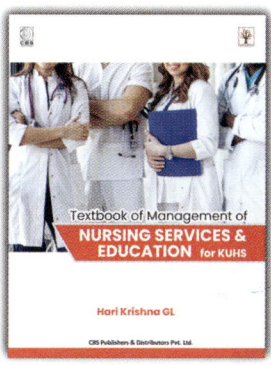

Textbook of
Nursing Management
for BSc Nursing (As per KUHS)
Hari Krishna GL et al.
978-93-90619-39-9
1/e, 2022
MRP: ₹695/-

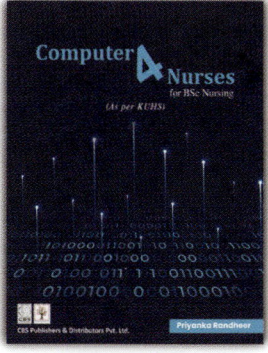

Computer 4 Nurses
for BSc Nursing (As per KUHS)
Priyanka Randheer
978-93-90619-62-7
1/e, 2022
MRP: ₹370/-

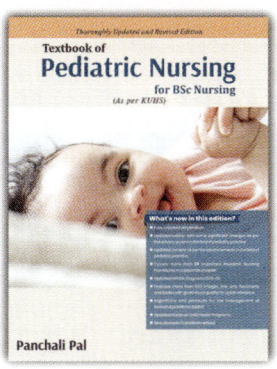

Textbook of
Pediatric Nursing
for BSc Nursing (As per KUHS)
Panchali Pal
978-93-90619-80-1
1/e, 2022
MRP: ₹795/-

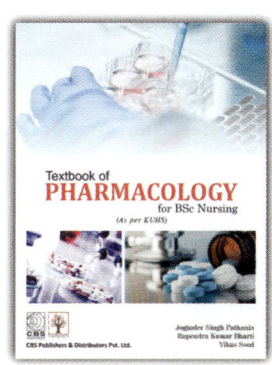

Textbook of
Pharmacology
for BSc Nursing (As per KUHS)
Joginder Singh Pathania et al.
978-93-90619-28-3
1/e, 2022
MRP: ₹650/-

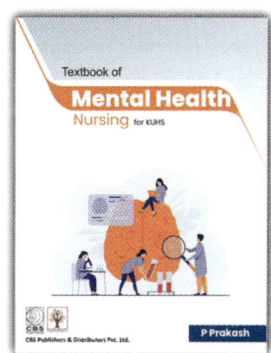

Textbook of
Mental Health Nursing
for BSc Nursing (As per KUHS)
P Prakash
978-93-90619-81-8
1/e, 2022
MRP: ₹625/-

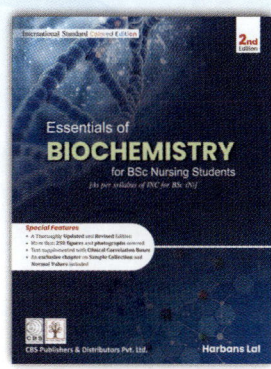

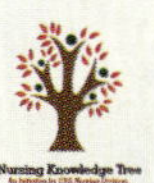

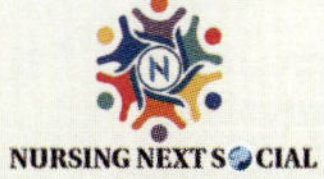

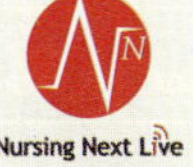